中医浊毒论

（汉英对照）

On Turbid Toxin of Traditional Chinese Medicine

(Chinese-English Version)

顾问 张伯礼 王 琦 王永炎 张大宁 孙光荣 吴以岭

Counselors Zhang Boli Wang Qi Wang Yongyan Zhang Daning
Sun Guangrong Wu Yiling

主编 李佃贵 姜建明 杨 倩 梅建强 杜艳茹

Chief Editors Li Diangui Jiang Jianming Yang Qian Mei Jianqiang Du Yanru

中国中医药出版社

中国•北京

China Press of Traditional Chinese Medicine

Beijing PRC

图书在版编目（CIP）数据

中医浊毒论：汉英对照 / 李佃贵等主编 . -- 北京：
中国中医药出版社，2024.6
ISBN 978-7-5132-8601-5

Ⅰ.①中… Ⅱ.①李… Ⅲ.①解毒—汉、英 Ⅳ.
① R256

中国国家版本馆 CIP 数据核字 (2023) 第 235485 号

中国中医药出版社出版

北京经济技术开发区科创十三街 31 号院二区 8 号楼
邮政编码　100176
传真　010－64405721
万卷书坊印刷（天津）有限公司印刷
各地新华书店经销

开本 787×1092　1/16　印张 23.75　字数 880 千字
2024 年 6 月第 1 版　2024 年 6 月第 1 次印刷
书号　ISBN 978－7－5132－8601－5

定价　149.00 元
网址　www.cptcm.com

服 务 热 线　010-64405510
购 书 热 线　010-89535836
维 权 打 假　010-64405753

微信服务号　zgzyycbs
微商城网址　https://kdt.im/LIdUGr
官 方 微 博　http://e.weibo.com/cptcm
天猫旗舰店网址　https://zgzyycbs.tmall.com

如有印装质量问题请与本社出版部联系（010－64405510）

《中医浊毒论（汉英对照）》编委会
Editorial Committee of *On Turbid Toxin of Traditional Chinese Medicine*

中医药文化源远流长，中医理论博大精深。中医药学已有几千年的历史，为保障民族繁衍昌盛、维护人民健康做出了重要贡献，至今仍然发挥着重要作用。中医药学为什么能够历久弥新、学术长青呢？这与中医药学在保持哲学思维和基础理论相对稳定的基础上，丰富的临床实践促使理法方药不断与时俱进相关。这也是中医药学发展的内生动力，燕赵医学可为佐证。

燕赵大地作为中华医药的重要发祥地之一，历代名医辈出，医家流派纷呈。扁鹊述《难经》而统四诊，张元素辨脏腑而创易水派，刘完素重热邪而创寒凉派，李东垣善脾胃而创补土派，王清任创新应用活血逐瘀法则，张锡纯开中西医汇通之先河……他们都为中医药的发展做出了重要贡献。

国医大师李佃贵教授数十年致力于中医临床事业，善于思考，勤求古训，精研勤学，学验俱丰。他创造性地提出"浊毒理论"，将其广泛应用于临床，尤其在治疗慢性萎缩性胃炎伴肠上皮化生和（或）不典型增生等胃癌前病变方面，临床疗效确切，打破了多年来"胃癌前病变不能逆转"的认知束缚，得到业界和社会的广泛认可，也让"浊毒理论"受到重视。

历代医家虽然对"浊""毒"都有记载，但是均未开展对浊毒系统的理论论述。浊毒论中所提出的"浊毒"，虽然吸纳和借鉴了古代关于"浊"与"毒"的概念含义，但并不仅仅是"浊"与"毒"的词义简单叠加，而是赋予了其丰富的时代内涵。李佃贵教授把所有对人体有害的不洁之物和不良的精神神志刺激均称之为"浊毒"。他带领团队围绕"浊毒"进行了理、法、方、药的系统理论构建，创新了新的发病观——浊毒化，以及新的治疗观——化浊毒，依照天人合一的整体观念分别称之为"天之浊毒""地之浊毒""人之浊毒"，并首倡当代人类的健康观为"净化人体内环境"。浊毒理论是新时代中医药的重要理论创新，是契合当代人类生态健康的中医治疗新理念。

由李佃贵国医大师、姜建明教授等主编的《中医浊毒论（汉英对照）》即将付梓。该书理论创新结合临床实践，既包括浊毒论在慢性胃炎、消化性溃疡、溃疡性结肠炎、胃癌、结肠癌、肝癌、肝纤维化等脾胃肝胆疾病中的应用，还包括肾病、代谢性疾病、眼病等领域，同时还有浊毒论在新冠病毒感染中的应用，从而形成了以"化浊解毒"为特色的理论体系和诊疗方案，创新了中医病因病机学，丰富了中医临床证治学内容。

"浊毒学说"是守正创新的生动实践，其来源于临床实践，又在理论上有所发现，有所创新，并在临床实践中得以验证。衷心希望浊毒论为传承创新发展中医药事业、维护人民健康事业做出更大的贡献。

中国工程院院士
国医大师
中国中医科学院名誉院长
天津中医药大学名誉校长
2023年12月于天津静海团泊湖畔

Traditional Chinese Medicine culture has a long history, and the theory of Traditional Chinese Medicine is extensive and profound. With a history of thousands of years, Traditional Chinese Medicine has made important contributions to promoting national reproduction and safeguarding people's health, and it still plays an important role today. Why can Traditional Chinese Medicine be durable and academically sustainable? Because the rich clinical practice of Traditional Chinese Medicine makes its principle, method, prescription and medicine keep pace with the times on the basis of relatively stable philosophical thinking and basic theory, which is also the endogenous driving force for the development of Traditional Chinese Medicine, as evidenced by Yanzhao medicine.

As one of the important birthplaces of Chinese medicine, Yanzhao has produced a large number of famous doctors and various schools of doctors. Bianque dictated *Nan Jing* and summarized four diagnosis, Zhang Yuansu told the differences of zang and fu and created of School of Yishui, Liu Wansu focused on fire diseases and created School of Cold and Cool, Li Dongyuan was good at treating spleen and stomach diseases and created School of Spleen Invigorating, Wang Qingren summarized and innovated the rule of activating blood flow to remove blood stasis, Zhang Xichun started the integration of Chinese and Western medicine ... They made positive contributions to the development of Traditional Chinese Medicine.

Professor Li Diangui who has been committed to the clinical cause of Traditional Chinese Medicine for decades is good at thinking, diligent in seeking ancient teaching, persistent in studying and researching, rich both in learning and experiences. He creatively proposed the "turbid toxin theory" and applied it widely in clinical practice, especially in the treatment of chronic atrophic gastritis accompanied by intestinal metaplasia and (or) atypical hyperplasia and other precancerous lesions of gastric diseases. It has broken the theoretical shackle as "the precancerous lesions of gastric diseases cannot be reversed" for many years, and has been widely recognized by the industry and society.

Although doctors of previous dynasties have scattered records of "turbidity" and "toxin", they have not systematically discussed turbid toxin. The "turbid toxin" mentioned in the theory of turbid toxin which absorbs and draws on the meanings of "turbidity" and "toxin" in ancient Chinese medicine is not only a simple superposition of "turbidity" and "toxin", it has rich connotation of the times. Professor Li Diangui calls all unclean things and bad mental stimulation harmful to human health as "turbid toxin". He led the team to build a systematic theoretical architecture of theory, method, prescription and medicine around "turbid toxin", respectively divides turbid toxin into "sky turbid toxin", "earth turbid toxin" and "human turbid toxin" according to the overall concept of the unity of heaven and man, and refreshes the cause of disease to be turbid toxin pollution , the process of diseases treatment to be turbid toxin removing, and firstly points out that the purpose of contemporary human health is "to purify internal environment of human body". Turbid toxin theory which is more in line with contemporary human health is an important theoretical innovation of traditional Chinese medicine in the new era .

On Turbid Toxin of Traditional Chinese Medicine (Chinese - English Version) edited by TCM master Li Diangui and Professor Jiang Jianming will be published soon. It combines theoretical innovation with clinical practice, covering the application of turbid toxin theory in treatment of spleen, stomach, liver and bile diseases such as chronic gastritis, peptic ulcer, ulcerative colitis, gastric cancer, colon cancer, liver cancer, liver fibrosis, the application of turbid toxin theory in treating other diseases like kidney disease, metabolic diseases, eye disease, and the application of turbid toxin theory in treatment of COVID-19. Thus, a theoretical system and diagnosis and treatment scheme characterized by "dissipating turbidity and removing toxin" has been formed, which has enriched TCM clinical syndrome and innovated TCM etiology and pathogenesis.

"Turbid Toxin theory" is a vivid practice of keeping the right while innovating the improper, it comes from clinical practice making innovation in theory and has been verified in clinical practice. I sincerely hope that turbid toxin theory will make greater contributions to the inheritance, innovation and development of TCM and the maintenance of people's health.

Zhang Boli
Academician of Chinese Academy of Engineering,
TCM Master
Honorary President of China Academy of Chinese Medical Sciences
Honorary President of Tianjin University of Traditional Chinese Medicine
December, 2023, Tuanbo Lake, Jinghai, Tianjin

中医学自诞生之日，即以创新为任。古之神农尽尝百草，创中药之先；华佗立疮科，组麻沸散剂，剔骨疗疾，创中医外科之先。今逢盛世中国，中医复兴之路即于足下。幸党和政府对中医药事业扶持力度的日益加大，以及业界同仁自身的努力，中医药事业有了长足的进步与发展。一些新理论、新观点和新技术应运而生，不断充实和完善了中医学体系，而浊毒理论便是其中的代表之一。

任何一种学术思想的形成都有其深刻的自然与社会因素。如刘河间行医时，正值火症大疫流行之际，提出"五运六气有所更，世态居民有所变，天以常火，人以常动，内外皆扰"，将理论与实践相结合，以火热立论，力挽时弊。而李东垣行医之时，正是金元之交，战乱频仍，饥困劳役，人们怒忿悲思恐惧，损伤元气，所以脾胃受困，内伤之病尤多，故而产生了内伤脾胃学说。由此可见，任何一门科学必须随着时代的发展而不断地完善，由此适应时代的需要。

近一百多年来，随着生态环境的不断恶化和生活方式的改变，人类的疾病谱发生了深刻变革，"浊毒"物质充斥全球每个角落以及人体之中，它们都不同程度地对人体造成了损害。毒之为毒，其义甚广，其害甚深，既是一个具有物质属性的概念，又是一个具有病理属性的概念。古之典籍论述毒者甚多，如风毒、火毒、湿毒、痰毒、瘀毒等五十余种，而独不见"浊毒"一词。其实浊毒证作为中医临床的一种证候表现，自古有之，但缺乏系统的研究。李佃贵教授是我国著名的脾胃病专家，在治疗慢性萎缩性胃炎及其癌前病变方面疗效显著。他依据多年的临床经验，结合古代典籍的经典论述和现代病谱的深刻变化，提出了浊毒理论。虽然该理论仍有一些需要完善的地方，但瑕不掩瑜，值得我们去深入研究和探讨。

幽幽燕赵，名医辈出，且不乏改革创新之先行者。伏羲神参日月，创八卦而明阴阳；黄帝明堂问道，著《灵》《素》而明医论；扁鹊负笈行医，述《难经》而统四诊；及至金元，张元素明脏腑而创易水派，刘完素重火热而创寒凉派，李东垣善脾胃而创补土派；到了近代，王清任勇于实践，将活血化瘀扩而广之，张锡纯学贯中西，开中西汇通之先河。诚望李佃贵教授能精研仁术，比肩先贤，而为新时代之创新先行者！

佳作已成，幸即付梓，邀余为序，有感编委会同仁的信任与鼓励，乐为之，以共勉。

王永炎

中国工程院院士

2023年10月

Traditional Chinese Medicine has been continuously innovated ever since its birth. The ancient Shennong started the practice of Chinese Medicine by tasting all kinds of herbs; Hua Tuo created traditional Chinese surgery by starting ulcer division, inventing the (anesthetic) prescription of Mafei Powder, treating the disease by scraping bones. We are lucky to live in prosperous China on the way to revive Traditional Chinese Medicine. Thanks to the increasing support of the Party and the government for the cause of Chinese medicine, as well as the efforts of the industry colleagues themselves, the cause of Chinese medicine has made considerable progress and development. Some new theories, new ideas and new technologies which have emerged at the right moment continuously enriched and improved the TCM system, and turbid toxin theory is one of the representatives.

The formation of any kind of academic thought has its profound natural and social factors. For example, when Liu Hejian practiced medical treatment at the time of the epidemic with dominated fire, he proposed that "while the five movements and six climates are taking turns, the world situation and its residents are changing, the sky is always on fire, the people are always moving, human body are disturbed from both inside and outside". He combined theory with practice, created fire disease theory trying to solve the problems of the time. Li Dongyuan practiced medical treatment at the alternative time of Jin and Yuan dynasties, when the war was frequent, hunger, fatigue, overwork, military service filled people with anger, sorrow, worry and fear, and damaged the vitality, so the spleen and stomach were trapped, and the diseases of internal injury were more frequent, so the theory of internal injury to the spleen and stomach was proposed. It can be seen that any science must be continuously improved along with the development of the times so as to meet the needs of the people.

In the past more than 100 years, the spectrum of human diseases has undergone profound changes along with continuous deterioration of the ecological environment and the change of life style, "turbid toxin" substances have filled every corner of the world and human body causing various degree of damages to human health. Toxin as a poisonous substance with wide connotation and serious harm is not only a concept of material property, but also a concept with pathological property. There are more than 50 kinds of toxin discussed on the ancient books, such as wind toxin, fire toxin, wet toxin, phlegm toxin, blood stasis toxin and so on, but the word "turbid toxin" has not been found in any of the above books. In fact, turbid toxin syndrome had existed as a clinical manifestation of TCM since ancient times, but systematic research was still absent. Professor Li Diangui is a famous expert in spleen and stomach diseases in China. He has a remarkable effect in the treatment of chronic atrophic gastritis and its precancerous lesions. Based on many years of clinical experience, he put forward the theory of turbid toxin in combination with the classical exposition of ancient books and the profound changes of modern disease spectrum. Although the theory still has some areas to be perfected, but the defects cannot obscure the virtues, it is worth our in-depth study and discussion.

Secluded Yanzhao produced large numbers of famous doctors in history out of which pioneers of reform and innovation appeared. Fuxi created eight diagrams and Yin and Yang through deep study of sun and moon; Huangdi wrote *Simple Conversation and Spiritual Pivot* and built medical theory through dialogue with his teacher Qibo; Bianque as a walking doctor dictated *Nan Jing* and regulated four diagnoses; in Jin and Yuan times, Zhang Yuansu proposed zang fu and created Yishui School, Liu Wansu focused on fire diseases and created Cold and Cool School, Li Dongyuan who was good at spleen and stomach diseases and created Spleen Invigorating School; in modern times, Wang Qingren had the courage to practise and promoted blood flow activating and blood stasis removing, Zhang Xichun learned from both TCM and West medicine, and started the cause of Sino-West integration.

I sincerely hope that Professor Li Diangui can become the forerunner of innovation in the new era through deep-study of medical science and the achievement of the past greats.

As the book has been completed and ready to be published, I am very happy to write the preface as above for mutual encouragement to the writer and myself. Thanks for the confidence and invitation from the editorial committee.

Wang Yongyan

Academician of China Engineering Academy

October, 2023

欣闻李佃贵教授的《中医浊毒论（汉英对照）》即将出版，甚为愉悦。我与李佃贵教授相识已有四十余年，其间经常互通书话。作为一名中医工作者，他既妙手仁心，躬身临床，普救许多含灵之苦；又善于钻研，勤求博采，首创中医"浊毒论"，充实了中医理论，为临床一些疑难杂症的诊疗开辟了新的思路和方法！

纵观中医历代各家，每一学术思想的形成都有其深刻的社会自然因素。如仲景之时，社会动荡，瘟疫流行，遂创六经辨证，开辨证论治之先河。河间之时，火症流行，遂以火热立论，力挽时弊。东垣之时，战乱频仍，饥困劳役，内伤脾胃，乃有补土一派。子和之攻下，丹溪之滋阴，莫不如此。由此可见，任何一门科学必须随着时代的发展而不断完善，才能适应时代的需要。

近年来，人们的生活方式发生了很大变化，生态环境也曾一度持续恶化，"浊毒"物质充斥于人体内外，它们都不同程度地对人体造成了损害，使得我国居民的疾病谱发生了深刻变化。"浊毒论"试图更深刻、直接地揭示疾病的病因和疾病发展的内在规律，将传统中医学的预防原则和现代预防医学的具体措施结合为一个整体，从而指导中医临床。该理论虽然仍有一些需要完善的地方，但瑕不掩瑜，由于其在指导中医临床多学科、多病种的显著疗效，所以值得我们去深入地研究和探讨。

《中医浊毒论（汉英对照）》是继《中医浊毒论》之后，李佃贵教授的又一倾力之作。该书以"浊毒论"贯其始终，重点突出，特色鲜明。其既溯源探流，深入挖掘历史理论渊源，具有传承性，又系统详尽阐述"浊毒论"这一中医新理论的核心内容，具有创新性；既旁征博引，兼采中西医相关之精华，具有权威性，又紧贴临床，注重实效，具有实用性，是中医临床工作者的有益参考。

实践是检验真理的唯一标准。对于医学而言，疗效是检验医学理论正确与否的唯一标准。李佃贵教授的"浊毒论"来源于临床实践，又在临床实践中得以验证。衷心希望"浊毒论"能够继续在临床中不断地完善和发展，为中国乃至世界人民的健康事业做出更大的贡献。

张大宁

国医大师

2023年10月

I am delighted to hear that Professor Li Diangui's book *On Turbid Toxin of Traditional Chinese Medicine* (*Chinese - English Version*) is about to be published. Professor Li Diangui and I have known each other and kept contact through letters and calls for more than forty years. As a Traditional Chinese Medicine worker, he is not only a smart hand with benevolent heart, deeply involved in clinical practice, rescue many patients from illness and suffering, he is also good at studying and seeking extensive learning. He first proposed TCM "turbid toxin theory", provides new ideas and methods for the diagnosis and treatment of some difficult diseases in clinical practice while enriching the theory of Chinese medicine.

Throughout the history of traditional Chinese medicine, the formation of each academic thought has its profound social and natural factors. For example, Zhang Zhongjing created the theory of six channel- syndrome differentiation and started the practice of syndrome differentiation treatment with the background of social turmoil and plague epidemic. Liu Hejian created fire disease theory to stop the disaster when the fire disease was prevalent. Li Dongyuan created the School of Spleen Invigorating when the war was frequent, hunger, fatigue, overwork, military service internally hurt the spleen and stomach. Zhang Zihe created Purgationist School, Zhu Danxi created Yin Nourishing School in related social and natural background. It can be seen that any science must be continuously improved in order to meet the needs of social development.

In recent years, the ecological environment has been continuously deteriorated along with the changing of people's life style, "turbid toxin" substances from inside and outside of the human body have caused damages to the human body to various degrees, profoundly changed the spectrum of diseases of our residents. The turbid toxin theory attempts to reveal the causes of diseases and the internal rules of disease development more profoundly and directly, and combines the preventive principles of traditional Chinese medicine with the specific measures of modern preventive medical science to guide the clinical practice of traditional Chinese medicine. Although there are still some spaces to be improved, the defects cannot obscure the virtues. Its remarkable effect in guiding multi-division and multi-disease treatment of TCM clinical practice, is worth our in-depth research and discussion.

On Turbid Toxin of Traditional Chinese Medicine (*Chinese - English Version*) is another masterpiece of Professor Li Diangui after *On Turbid Toxin Diseases of Traditional Chinese Medicine*. The book is consistent with "turbid toxin theory", with prominent emphasis and distinctive features. With the feature of inheritance, it traces back to the source and digs deeply into the historical theoretical origin, at the same time it systematically elaborates the core content of the new theory of TCM which forms the feature of innovation. It is authoritative by quoting extensively and drawing on the essence of traditional Chinese and western medicine, and practical by standing closely to the clinical practice and emphasizing on medical effect. Therefore it becomes a useful reference book for clinical workers of Traditional Chinese Medicine.

Practice is the sole criterion for testing truth. For medicine, curative effect is the only criterion to test the correctness of medical theory. Professor Li Diangui's "turbid toxin theory" is originated from and has been verified in clinical practice. I sincerely hope that "turbid toxin theory" can be continuously improved and developed in clinical practice, and make greater contribution to the health cause of people in China and even the world.

Zhang Daning
TCM Master
October, 2023

　　医之为道，在扶正祛邪，在平衡阴阳，使人体渐至"中和"之臻境。古今医家，概莫能外。昔在远古，伏羲制九针，神农尝百草，黄帝创医论，而并为医之祖也！及至秦汉，《内经》《本草》问世，为万世立法；仲景"勤求古训，博采众方"而著《伤寒杂病论》，开理法方药之先河。晋唐七百年，儒、道、佛三教渐浸岐黄，以厚其根基。宋元四百年，理学渐浸岐黄，以繁其枝叶，尤其刘、朱、李、张四君继出，各执牛耳，精彩纷呈。而明清五百年，温病理法日趋完善，国医之道，始臻完备。及至民国，张君锡纯等辈贯通中西，创新理论，堪为近代之楷模。而后西医渐兴，国医渐衰，岐黄之道，日益陵替。

　　三千年之国粹，九万里之福音，中医药学传至今日，虽历尽波折，但由于其效果显著，仍彰显着顽强之生命力。弘扬中医是杏林中人义不容辞之责任！而要弘扬中医，既要志存高远，又要医技精湛；既要善于继承，又要勇于创新。志存高远而医技不精，则好高骛远，于事无益；医技精湛而胸无大志，则安于现状，难成大业。继承而不创新，则继承便缺乏活力；创新而不继承，则创新便缺乏基础。李佃贵教授业医数十余年，常以振兴中医为己任，精研勤学，学验俱丰，在查阅大量文献和多年临床经验之基础上，首创"浊毒"学说，并以之指导临床，在治疗慢性萎缩性胃炎伴肠上皮化生和（或）不典型增生等胃癌前病变方面，疗效显著，打破了多年来"胃癌前病变不能逆转"的理论束缚，为中医药治疗本病及其他许多疑难杂症开辟了一条新路。

　　"浊毒"一词，古籍未见记载，然其始动因素"浊"却早在《黄帝内经》时代已广泛应用。在《黄帝内经》中，清浊是经常被使用的词语，几乎与寒热、气血、阴阳一样属于基本概念，浊有生理之"浊"，有病理之"浊"，浊毒当为病理"浊"之甚者。其既是致病因素，又是病理产物，通过化浊解毒，使人体邪去正安，阴平阳秘，达到"中和"的理想状态。深刻研究浊毒的病因病机及浊毒证的治则方药，对于中医多学科的临床和科研工作都将会产生积极而深远的影响。

　　张锡纯曰："夫事贵师古者，非以古人之规矩、准绳限我也，惟藉以瀹我性灵，益我神智。迨至性灵神智，洋溢活泼，又贵举古人之规矩、准绳而扩充之、变化之、引伸触长之，使古人可作，应叹为后生可畏。凡天下事皆宜然，而医学何独不然哉！"今日之中医，实乏创新之人才及实用之理论，"浊毒"学说，虽未臻至善，但以之遣方处药，效如桴鼓，可谓济世之良器也！

　　值此《中医浊毒论（汉英对照）》即将出版之际，欣然为之序！

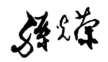

国医大师

2023年10月

The art of healing is to promote health and dispel evil, to balance Yin and Yang, and to make human body gradually achieving "harmony". Ancient and modern doctors do the same without exception. In ancient times, Fuxi invented nine needles, Shennong tasted all kinds of herbs, and Huangdi created the theory of medicine, and they were the ancestors of Chinese medicine. In Qin and Han dynasties, *Medical Classic of the Yellow Emperor* and *Shennong's Classic of Materia Medica* were published and set the fundamental principle for later generations. Zhang Zhongjing "deligently seek the ancient teaching and widely absorbing all kinds of prescriptions" and wrote *Treatise on Typhoid and Miscellaneous Diseases* and started the time of theory, method, prescription and medicine. In the seven hundred years of Jin and Tang dynasties, the three religions of Confucianism, Buddhism, and Taoism were gradually immersed into TCM to deepen their foundation. During the four hundred years from Song to Yuan dynasty, neo-Confucianism gradually immersed into TCM, multiplied the branches and leaves of TCM, especially Liu Hejian, Zhu Danxi, Li Dongyuan, Zhang Zihe four gentlemen appeared stage after stage leading their own school of academy, wonderfully enriched and promoted the development of TCM. In the five hundred years of Ming and Qing dynasties, the theory and method of warm diseases became more and more perfect, and the system of TCM began to be perfect. Until the time of Republic of China, Zhang Xichun and other predecessors connected TCM with Western Medicine, innovated the related theory, were regarded as the model of the times. Then Western medicine was gradually prospered in China, Chinese medicine was gradually declined, and the healing art of Qihuang was gradually replaced.

As the quintessence of China for three thousand years and the Gospel across ninety thousand miles, today traditional Chinese medicine still demonstrates the tenacious vitality because of its remarkable effect after various kind of twists and turns. It is the bounden duty of the people of apricot forest to promote Chinese medicine. To carry forward TCM, we should not only aim high, but also have excellent medical skills. We should not only be good at inheriting, but also have the courage to innovate. High aim without fine medical skills is useless in clinical practice; self-satisfied with fine skills at present without further ambition is difficult to make great achievements. Inheritance without innovation, inheritance will lack vitality; innovation without inheritance, innovation will lack the foundation. Professor Li Diangui has been practicing medicine for decades of years, taking the rejuvenation of traditional Chinese medicine as his own responsibility. He is persistent in researching and diligent in learning with rich experience of teaching and clinical practice. Based on referencing large number of medical literature and many years of clinical experience, he created turbid toxin theory and practise it in clinical treatment. The theory has broken many years of theoretical shackles that "gastric precancerous lesions cannot be reversed", and opened a new way for the treatment of this disease and many other difficult and complicated diseases by traditional Chinese medicine.

The word "turbid toxin" has not been recorded in ancient books, but its initial factor "turbidity" has been widely used as early as the era of *Medical Classic of the Yellow Emperor*. In *Medical Classic of the Yellow Emperor*, cleanness and turbidity are frequently used words, almost as basic as coldness and heat, Qi and blood, Yin and Yang. Turbidity can be divided into physiological "turbidity" and pathological "turbidity". Turbid toxin should be pathological "turbidity" with serious pathogenic factor. It is the cause of diseases as well as pathological product. The aim of turbid toxin theory is to dissipate the turbid toxin, drive out the evilness and protect the goodness of the human body to smooth Yin and save Yang so as to achieve the ideal state of "harmony". The profound study on the etiology, pathogenesis and treatment of turbid toxin will have positive and far-reaching influence on clinical practice and scientific research of TCM.

Zhang Xichun said, "To learn the experience of the former generations does not mean to limit ourselves by the rules and criteria of the ancients, but to change our spirit and benefit our sanity. Until the spirit and consciousness is permeated with vivacity, we refer to the rules and criteria of the ancients, expand it, change it, extend it, so that if the ancients can make sound, they should sigh that the future generation is terribly innovative. Everything in the world is appropriate for this, no exception for medicine." Today's Chinese medicine, is still short of innovative talent and practical theory, "turbid toxin" theory although not perfect, but when it is used in clinical prescription it makes sound effect like the drumstick struck the drum, and can be regarded as a good tool to help the world.

On the occasion of the forthcoming publication of *On Turbid Toxin of Traditional Chinese Medicine (Chinese - English Version)*, I am glad to preface it!

Sun Guangrong

TCM Master

October, 2023

作为中华传统文化的重要组成部分，中医学经历了漫长的历史演变过程，从春秋时期《黄帝内经》的出现，标志着中医学理论体系的形成，至张仲景《伤寒论》开脏腑辨证之先河、辨证论治体系之肇始；从晋代王叔和编撰中医学首部脉学专著《脉经》，隋代巢元方撰写第一部病因证候学专著《诸病源候论》，至金元时期四大医家的出现；从清代叶天士、吴又可、吴鞠通、王孟英等温病学派对外感病和内伤杂病的认识及治疗，至近代王清任的《医林改错》对瘀血、张锡纯的《医学衷中参西录》对中西医汇通的认识，都经过了诸多医家的不同学说、不同流派对经典文献的挖掘整理、继承发挥，进一步促进、丰富和发展了中医学的理论体系，彰显了中医学的发展和学术争鸣的繁荣景象。纵观中医学发展的历史，中医学术水平的提高，无一不是医家在学习总结先贤理论和经验的基础上，经过长期的临床实践，又不断发现，不断充实，不断提高，逐步发展完善的，而每位医家的学术思想，又无一不是经过争论、争鸣，最终结出的果实。《中医浊毒论（汉英对照）》的出版可以说是在此基础上孕育而生的。

燕赵自古名医辈出，而且每位医家都为中医学历史的发展留下了浓重的一笔。从邢台内丘的扁鹊，到肥乡的窦默，从易水学派鼻祖张元素，到金元四大家中寒凉派的刘河间、补土派的李东垣，以及藁城的罗天益、赵县的王好古，从倡导活血化瘀的玉田县的王清任，到首创中西汇通的盐山县的张锡纯等，都为燕赵大地积淀了厚重的中医学发展创新的底蕴。现为河北省十二大名中医之一的李佃贵教授，正是遵循中医学发展的规律，溯本求源，通过查阅大量文献，结合自己多年的临床实践经验，首次提出中医创新理论——浊毒论，并将其应用于慢性胃炎、肠上皮化生、异型增生等胃癌前病变，以及慢性肝病、肝纤维化、溃疡性结肠炎等疾病，取得了可喜的临床疗效。

在河北省首届中医药发展高峰论坛上，国医大师陆广莘对浊毒论给予了高度评价。近年来，浊毒证的研究，在以李佃贵教授为首的学术团队的共同努力下，取得了可观的成就，诸多学术论文发表在国家级杂志上，相关研究成果多次在全国学术大会上进行交流并获得多项省部级科技进步奖。同时，培养出一大批诸如博士、硕士、全国和省级优秀临床人才等中医学高级人才，为浊毒证的研究乃至中医学事业储备了人才，注入了新鲜血液。浊毒理论研究受到了高度重视，国家中医药管理局批准建立了浊毒证（慢性胃炎）重点研究室，在研究室的申报、建设和验收过程中，多位专家对浊毒证研究提出了建设性意见和厚望。河北省中医院脾胃病科又以浊毒证研究为基础，先后成功申报了国家临床重点专科，国家中医药管理局重点学科、重点专科，河北省科学技术厅重点实验室，河北省中医药管理局慢性肝病浊毒证重点研究室、溃疡性结肠炎浊毒证重点研究室等，为浊毒证研究搭建了医、教、研"三位一体"的水平更高、辐射面更广的学术平台。

《中医浊毒论（汉英对照）》集浊毒理论研究之大成，凝聚了多年来李佃贵教授学术团队的研究成果。"浊"和"毒"的概念肇始于《黄帝内经》，又散见于诸多朝代的医籍中，但都是分而谈之，并未见有"浊毒"之说。中医学的特点决定了浊毒论的产生与时代的发展密不可分，浊毒的形成是社会、经济、人文、科学、自然环境发生巨大变化后机体的致病因素随之发生相应改变的重要结果之一。因此，浊毒对人体的影响既有内因，又有外因，必然产生不同于传统外感六淫、七情损伤等病因。同样，浊毒作用于人体，使之发生的病理变化又有其特异性。本书从古代文献溯源浊毒的概念、病因、病机的源头，探讨其历史演变过程，以及在临床各科的应用，系统总结并初步构建了浊毒理论的学术体系，具有较高的学术价值和学术地位。

《中医浊毒论（汉英对照）》的出版，势必为浊毒证研究注入强劲的动力，进一步推动本研究的深入，同时一定对推动中医学理论的丰富、创新和发展起到重要的启迪作用，故乐为之序。

中国工程院院士
2023年10月

As an important part of traditional Chinese culture, TCM has experienced a long historical evolution process. The emergence of *Medical Classic of the Yellow Emperor* in the Spring and Autumn Period marked the formation of the theoretical system of TCM. Zhang Zhongjing's *Treatise on Febrile Diseases* first started the time of ZangFu syndrome differentiation. The formation of the syndrome differentiation treatment system experienced classical literature excavation, collation, inheritance and development by doctors of different theories and schools. In Jin dynasty, Wang Shuhe compiled *Pulse Classic* — the first monograph of TCM pulse. In Sui dynasty, Chao Yuanfang completed *On Sources Of All Kinds Of Diseases* — the first monograph on etiology and syndromes. The understanding and treatment of external diseases, internal injuries and other febrile diseases of Liu Wansu, Zhang Yuansu, Li Dongyuan, Zhu Danxi, Four major physicians of Jin and Yuan dynasties, and Ye Tianshi, Wu Youke, Wu Jutong, Wang Mengying of Qing dynasty, Wang Qingren's understanding of blood stasis in *Error Correction of Medical Forest*, Zhang Xichun's understanding of integrating TCM with Western Medicine in *Records of Practising TCM in combination with Western Medicine*, further promoted, enriched and developed the theoretical system of TCM, reflecting the prosperity of TCM cause and academic contention among different schools. The history of the development of traditional Chinese medicine shows that the improvement of the academic level of traditional Chinese medicine relies on learning and summarizing the theory and experience of the sages, relies on sustainable discovering, enriching, improving, developing and perfecting in long - time clinical practice by physicians of different generations. Every medical academic thought is formed through debating, contention, and finally bear fruit. The academic thoughts of every physician are all the fruit of debating and contention. The publication of *On Turbidity Toxin of Traditional Chinese Medicine* (*Chinese - English Version*) is completed on similar basis.

Yanzhao has produced a large number of famous doctors since ancient times, and each doctor has left a remarkable record for developing traditional Chinese medicine. Bianque of Xingtai, Dou Mo of Feixiang County, Zhang Yuansu — the originator of the Yishui School, Liu Hejian, one of the Four Gentlemen of Jin and yuan dynasties, Li Dongyuan — the creator of Spleen Invigorating School, Luo Tianyi of Gaocheng, Wang Haogu of Zhao County, Wang Qingren of Yutian County who focused on promoting blood circulation to remove blood stasis, and Zhang Xichun of Yanshan County who pioneered on integrating Chinese and Western medicine, have paved profound heritage in developing and innovating traditional Chinese medicine in Yanzhao. Professor Li Diangui, one of the 12 famous Chinese medicine practitioners in Hebei Province, follows the law of the development of Chinese medicine, traces back to the source, after consulting a large number of literature in combination with his many years of clinical practice experience, first proposed the innovative theory of Chinese medicine turbid toxin theory, and applied it in treatment of chronic gastritis, intestinal metaplasia, dysplasia and other gastric precancerous lesions, as well as chronic liver disease, cirrhosis, ulcerative colitis and other diseases, has achieved gratifying clinical effects.

At the first TCM Development Summit Forum in Hebei Province, TCM master Lu Guangxin spoke highly of turbid toxin theory. In recent years, owing to the joint efforts of the academic team headed by Professor Li Diangui, the research of turbid toxin syndrome has achieved considerable achievements, many academic papers have been published in national journals, the relevant research results have been exchanged in national academic conferences for many times and won a number of provincial and ministerial science and technology progress awards. At the same time, a large number of Chinese Medicine senior talents such as doctors, masters, national and provincial outstanding clinical talents have been cultivated, which has reserved talents and injected fresh blood for the research of turbid toxin syndrome and even the cause of Chinese medicine. The study of turbid toxin theory has been highly valued. The State Administration of Traditional Chinese Medicine approved the establishment of a key research office of turbid toxin syndrome (chronic gastritis). In the process of application, construction and acceptance of the laboratory, a number of experts put forward constructive suggestions and high hopes for the study of turbid toxin syndrome. Based on the study of turbid toxin syndrome, the Spleen and Gastric Diseases Department of Hebei Provincial Hospital of Traditional Chinese Medicine has successfully applied for national clinical key specialties, key disciplines and key specialties of the State Administration of Traditional Chinese Medicine, key laboratory of Hebei Provincial Department of Science and Technology, Key Laboratory of Chronic Liver Disease Turbid Toxin Syndrome of Hebei Provincial Administration of Traditional Chinese Medicine, Key Laboratory of turbid toxin syndrome of ulcerative colitis, etc. It has built an academic platform with higher level and wider radiation for the study of turbid toxin syndrome, which is the trinity of medicine, teaching and research.

On Turbid Toxin of Traditional Chinese Medicine (Chinese - English Version) collects the great achievements of the study of turbid toxin theory, and embodies the research results of Professor Li Diangui's academic team over the years. The concept of "turbidity" and "toxin" is originated in *Medical Classic of the Yellow Emperor*, and scattered in many medical books of the dynasties, but they were all discussed separately, and there was no expression as "turbid toxin". The characteristics of traditional Chinese medicine determine that the emergence of turbid toxin theory is closely related to the development of the times. It is one of the important results of corresponding changes in the pathogenic factors of the body after great changes of society, economy, humanity, science and natural environment. Therefore, the influence of turbid toxin on human body has both internal and external causes, which will inevitably produce disease cause different from the traditional exogenous hurt of six evils and internal injuries of seven kinds of emotions. Similarly, how turbid toxin acts on the human body and causes the pathological changes has its own characteristic. This book traces the concept, etiology and pathogenesis of turbid toxin from ancient literature, discusses its historical evolution and its application in clinical departments, systematically summarizes and initially constructs the academic system of turbid toxin theory, which has high academic value and academic status.

The publication of *On Turbid Toxin of Traditional Chinese Medicine* (*Chinese - English Version*) is bound to inject strong impetus into the study of turbid toxin syndrome, further promote the depth of this study, and it will surly play an important inspiring role in promoting the enrichment, innovation and development of traditional Chinese medicine theory. Therefore, I am delighted to preface it.

Wu Yiling

Academician of China Engineering Academy

October, 2023

前 言
Introduction

中医学是中国传统医学的重要组成部分，其几千年的辉煌历史为中国乃至世界人民的繁衍昌盛及身心健康做出了不可磨灭的贡献。中医历代名医名家辈出，学术思想不断创新，诊疗方法不断完善，为后世留下了宝贵的文化遗产。

国医大师李佃贵教授亦是发展中医临床文化，创新中医学术思想的典型代表。他遵循中医学的发展规律，溯本求源，通过查阅大量文献，结合自己数十年的临床实践经验，尤其在治疗慢性萎缩性胃炎伴肠上皮化生和（或）不典型增生等胃癌前病变方面，打破了多年来"胃癌前病变不能逆转"的理论束缚，守正创新，首次提出中医创新理论——浊毒论，得到了业界的高度评价。

目前，随着生态环境的变化和生活方式的改变，人类的疾病谱发生了巨大变化。中医浊毒论深刻地揭示了疾病的病因和疾病发展的内在规律，并与现代病因学接轨，将传统中医学的预防原则和现代预防医学的具体措施结合为一个整体，对预防疾病的发生和阻止疾病的发展有重要的指导作用。为了让中医浊毒论走向国际，进一步推动中医药的全球化进程，国医大师李佃贵教授团队历时近三年，编写而成《中医浊毒论（汉英对照）》。本书共分十二章，阐述了浊毒概论和相关疾病的浊毒理论，内容涵盖慢性胃炎浊毒论、消化性溃疡浊毒论、肝纤维化浊毒论、胃癌浊毒论、肝癌浊毒论、溃疡性结肠炎浊毒论、结肠癌浊毒论、肾病浊毒论、代谢性疾病浊毒论、眼病浊毒论及新冠病毒感染浊毒论等内容。

本书可供致力于或关注浊毒论工作的国内及国外中西医临床、科研、教学人员阅读，也可供中西医高等医学院校研究生和大学生学习、参考。

编者
2023年11月

As an important part of world traditional medicine, Traditional Chinese Medicine with glorious history of thousands of years has made indelible contributions to the prosperity and physical and mental health of people in China and even the world. TCM has produced a large number of famous doctors in the past dynasties, made continuous innovation in academic thinking and improvement in diagnosis and treatment methods, left valuable cultural heritage for later generations.

TCM master, Professor Li Diangui as a typical representative in developing TCM clinical culture and innovating TCM academic thought is especially good at treating gastric precancerous lesion such as chronic atrophic gastritis accompanied by intestinal metaplasia and/or atypical hyperplasia. He follows the development rule of TCM and traces back to the origin, upholds fundamental principles and breaks new ground, put forward the innovative theory of traditional Chinese medicine — turbid toxin theory for the first time after consulting a large number of literature and combining his decades of clinical practice. The theory has broken the theoretical bondage of "gastric precancerous lesions cannot be reversed" for many years and has been highly praised by the industry.

At present, along with the changes of ecological environment and life style, the spectrum of human diseases has undergone great changes. The turbid toxin theory of traditional Chinese medicine which deeply reveals the etiology of diseases and the internal rule of disease development and integrates the preventive principles of traditional Chinese medicine with the specific measures of modern preventive medicine as a whole has an important guiding role in preventing the occurrence and development of diseases. In order to make the theory of TCM turbid toxin go international and further promote the process of TCM globalization, the team of TCM master Professor Li Diangui spent nearly three years to write *On Turbid Toxin of Traditional Chinese Medicine* (*Chinese - English Version*). The book is divided into 12 chapters introducing the turbid toxin concept and the application of turbid toxin theory in related diseases treatment including chronic gastritis, peptic ulcer, liver fibrosis, gastric cancer, liver cancer, ulcerative colitis, colon cancer , kidney disease, metabolic disease, eye disease and novel coronavirus pneumonia.

This book is adapted to domestic and foreign clinical, researching and teaching personnel who are committed to or concerned about the work of turbid toxin, and can also be studied and referred to by postgraduates and college students in medical colleges of traditional Chinese and Western medicine.

Editors
November, 2023

译者的话
Translator's words

《中医浊毒论（汉英对照）》翻译是我四年跟师学习的一个小结，也是我在中医之路上执着前行的一个新的起点。作为恩师李佃贵教授的弟子，有幸在临床一线直面形形色色的疑难疾患，我见证了恩师的浊毒理论及其理法方药在缓解患者疾苦，逆转癌前病变方面创造的诸多惊喜与奇迹。如果说新冠让全球再次发现了中医在应对重大疫情方面的积极作用，那么，李佃贵教授创立的浊毒理论则是打开癌前病变防治之门的一把钥匙。

桃李不言，下自成蹊。期待本书的出版能为医学中人和国内外患者提供实用有效的理论指导和治疗帮助，为中医走向世界和全球医学事业的发展进步有所贡献。

翻译是对原著的跨语言、跨文化解读与再创作，但中医本身是哲学、医学和科学的高度综合，中国人学中医都需要克服古汉语和通俗汉语之间，专业术语和日常用语之间的表达和理解屏障，译成英文给全球英语读者去领会和理解自然会面临更大的困难和挑战。感恩恩师的信任和编委会、出版社领导和编辑的包容与支持，使本书翻译顺利完成，感谢中医翻译界前辈特别是李照国老师翻译《黄帝内经》、编纂《汉英中医药大词典》并拟就中医英译规范与标准，使本书译者得以有效参考。

张振祥

2023年12月

Translation of *On Turbid Toxin of Traditional Chinese Medicine* (*Chinese - English Version*) is a summary of my four years of learning from teacher in clinical practice, and also a new starting point for my persistent progress on the road of traditional Chinese medicine. As a disciple of TCM Master, Professor Li Diangui, I had the honor to face all kinds of difficult diseases in the clinical front line, and witnessed many surprises and miracles created by my teacher's turbid toxin theory with its principles, methods, prescriptions and medicines in alleviating patients' suffering and reversing precancerous lesions. I believe as the new coronavirus has made the world once again discover the positive role of Traditional Chinese Medicine in dealing with major epidemics, the turbid toxin theory created by Professor Li Diangui will be and has already become a key to open the door for prevention and treatment of precancerous lesions.

Peach and plum blooms need not blow their own horns, spontaneously sightseers come to them in droves. It is expected that the publication of this book can provide practical and effective theoretical guidance and treatment help for medical practitioners and patients at home and abroad, and contribute to the development and progress of TCM to the world and the global medical cause.

Translation is a cross-language and cross-cultural interpretation and re-creation of the original work. However, TCM itself is highly integrated in philosophy, medicine and science, even Chinese people learning TCM need to overcome the barrier of expression and understanding between ancient Chinese and popular Chinese, between professional terms and daily expressions. Therefore, translating turbid toxin theory into English for global English readers will naturally face greater difficulties and challenges. Thanks to the trust of my teacher Professor Li Diangui, and the tolerance and support of the editorial board, the leaders of the publishing house and the editors, the translation of this book has been successfully completed. Thanks to the predecessors in the field of TCM translation, especially Teacher Li Zhaoguo for translating *Medical Classic of the Yellow Emperor*, compiling the *A Comprehensive Chinese-English Dictionary of Traditional Chinese Medicine*, and preparing the norms and standards for the translation of TCM into English, so that the translator of this book can have an effective reference.

Zhang Zhenxiang

December, 2023

目　录
CONTENTS

目 录
Contents

"浊毒理论"是由我国著名中医脾胃病专家、国医大师李佃贵教授提出的中医新理论，最初用于指导慢性萎缩性胃炎伴肠上皮化生、异型增生等胃癌前病变的治疗，形成了以"化浊解毒"为特色的理论体系和诊疗方案。之后，该理论不断丰富发展，不仅应用于脾胃、肝胆系疾病，还广泛用于指导内科、外科、妇科、儿科、皮肤科、五官科等多学科疾病的诊疗。它充实了中医证候学，创新了中医病因病机学。

"Turbid toxin theory" is created by Chinese Professor Li Diangui, National TCM master, and famous professional expert in spleen and stomach diseases. Turbid toxin theory was firstly used to instruct the treatment of chronic atrophic gastritis, intestinal metaplasia, dysplasia and other gastric precancerous lesions. Then it formed systematic theory and medical solution characterized by turbidity resolving and toxin removing. Later on utilization of the theory was widely expanded from the treatment of spleen and stomach diseases, hepatobiliary diseases into the treatment of internal diseases, surgery diseases, gynecology, pediatrics, dermatology, ent and other multidisciplinary diseases. It enriched TCM syndrome and innovated TCM etiology and pathogenesis.

任何一种学术思想的形成都有其深刻的社会、自然因素。如张仲景行医之时，正值伤寒肆虐，宗族二百余人，"犹未十稔，其死亡者三分有二，伤寒十居其七"，于是，"勤求古训，博采众方"，撰写了《伤寒杂病论》。刘河间行医时，正值火症大疫流行之际，提出"五运六气有所更，世态居民有所变，天以常火，人以常动，内外皆扰"，理论结合实践，以火热立论，力挽时弊。而李东垣行医之时正是金元之交，战乱频仍，饥困劳役，人们怒忿悲思恐惧，损伤元气，所以脾胃受困，内伤之病尤多，故而形成了内伤脾胃学说。

The formation of any professional thought has specific social and natural background. For example, Zhang Zhongjing wrote *On Febrile Miscellaneous Diseases* on the basis of learning from history and integrating all kinds of prescriptions of fellow colleagues, because he lived in the years of typhoid fever. "two thirds of my 200 family members died in less than 10 years, seven tenths of which died of typhoid fever." Liu Hejian pointed out "weather and lifestyle changes, weather is filled with constant fire, while people move in constant motion. Health is troubled with inner and outer pathogenic factors." Combining theory with practice, he created fire theory to defeat the bizarre. Li Dongyuan created spleen and stomach diseases theory, because he lived Jin and Yuan time, when people were troubled more with inner diseases, especially spleen and stomach diseases because of constant war, hunger, overdue work, anger, worry and fear.

随着近代工业文明的兴起和城市的发展，人类在创造巨大财富的同时，也把数十亿吨计的废气和废物排入天地之间，生态环境受到严重污染，加之人们生活方式的深刻变革，疾病谱也发生了深刻变化，传统中医理论在指导某些疾病的诊疗时，日益暴露了一些局限性。正如张元素所言："运气不齐，古今异轨，古方新病，不相能也。"在继承前人的基础上，依据当代人类疾病谱的深刻变革和对健康的新需求，不断地丰富中医学知识体系的关联及其所形成的多维、多层级结构，以创新适应时代需求的理论体系，是中医学不断蓬勃发展的内在动力，也是遵循中医药学自身发展规律，不断传承精华，守正创新的生动实践。

The rise of modern industrial civilization and the development of urbanization created enormous wealth, at the same time produced billions of tons of waste gas in the air and solid waste down to the earth. The seriously polluted ecological environment profoundly changed people's lifestyle together with the disease spectrum. Traditional Chinese Medicine theory is frequently exposed to some limitations in guiding diagnosis and treatment of some diseases. As Zhang Yuansu said: "The weather in modern times is different with that in ancient times, some new diseases can not be cured by old prescriptions." Considering the deep changes of the contemporary human diseases and the new demand for health, to constantly improve the associated multidimensional and hierarchical structure of TCM knowledge system and innovate the theoretical system on the basis of inheriting predecessors' experiences becomes the inner motivation and vivid practice for us to inherit essence, uphold integrity and make innovation according to the developing rules of TCM.

历代医家虽然对"浊""毒"有零散记载，但是均未对浊毒进行系统的论述，而浊毒理论所说的"浊毒"，虽然吸纳和借鉴了中医古代关于"浊"与"毒"的含义，但并不仅仅是"浊"与"毒"的简单叠加，而是赋予了其丰富的时代内涵。李佃贵教授考据《说文解字》"浊者，清之反也"，《康熙字典》"毒，恶也，害也，苦也"，因此，就把所有对人体有害的不洁之物和不良的精神神志刺激均称之为"浊毒"。他带领团队围绕"浊毒"进行了理、法、方、药的系统理论构建，创新了新的发病观——浊毒化，以及新的治疗观——化浊毒，并首倡当代人类的健康观为"净化人体内环境"。浊毒理论是新时代中医药的重要理论创新，是更契合当代人类健康的中医新理论。

Physicians of different times left scattered records of "turbidity" and "toxin", but turbid toxin has never been systematically discussed in history. Although the turbidity toxin theory absorbed and referred to the implication of "turbidity" and "toxin" in ancient TCM, but the theory is not just a simple line-up of the two words, it contains rich connotation of the era. Professor Li Diangui found in the ancient dictionary of *Shuowen Jiezi*, "turbid", means contrary to clear. Then in *Kangxi Dictionary*: "toxin, means evil, harm and bitter", therefore, he summarizes all unclean materials harmful to human body and harmful mind and mental stimulation generally called "turbid toxin". He lead his team to construct the systematic "turbid toxin theory" with principle, method, prescription and medicine, refreshed the outlook of diseases as "turbid-toxin change" and the view of treatment as "turbidity resolving and toxin removing" and firstly refreshed the contemporary human health perspectives as "purifying the inner environment of human body". Turbid toxin theory is an important theoretical innovation of the new era of Traditional Chinese Medicine, which is more suitable for contemporary human health.

第一章 浊毒概论
Chapter 1 Overview of Turbid Toxin

第一节 浊毒的基本内涵
Section 1 The Basic Connotation of Turbid Toxin

一、浊毒的基本含义
1. The basic meaning of turbid toxin

（一）广义浊毒
1.1 Broad sense of turbid toxin

广义的浊毒，泛指一切对人体有害的不洁物质和不良情志，可分为外浊毒和内浊毒，外浊毒又分为"天之浊毒"和"地之浊毒"，内浊毒主要指"人之浊毒"。

In a broad sense, turbid toxin refers to all unclean substances and bad feelings harmful to human body, which can be divided into external turbid toxin and internal turbid toxin. External turbid toxin is divided into "turbid toxin of heaven" and "turbid toxin of earth", and internal turbid toxin mainly refers to "turbid toxin of human".

1.天之浊毒 《灵枢》曰："人与天地相参也，与日月相应也。"人类生活在自然界，自然界有着人类赖以生存的必要条件。人体生命活动受自然规律的支配和约束，天地大自然的各种变化时时影响着人的功能活动。传统中医认为，自然界风、寒、暑、湿、燥、火六气太过成为"六淫"，或非其时而有其气形成的自然灾害，均可影响脏腑气血功能而致疾病发生。近代随着生态环境的不断恶化，外感六淫已经无法涵盖外在的致病因素，所谓天之浊毒，除包括传统的六淫之外，还包括以下因素：

1.1.1 Turbid toxin of the sky *Spiritual Pivot* says, "Man interacts with heaven and earth, sun and moon." Human beings live in nature which provides necessary conditions for survival. The life activities of people are governed and constrained by rules of nature, the various changes of heaven, earth and nature always affect the functional activities of human beings. According to Traditional Chinese Medicine, the excessive wind, cold, heat, dampness, dryness and fire from nature become "six evils", the natural disasters caused by abnormal weather in wrong time can affect the function of breath and blood of viscera organs and cause diseases. The constant deterioration of the ecological environment in modern times produced the following factors which causes diseases beside the traditional six evils:

（1）空气中污染物：包括悬浮颗粒物、飘尘、二氧化硫、一氧化碳、碳氢化物、氮氧化物、碳烟等。这些物质不仅是构成或加重人类呼吸疾病的重要原因，还可直接产生或诱发多种疾病。

1.1.1.1 The pollutants in the air: they include suspended particulate matter, floating dust, sulfur dioxide, carbon monoxide, hydrocarbons, nitrogen oxides, carbon smoke, etc. These substances are not only important causes that constitute or aggravate human respiratory diseases, but also can directly produce or induce a variety of diseases.

（2）大量的致病微生物：随着全球气候变暖，生态环境恶化，大量致病微生物生成繁殖，致使瘟疫频发。有研究表明，温暖的气候与瘟疫爆发之间有联系，更为湿润和温暖的气候条件意味着比正常情况下更适合细菌和病毒生存，而这些病菌传播到人身上的危险性也更大。气候变化还会使人的抵抗能力和免疫能力下降，这些因素综合在一起，就会增加瘟疫流行的概率。

1.1.1.2 Large quantity of pathogenic microorganisms: along with global warming and the deterioration of ecological environment, a large number of pathogenic microorganisms generate and reproduce, resulting in frequent plague. Studies have shown that a warm climate is linked to plague outbreaks, wetter and warmer climates are more suitable to survive bacteria and viruses, at the same time increase the danger of pathogen transmission to people. Climate changes also reduce human resistance and immunity, which, taken together, can increase the probability of a plague epidemic.

（3）噪声、电磁辐射、光辐射等：随着现代化、城市化的进程，各种噪声、电磁、辐射物质及光等无形的辐射增加，它们弥漫于空中，虽然看不见、摸不到，但又的确是客观存在的，并且逐渐成为人类无形的杀手。研究证实，长期接受噪音干扰和电磁辐射会造成人体免疫力下降、新陈代谢紊乱，甚至导致各类癌症的发生。

1.1.1.3 Noise, electromagnetic radiation, light radiation, etc. :the process of modernization and urbanization produce and increase all kinds of noise, electromagnetic, radiation materials, light and other invisible radiation. They diffuse in the air, although invisible, cannot be touched, but exist objectively, and gradually become the invisible killer of human beings. Studies have confirmed that long-term exposure to noise interference and electromagnetic radiation can reduce human immunity, induce metabolic disorders and increase the occurrences of all kinds of cancers.

2.地之浊毒　《素问》曰："天食人以五气，地食人以五味。"人类的生存除了依赖"天之五气"，还离不开"地之五味"，地之浊毒主要是指受污染的水和食物。水是一切生命赖以生存的基础，水污染使食物的质量安全难以得到保障。污染水中的重金属通过水、土壤，在植物的生长过程中逐步渗入其中。食用吸收了含有的过量重金属元素污染的动植物后会对人体产生危害，还有当水中含有的放射性物质较多时，一些对某些放射性核素有很强的富集作用的水产品，如鱼类、贝类等，就会使得食品中放射核素的含量可能显著地增加，对人体造成损害。水中含有的有机污染物对食物安全影响更大。一些有机污染物的分子比较稳定，通过水的作用很容易在动植物内部蓄积，损害人体健康。而农药化肥的滥用也是农作物污染的重要因素。这些被污染的水和食物首先经口进入人体的消化系统，损伤脾胃，使后天之本受损，变生浊毒，以致百病丛生。

1.1.2 Turbid toxin of earth　*Simple Conversation* said: "The sky feed people with five gases, and the earth feed people with five tastes." Human survival not only depends on the "five gases of heaven", but also depends on the "five tastes of earth". The turbid toxin of earth mainly refers to the polluted water and food. Water is the basis of all life, water pollution makes it difficult to guarantee the quality and safety of food. Heavy metals in contaminated water pass through water and soil, and gradually penetrate into the plants during the growth of them. Edible absorption of plants and animals containing excessive heavy metal element will harm human body. When water contains more radioactive substances, the content of radionuclides in aquatic products such as fish, shellfish, may be significantly increased, which cause damages to human body. Organic pollutants contained in water have a greater impact on food safety. The molecules of some organic pollutants are relatively stable, and will be accumulated in plants and animals through the action of water, damage human health. The abuse of pesticides and fertilizers is also an important factor in crop pollution. These polluted water and food first enter the human digestive system through the mouth, damage the postnatal basis of spleen and stomach, produce turbid toxin, which bear all kinds of diseases.

3.人之浊毒　即狭义之浊毒，为现阶段浊毒理论研究的重点，下文关于浊毒的论述大多是指人之浊毒。

1.1.3 Turbid toxin of human　Human turbid toxin is the narrow sense of turbidity toxin, which is the focus of study on the turbid toxin theory at the present stage. The following discussion on turbid toxin mostly refers to human turbid toxin.

（二）狭义浊毒

1.2 The narrow sense of turbid toxin

狭义浊毒即人之浊毒，主要由情志不畅、神志不清、饮食不节（洁）、起居失常以及代谢障碍所形成，又可分为"身之浊毒"和"心之浊毒"。

The narrow sense of turbid toxin, so-called the turbid toxin of people, mainly refers to depression and confusion in mind, excess of diet, irregular lifestyle, and metabolic disorders, and can be divided into "the turbid toxin of the body" and "the turbid toxin of the mind".

1.身之浊毒　它既是致病因素，又是病理产物。其常由多种因素导致脏腑功能紊乱、气血运行失常机体内产生的代谢产物不能及时正常排出，蕴积体内而化生，又可以对人体脏腑经络及气血阴阳均能造成严重损害。按其所在部位可分为脏浊毒、腑浊毒、经浊毒、络浊毒、气浊毒、血浊毒、津浊毒、液浊毒等，按其属性的不同，又可分为湿浊毒和谷浊毒两种。

1.2.1 The turbid toxin of the body　It is both a pathogenic factor and a pathological product. It is born of retained and accumulated metabolites in human body which can not be discharged normally in time due to dysfunction of the viscera, abnormal operation of breath and blood, and can cause serious damage to the human viscera, meridians, breath, blood, Yin and Yang. According to its location, turbid toxin can be divided into turbid toxin of storing organ, turbid toxin of transforming organ, turbid toxin of channel, turbid toxin of collateral, turbid toxin of breath, blood toxin, turbid toxin of sweat, turbid toxin of liquid of body. According to its different properties, turbid toxin can be divided into wet turbid toxin and grain turbid toxin.

（1）湿浊毒：人体从饮食中摄入的水谷精微应细分为"水精微"和"谷精微"，相应地，饮食在人体的代谢失常所产生的病理产物也应分为"湿浊"和"谷浊"。湿浊是人体水液代谢失常所形成的病理产物的统称，包括水湿、痰饮等。关于水液在人体内的代谢过程，《黄帝内经》已有精辟论述。《素问·经脉别论》曰："饮入于胃，游溢精气，上输于脾，脾气散精，上归于肺，通调水道，下输膀胱，水精四布，五经并行。"水饮摄入人体后，经胃、小肠、大肠的消化吸收，脾脏的运化转输，上归于肺，通过肺气通调水道的作用，一方面把水液经肺气宣发，心脉运载，而输布全身，调养脏腑腠理皮毛等各组织器官，一部分变成汗液排出体外；另一方面水液沿着水道，经肺气的肃降，肝脏的疏利，三焦的通调，水液下降至肾，肾脏分别清浊，清者又上输于肺，敷布全身，浊者形成尿液，下输膀胱，经气化而把尿液排出体外。如此推陈出新，循环不息。无论是外罹天之浊毒、地之浊毒，还是七情、劳倦、饮食内伤，致使人体脏腑功能失调，或肺失于宣肃，或脾失于运化，或肾失于气化，皆可产生湿浊毒。尤其是脾运化水湿的功能失调，由于脾位于中焦，为人体气机升降的枢纽，脾失健运，则水液既无法上输于肺，又无法下达于肾，则水液停滞于体内，变生水湿、痰饮等湿浊。浊毒的生成一般遵循湿—热—浊—毒的演变过程。湿本是自然界的六气之一，《素问·五运行大论》曰："燥以干之，暑以蒸之，风以动之，湿以润之，寒以坚之，火以温之。"正常的湿气是万物赖以滋养繁茂的重要因素。如果湿气太过或非其时而有其气，则为湿邪。湿邪既有内外之分，又有清浊之别。就自然界来说，清湿者，地气轻清上升所致，雾露雨雪，皆为其象；浊湿者，重浊污秽，淫雨泥水皆为其象。就人体而言，或因外感湿邪，或因脾胃受损，水湿不化，久蕴体内，多从热化，多自热生。刘完素《河间六书》曰："湿本土气，火热能生土湿，故夏热则万物湿润，秋凉则湿复燥干也。湿病本不自生，因于火热怫郁，水液不能宣行，即停滞而生水湿。故湿者多自热生。"浊即湿久蕴热所致，叶天士谓"湿久浊凝"。朱丹溪谓："浊主湿热，有痰有虚。""血受湿热，久必凝浊。"浊邪进一步发展即为浊毒，浊毒为浊邪之极，浊邪为浊毒之渐。

1.2.1.1 Wet turbid toxin: the micro essence of water and grain consumed by people from diet should be subdivided into "micro water essence" and "micro grain essence", accordingly, the pathological products produced by the metabolic disorder of diet in human body should also be divided into "wet turbidity" and "grain turbidity". Wet turbidity is a general term for the pathological products formed by the disorder of human water fluid metabolism, including water dampness, sputum drinking, etc. The metabolic process of water fluid in the human body has been brilliantly discussed in *The Medical Classic of the Yellow Emperor. Simple Conversation-Special Discussion on Channels and Vessels says*, "Beverages are drunk into stomach, the vital essence in the beverage rises into spleen, spreading the essence through the spleen and then into lung, regulating waterways, and the remaining part settles down as urine into bladder. Water and essence are distributed to the whole body, running through the five meridians simultaneously." After the water drink is ingested into human body, it is digested and absorbed by stomach, small and large intestine, and then the essence is transported into spleen spreading over the whole body through lung movement. Lung has the function of dredging and regulating the waterway. Part of the water essence are transported to the body through heart meridian nourishing the viscera, fur, tissues and organs. The other part of the water essence is turned into sweat leaving the body through sweating pores. On the other hand, along the waterway, the water fluid drops into kidney viscera after being purified and descended by lung, promoted by liver, dredged and regulated by the triple energizer. The kidneys separate the settled water into clean and turbid water respectively. The clear ones are transmitted to the lung and spread again all over the body. The turbid ones are turned into urine, which is transmitted to the bladder, and discharged from the body through bladder vaporization. In this way, the metabolism continues in an endless cycle. Dampness and turbidity toxin can be produced either from the external turbidity toxin of heaven and earth, or from the internal turbid toxin of seven emotions, fatigue and internal injury of diet, which lead to the dysfunction of human viscera, such as the dysfunction of purification and descending of the lung, the dysfunction of transporting and transformation of spleen, or the dysfunction of vaporization of kidney. In particular, the dysfunctional of water and dampness transporting of spleen will block the water channel to lung and kidney, and the polluted water will stagnate in the body, resulting in dampness, phlegm and other kind of damp turbid toxin, because the spleen is located in the middle coke of the body, and is the pivot for air rising and fall of human body. The generation of turbid toxin generally follows the evolution process of dampness, heat, turbid, and toxin. Dampness is one of the six evils in nature. *Simple Conversation-Five Movement Theory* says: "Dryness is to dry, heat is to steam, wind is to move, dampness is to moist, cold is to firm, and fire is to warm." Normal moisture is an important factor for all things to nourish and flourish. If the moisture is too much or not at the right time, it is called dampness toxin. Dampness toxin can be divided into internal and external, as well as clear and turbid. In nature, clear dampness is produced by the light rise of soil vapor such as fog, dew, rain and snow and other climate phenomenon; turbid dampness is produced from heavy turbidity and filthy such as obscene rain, and mud water. In human body, the damp turbid toxin is caused either by exogenous dampness evil, or by internal heat brewed from the long-time accumulated remaining water due to the dysfunction of spleen and stomach, *Hejian Liu Shu (Liu Wansu's Six Medical Books)* says: "Dampness is originally soil vapor, and fire can heat the soil vapor to rise up. Therefore, in hot summer, everything is wet, and in cool autumn, even wet things turn to be dry. Diseases of dampness are not born by themselves, they are born from internal heat of human body. Because boiling and depression of inner fire and heat, block the fluent spreading of water and liquid, therefore, brews the water dampness. Therefore, dampness was most probably born from heat." Turbidity is caused by accumulated heat brewed from stagnated dampness, and Ye Tianshi said: "Turbidity is born from stagnated dampness." Zhu Danxi said: "Turbidity dominates damp heat, phlegm and deficiency","blood attacked by damp heat will certainly brew turbidity in future." The further development of turbid evil is turbid toxin. Turbid toxin is the future of turbid evil, turbid evil is the past of turbid toxin.

（2）谷浊毒：谷浊即谷精微在人体内运化失常所致。谷精微的化生和转运，主要是脾胃和大小肠共同作用的结果。《灵枢·海论》说："胃者，水谷之海。"《灵枢·本输》也说："胃者，五谷之腑。"指出了胃的受纳功能。杨上善说："胃受五谷成熟，传入小肠。"指出了胃的腐熟功能。后世概括认为胃是对水谷进行初步消化的器官，具有受纳水谷，继而腐熟水谷成糊状食糜的功能。对于小肠的功能，《素问·灵兰秘典论》认为"小肠者，受盛之官，化物出焉"，后世概括为主受盛化物，泌别清浊，即指经胃初步消化的饮食物，在小肠内必须有相当时间的停留，以利于进一步彻底消化，将水谷分化为精微与糟粕两部分。脾则将这些谷食之精气化为营气和卫气，转运输送于上焦，大肠则将糟粕排出体外。《素问·经脉别论》曰："食气入胃，散精于肝，淫气于筋。食气入胃，浊气归心，淫精于脉。脉气流经，精气归于肺，肺朝百脉，输精于皮毛。毛脉合精，行气于腑。"在这一系列的过程中，任何一个环节出现障碍，都会使谷精微运化失常而化生为谷浊。或因胃失和降，腐熟受纳功能障碍，致使水谷滞留中焦，化为浊毒，如朱丹溪所谓"故五味入口，即入于胃，留毒不散，积聚既久，致伤冲和，诸病生焉"；或小肠受盛泌别失常，清浊不分；或脾气虚弱，无力将水谷精微输布全身，滞留脉道日久而为浊（包括脂浊、糖浊等）；或大肠传导失司，糟粕郁于肠内而生浊。上述各项虽本是精微物质或正常代谢产物，但是过量聚集或失于运化，均可对人体脏腑气血造成损害，我们称之为谷浊毒，它既是病理产物，又是致病因素。

1.2.1.2 Grain turbid toxin: grain turbid toxin is caused by the abnormal transportation of grain essence in human body. The energy- transformation and transportation of grain essence are mainly the result of the joint action of spleen, stomach, large and small intestines. *Spiritual Pivot-Discussion on Seas* says "The stomach is the sea of water and grains", and *Spiritual Pivot-Discussion on Acupoints* also says: "The stomach is the house of five grains." The receiving function of stomach is pointed out. "The stomach matures the food and then send them to small intestine," Yang Shangshan said. The rotting function of stomach was pointed out. Later generations generally believed that stomach is an organ for preliminary digestion of water and grain, it receives water and grain and then rot them into pasty chyme. As for the function of the small intestine, *Simple Conversation-Linglan's Secret Treatise* holds that "the small intestine is the official of receiving, who receives the rotted food from the stomach and then separate it into subtle and dross". Later generations summarize that the small intestine mainly receives the rotted food and separate them into clear and turbid, that is, the diet primarily digested by stomach must stay in the small intestine for a considerable time, so as to be further digested and then be divided into two parts: subtle and dross. The spleen converts the essence of these cereal foods into nutrient qi and defensive qi, then transport them to the upper coke, and the large intestine expels the dross from the body. *Simple Conversation-Special Discussion on Channels and Vessels* says: "stomach receives foodstuff, disperses essence in liver and nourish the tendons with the essence. Stomach receives foodstuff, return essence to heart, and then indulge essence into the pulses. The driving force of pulse helps the operation of meridians. The essence of food returns to lung, which spread the essence over through all pulses including the pulses of skin and fur. The essence on skins and in pulses are combined and sent into viscera at last". In this series of processes, any obstacle in any link will lead to abnormal transportation of grain essence and transform it into grain turbidity. For example, if stomach force is not harmonized and restrained, rotting and receiving function does not work, the water and food will stay in the middle coke and become turbid toxin. Thus Zhu Danxi said that "The five flavors enter the mouth and stomach, stay the toxin for a long time, damage the harmony state in the middle coke, therefore all diseases arise". If the small intestine is abnormal to receive rotted food and separate the clear and turbid, or the spleen is weak, unable to transport the essence of water and grains to the whole body, water and grains will stay in pulses for a long time and become turbidity (including fat turbidity Sugar turbidity, etc.). If the conduction function of large intestine does not work, dross will stagnate in the intestine and produce turbidity. Although the above items are originally fine substances or normal metabolites, excessive accumulation or loss of transportation can cause damage to human viscera, breath and blood. We call it grain turbid toxin, which is a pathological product, as well as a pathogenic factor.

2.心之浊毒　主要是指对人体有害的不良精神意识思维活动和七情五志的异常。中医认为"心主神明"，所以人的精神意识思维活动为心所主，也就是"心主神志"。七情五志虽各有脏腑归属，但是心君主之官，为五脏六腑之大主，人对客观世界的感知活动及内心体验都是在心神主导之下进行的，故心神在情志活动中也发挥着重要作用，也就是"心主情志"。因此，我们把对人体有害的不良精神意识思维活动和七情五志的异常都称为心之浊毒。心之浊毒主要为情志之浊毒，曾国藩说："治心之道，先去其毒，阳毒曰忿，阴毒曰欲。"这里的毒就可以理解为心之浊毒的情志之浊毒。情志之浊毒也可以细分为阴浊毒、阳浊毒，阴浊毒包括大忧、大思、大悲，阳浊毒包括大怒、大恐、大惊等。

1.2.2 The turbid toxin of the mind　Mainly refers to the bad mental consciousness and thinking activities harmful to human body, and the abnormal seven emotions and five aspirations. Traditional Chinese Medicine believes that "the heart controls mental activities", so people's spiritual consciousness and thinking activities are controlled by heart, that is, "heart is the master of mental and emotional activities." Although the seven emotions and five aspirations are decided by different visceral organ, but heart is the master, or the monarch of all the viscera. People's perception and experiencing of the objective world are carried out under the leadership of the mind, so the mind also plays an important role in the activities of emotion, that is, "the mind controls spiritual and emotional activities". Therefore, all mental consciousness, thinking activities, and abnormal feelings and aspirations harmful to human body, are called the turbid toxin of the heart. The turbid toxin of the heart is mainly the turbid toxin of emotion, Zeng Guofan said: "To cure the heart, first remove its toxin, Yang toxin is anger, Yin toxin is desire." Here the toxin can be understood as the emotional turbid toxin of heart. The emotional turbid toxin can be subdivided into sunny turbid toxin and cloudy turbid toxin. Cloudy turbid toxin includes excessive worry, consideration and sad; sunny turbid toxin includes excessive anger, fear and surprise.

二、净化人体内环境是浊毒理论的健康观和核心思想
2. Purifying the human body environment is the health view and the core idea of the turbidity toxin theory

未来最好医学的标准，不是治好病的医学，而是使人不生病的医学；未来医学的研究方向，不应继续以疾病为主要研究领域，而应以人类健康作为医学的主要研究方向；未来医学的目标，应逐步向预防疾病、维护健康、防止损伤调整。而未来医学的标准、方向和目的，归根到底就是我国2000多年前中医经典《黄帝内经》里所提倡的三个字——"治未病"。"治未病"将引领未来医学发展。"治未病"的含义主要包括三个方面：未病先防，已病防变，既愈防复。但同样是治未病，当下的治未病已经和2000多年前的治未病有很大的差异。因为人们所处的生态环境、生活方式、疾病谱都发生了很大的不同！正如张元素所言："运气不齐，古今异轨，古方新病，不相能也。"浊毒理论赋予治未病思想新的内涵：未病先防——预防浊毒内生和外感；已病防变——及早发现并祛除浊毒；既愈防复——扶正固本，根除浊毒之源。

The standard of the best medical science in future is not to cure diseases, but to defend people against the harm of diseases. The future research direction of medical science should not focus on diseases, but focus on human health. The goal of future medical science should be adjusted to prevent disease, maintain health and reduce injury. Summarizing the above, it was advocated in *The Medical*

Classic of the Yellow Emperor more than 2,000 years ago that the standard, direction and purpose of future medical science is "to cure future disease". "To cure future disease" will lead the future development of medical science. The meaning of "to cure future disease" mainly includes three aspects: preventing human body from disease occurrence; preventing disease of human body from malignant transformation; preventing recovered disease from recurrence. But "to cure future disease" today is very different from that of more than 2,000 years ago, because people's ecological environment, lifestyle, disease spectrum are very different! As Zhang Yuansu said: "Climate, weather and even rules of nature of ancient and modern time are quite different, therefore ancient prescriptions may not cover all the diseases today." The theory of turbid toxin gives new connotation to the idea of curing future disease: to prevent disease by preventing endogenous generation and external infection of turbid toxin; to prevent transmission and deterioration of disease by detecting and removing turbid toxin as early as possible; to prevent disease recurrence by strengthening the positive energy and eradicating the source of turbid toxin.

俄罗斯诺贝尔奖获得者梅契尼科夫曾提出人体自身中毒学说，认为人体自身代谢的垃圾不能及时排出，是导致人类多种疾病和早衰的首要原因，这与浊毒理论的观点不谋而合。而从中医整体观来看，不能忽视外界因素，即天之浊毒和地之浊毒对人类健康的影响。当前生态环境恶化已是全人类健康的公敌，浊毒物质充斥全球，人类已成为时代产物的"浊毒垃圾桶"，而这也是影响人类健康的根源所在。因此，浊毒理论提出新时代的健康观是"净化人体内环境"，这也是浊毒理论的核心思想。即通过人体净化浊毒系统协同作用，使人体清净明亮，健康长寿，并以此指导临床诊疗和养生保健。

The Russian Nobel Prize winner Mechnikov has put forward the theory of self-poisoning theory, which coincides with the view of turbid toxin theory. It is believed that the garbage metabolites in human body which cannot be discharged in time, is the primary cause of various human diseases and premature aging. From the perspective of the overall view of TCM, external factors including the influence of the turbid toxin of sky and earth cannot be ignored. At present, the deterioration of ecological environment has become the public enemy of human health, toxic substances fill the world. Human beings have become the "toxic trash can" produced by the times, which is also the basic cause of human health. Therefore, the theory of turbid toxin proposes that the health view in the new era is to "purify the internal environment of human body", which is also the core idea of the turbid toxin theory. The coordinated work of turbid toxin purification system of internal environment make the human body clean and bright, healthy and longevity. This view and idea will guide the clinical diagnosis, treatment and health care.

三、浊毒化是浊毒理论的发病观
3. Turbid toxin change is the pathogenesis of turbid toxin theory

浊毒理论从"浊毒"角度研究疾病发生发展的规律，认为浊毒有内外之分，有轻重之别，有有形之浊毒，有无形浊毒，有在经络，有在脏腑，可上犯清窍，可下注二阴。疾病的发生很多都是浊毒病邪胶结作用于人体，导致人体细胞、组织和器官的浊化，即致病过程；浊化的结果导致细胞、组织和器官的浊变，即形态结构的改变，包括现代病理学中的肥大、增生、萎缩、化生和癌变，以及炎症、变性、凋亡和坏死等变化。浊变的结果是毒害细胞、组织和器官，使之代谢和功能失常，乃至功能衰竭。

The theory of turbid toxin studies the rule of disease occurrence and development from the perspective of "turbid toxin". It thinks turbid toxin may be divided into internal and external turbid toxin, light and serious turbid toxin, visible and invisible turbid toxin, channel and visceral turbid toxin, it can attack the seven upper orifices of the head, as well as two lower orifices. The occurrence of diseases, or the pathogenic process of disease are mostly caused by turbid transmission of cells, tissues and organs resulting from the stalemated reaction of of turbid toxin evil in human body. The result of turbid transmission is the turbid change, namely the structure and state change of human cells, tissues and organs, including hypertrophy, hyperplasia, atrophy, metaplasia and canceration, and changes in inflammation, degeneration, apoptosis and necrosis. The result of turbidity is to toxin cells, tissues and organs, causing dysfunction, and even functional failure of metabolism.

四、化浊毒是浊毒理论的方法论
4. Resolving turbidity and removing toxin is the methodology of turbid toxin theory

浊毒理论提倡张子和的"陈莝去而肠胃洁，癥瘕尽而营卫昌"。但在浊毒的治疗上，不是单纯的攻邪，更重要的是"化"，既固本以清源，又解毒以澄流。注重治未病，防治结合。浊毒理论提出了三清三调，所谓三清，即在体内浊毒壅盛时，清理体内浊毒的三个重要法则：透表化浊解毒——从汗液而排；通腑泄浊解毒——从大便而出；渗湿化浊解毒——从小便而去。所谓三调，即在体内浊毒尚未形成，或疾病缓解期时，扶正以绝浊毒之源的三个重要法则：宣肺化浊解毒——绝上焦浊毒之源；健脾化浊解毒——绝中焦浊毒之源；益肾化浊解毒——绝下焦浊毒之源。三清三调不是孤立的，而是相辅相成的，临床上当视疾病不同阶段，抓住疾病当下的主要矛盾，或以三清为主，辅以三调，或以三调为主，辅以三清，灵活运用，不可拘泥。

The turbid toxin theory advocates the saying of Zhang Zihe: "The retained metabolites go, stomach and intestines are clean; and the nourishing and defensive system is healthy without stagnation and stasis." But the treatment of turbid toxin is not only evil-attacking fight, it is more important to "change", to strengthen the positive energy and remove the source of disease, and detoxify the human body and recover the normal operation. Pay more attention to the treatment of future disease, associate prevention with treatment. The theory of turbid toxin put forward the saying of "three clearing", and "three regulating". "Three clearing" indicates three important principles to remove the abundant accumulation of turbid toxin in human body: to clear the surface turbid toxin through sweating; to clear the visceral turbid toxin through stool; to clear the wet infiltrated turbid toxin through urine. The so-called "three regulating" indicates three important principles to remove the source of turbid toxin by strengthening positive energy before the formation of turbid toxin or during the recovery period of disease, i.e to remove the source of turbid toxin in upper energizer by regulating lung, to remove the source of turbid toxin in middle energizer by regulating spleen, to remove the source of turbid toxin in lower energizer by regulating kidney. "Three clearing" and "three regulating" is not isolated, but supplementary to each other. In clinical practice, we should flexibly, not rigidly use the above principles according to the different stages of the disease, seize the main contradiction of the disease at present, either use "three clearing" supplemented by "three regulating", or use "three regulating", supplemented by "three clearing".

第二节　浊毒的病因病机
Section 2　The Etiology and Pathogenesis of Turbid Toxin

病因、病机是疾病动态演变过程中不可分割的两部分。"因"者，一为病因，即将浊毒视为一种致病因素，既可由表侵入，又能由里而生；二为导致浊毒生成的原因，涵盖了浊毒及在其基础上形成的与浊毒相关的病理产物。浊毒作为复合的病因、病机，其致病过程即机制演变贯穿于整个动态过程中，表现为易耗气伤血、壅结脉络，易阻碍气机、胶滞难祛，易积成形、败坏脏腑及迁延性、难治性、顽固性、内损性的特征。从现代医学视角探讨浊毒的致病机制，认为浊毒病邪胶结作用于人体，是通过"浊化—浊变—毒害"的病理演变，最终导致细胞、组织和器官代谢功能失常，乃至衰竭，其中包括现代病理学中的炎症、增生、萎缩、化生和癌变等变化。浊毒病邪常侵犯消化系统，是慢性萎缩性胃炎、消化性溃疡、溃疡性结肠炎、肝硬化、胰腺炎等疾病重要的致病因素。如在慢性萎缩性胃炎中，先有肝郁气滞，横犯中土，克脾伐胃，中土既虚，水湿停聚，继而积湿成浊，浊郁化热，热蕴成毒，浊毒之邪深伏胃络血分，最终形成慢性萎缩性胃炎繁杂难解的病理改变。将现代微生物学与浊毒理论相结合来看，"浊"是疾病状态下在人体内以微生态群的形式存在，与人体内微生态环境的变化密切相关，而"毒"则是致病因素达到的一种高度聚集或相对制约机制遭到破坏而成的病理状态。当人体微生态内环境失衡，即表现为"浊"，从而进一步产生"毒"。此外，浊毒还可侵及全身多系统，如呼吸系统、心脑血管系统、风湿免疫系统等，其致病常导致机体内部失调，发生脏腑组织器官等功能、代谢、形态结构上的变化。浊毒作为病理产物，在疾病发展、演变过程中亦有重要作用，如在慢性、难治性疾病病变过程中脏腑功能紊乱，气血运行失常后可产生浊毒，进一步损伤原发病灶，耗损气血，破坏形体。将浊毒作为该领域深入研究的切入点之一，在辨证、遣方用药方面考虑到浊毒的作用，对于提高临床疗效有一定的作用。

Cause and pathogenesis are two inseparable parts in dynamic evolution process of disease. As a compound of etiology and pathogenesis, turbid toxin is easy to consume energy and blood, obstruct pulses, hinder the breath, stiffly stagnated, easy to be clumped up to block, corrupt viscera, with characteristics as delaying, refractory, stubborn and internal damaging. From the perspective of modern medical science to explore the pathogenic function of turbid toxin, it is believed that evil of turbid toxin affect human body like cement through the process of pathological evolution as "turbid transmission- turbid change -toxification", eventually lead to dysfunction and even failure of metabolic function of cells, tissues and organs, including modern pathological changes like inflammation, hyperplasia, atrophy, metaplasia and canceration. The evil of turbid toxin often invades the digestive system and is an important pathogenic factor of chronic atrophic gastritis, peptic ulcer, ulcerative colitis, cirrhosis, pancreatitis and other diseases. For example, the arising and development process of chronic atrophy gastritis includes the following periods. First, liver depression and breath stagnation invades the mid-soil, affects the spleen and stomach. Second, when the mid-soil is deficient, water and wetness stays and retains. Third, wetness is accumulated into turbidity, then turbidity is stagnated into heat, heat is nurtured into toxin. Fourth, evil of turbidity and toxin goes deeply into stomach collateral and blood content, and finalizes the complex and difficult pathological change of chronic atrophy gastritis. Combining modern microbiology and turbid toxin theory, it is recognized that "turbidity" exists in the form of microecological group in human body, which is closely related to the changes of the microecological environment of human body. "Toxin" is a pathological state when pathogenic factors are highly clustered and relative restriction mechanism are damaged. In general, when human microecology environment is unbalanced, turbidity is manifested, then turbidity is further nurtured into "toxin". Further more, turbid toxin can invade different kinds of systems of human body, such as respiratory system, cardiovascular and cerebrovascular system, rheumatic immune system, etc. leads to internal disorders of human body, and makes changes in function, metabolism, morphology and structure of viscera, tissues and organs. As a pathological product, turbid toxin also plays an important role in the development and evolution of diseases. For example, in the process of chronic and refractory diseases, turbid toxin arises from dysfunction of viscera and abnormal operation of breath and blood, then further damage the disease focus, consume energy and blood, and destroy the body.

一、浊毒病因特点
1. The etiology and characteristics of turbid toxin

（一）外感淫疠毒邪
1.1. Exterior evil and pestilence

　　浊毒可由外而入，或从皮毛，或从口鼻，侵入机体，对人体脏腑、经络、气血、阴阳均能造成严重损害。"浊"者，不清也，浊与湿紧密相关，外感湿浊，由表入里。外界湿浊之邪侵入人体的途径大致有三条：一是通过呼吸由口鼻进入人体，先影响人体的上焦，进而影响到中焦、下焦。正如《医原·湿气论》所说："湿之化气，多从上受，邪自口鼻吸入，故先传天气，次及地气。"二是通过肌肉皮肤渗透进入人体，先客于肌表关节，次阻经络，最终深入脏腑。清代张璐说："湿气积久，留滞关节。"《素问·调经论》曰："风雨之伤人也，先客于皮肤，传入于孙脉，孙脉满则传入于络脉，络脉满则输于大经脉。"又曰："寒湿之中人也，皮肤不收，肌肉坚紧，荣血泣，卫气去，故曰虚。"三是湿邪中伤脾胃。《六因条辨·卷下》曰："夫湿乃重浊之邪，其伤人也最广……殆伤则伤其表，表者，乃阳明之表，肌肉也；中则中其内，内者，乃太阴之内，脾阴也，湿土也。故伤则肢节必痛，中则脘腹必闷。"当然外感湿浊之邪侵犯人体，可能只有一种途径，也可能两种或者三种途径同时存在。如湿温病初起多为卫气同病，为湿热之邪同时侵犯人体的肌表和脾胃所引起，因此在临床诊治时应灵活应用，不可教条。凡外感之邪，凡有湿性，即为浊毒之一种，即或无湿，侵袭人体，留止不去，易生浊化毒，必防浊毒之变。

　　Turbid toxin can enter from outside of the body, or from the fur, through mouth and nose, invade the body, seriously damage the viscera, breath and blood, Yin and Yang. "Turbid", means not "lucid", turbidity and wetness are closely related. External infected wetness and turbidity, invades the body from the surface by three ways, first, to enter the upper energizer of human body through breathing by way of mouth and nose, then affect the middle and lower energizer. As *The Source of Medical Science-Discussion On Moisture* says: "Wet vapor, is mostly accepted through the upper skin and fur, evil is accepted through mouth and nose inhalation, so the weather is accepted earlier, then the climate evil". Second, the turbidity and wetness penetrates into human body through muscle and skin, stays in the muscle surface and joint, obstruct meridians, and finally gets into the viscera. Zhang Lu of Qing dynasty said: "Long-time accumulated moisture usually retains in joints." *Simple Conversation-Discussion on Regulation of Channels* says: "Wind and rain hurt human body, first in skin, then into the fine collateral, then into collateral, then into meridians." "The attack by cold and dampness is marked by contraction of the skin, tenseness of the muscles, stagnation of blood, separation of defensive energy, that is why it is called 'deficiency'." Third, evil of dampness hurt the spleen and stomach. *Discussion On Six External Evils-The Third Volume* says: "Wet is heavy turbid evil, it hurt human health widely... It hurt muscles, the surface of Yangming; it attacks on the spleen, wet soil of Taiyin. When it hurts muscles, the limbs will be painful, when it attacks spleen, the abdomen will be stuffy." Anyhow, the evil of external dampness and turbidity might infringe the human body, by one way, or two and three ways. For example, when damp epidemic febrile disease arises at the beginning, the defensive energy and breath will be involved simultaneously, as the evil of dampness and heat invade the human's muscle surface and spleen and stomach at the same time. So in clinical practice of diagnosis and treatment, we should flexibly apply the principle, not dogmatically. The evil of exogenous with characteristic of wetness, is a kind of turbid toxin. Even without wetness, when the exogenous evil invade and retain in human body for a long time, it will produce turbidity and toxin, we must prevent the tendency of turbid toxin transmission.

另外，外来之毒邪侵袭人体，易极化为浊毒性质而致病。"外毒"是来源于人体之外的环境产生的有害于人体健康的致病物，结合现代医学的认识，外毒包括化学致病物、物理致病物、生物致病物等。化学致病物包括药毒、毒品、秽毒、各种污染等，废气污水、生物垃圾、化肥农药、装饰材料、烧烤粉尘等皆可为毒。物理致病物包括跌仆损伤等意外伤害，水、火、雷、电等自然灾害，气候、气温变化，噪声、电磁波、超声波、射线辐射对人体的干扰等。其中气候变化是引起疾病发生的因素之一。气候变化是毒邪、疫疠之毒产生和传播的重要条件。生物致病物包括温病毒邪、疫疠之毒、虫兽毒、食物中毒等。《诸病源候论》曰："诸生肉及熟肉，内器中密闭头，其气壅积不泄，则为郁肉，有毒，不幸而食之，乃杀人。其轻者，亦吐利，烦乱不安等。"《金匮要略》曰："六畜自死，皆疫死，则有毒，不可食之。"

In addition, the evil of "external toxin" is one kind of pathogenic agent derived from the environment outside the human body but harmful to human health. According to the understanding of modern medical science, external toxin includes chemical pathogenic agent, physical pathogenic agent, biological pathogenic agent and so on. Chemical pathogenic substances including drug toxin, drugs, filth, all kinds of pollution, waste gas sewage, biological waste, chemical fertilizer pesticides, decorative materials, barbecue dust and so on, are all toxic. Physical pathogenic substances include accidental injuries such as traumatic injuries, natural disasters such as disaster water, fire, thunder, electricity, climate, temperature changes, noise, electromagnetic waves, ultrasonic, radiation interference to human health. Climate change is one of the pathogenic causes of disease, providing important conditions for the emergence and spread of evil of toxin and epidemic diseases. Biological pathogenic substances include warm virus evil, epidemic virus, insect and animal virus, food toxin and so on. *Zhu Bing Yuan Hou Lun (Discussion on the Source of All Kinds of Diseases)* says: "Either raw meat or cooked meat, as they are kept in inner closed environment with abundant accumulation of gas undischarged, is depressed and toxic, may kill the people who unfortunately eat them. Even those people who eat the meat but fortunately escape from death, will constantly vomit and purge feeling upset and down". *Synopsis of the Golden Chamber* says, "If animals die themselves, or die of epidemic diseases, they are toxic and can not be eaten."

外来之浊与毒，侵入人体，影响人体的新陈代谢，导致气机失调，脏腑失用，从而浊毒内生，蕴于体内，百病丛生。

External turbidity and toxin invades human body, affects the metabolism, leads to imbalance of energy mechanism, viscera dysfunction, in result produces endogenous turbid toxin in human body, and causes various kind of diseases.

（二）饮食失节
1.2 Diet out of control

《素问·脏气法时论》指出："五谷为养，五果为助，五畜为益，五菜为充，气味合而服之，以补精益气。"这就要求我们以植物性食物为主，动物性食物为辅，并配合果、蔬，使饮食性味柔和，不偏不倚，以保证机体阴阳平衡，气血充沛。然而，随着人们生活水平的不断提高，传统的饮食习惯已被打破，过去偶尔食之的鸡鸭鱼肉等副食品已经成为人们的日常饮食，高热量、高蛋白、高脂肪的"西式快餐"被奉为美味佳肴，强食过饮现象非常普遍。而过食肥甘厚味，超出脾胃运化功能，则湿聚食积，化为痰饮，蕴郁日久，化为浊毒之邪。正所谓"肥者令人内热，甘者令人中满"（《素问·奇病论》），"多食浓厚，则痰湿俱生"（《医方论·消导之剂》）。

Simple Conversation- Discussion On the Association of the Zang-Qi with the Four Seasons points out: "The five kinds of grain are provided to feed and nourish people, five kinds of fruit are provided to help nourishing, five kinds of livestock are provided to benefit nourishing, and five kinds of vegetables are provided to enrich nourishing, smell and flavor can be taken together to replenish the essence and energy." This requires us to mainly depend on plant food, with animal food as assistance, fruit and vegetables as supplementation, make the diet tasty, soft, and impartial, in order to ensure the balance of Yin and Yang, and abundant provision of energy and blood. However, the traditional diet habit have been broken by continuous improvement of people's living standard. Chicken, duck, fish and other non-staple foods occasionally used in the past, have become people's daily diet. "Western fast food" with high calorie, high protein and high fat has been regarded as delicious food. The overdone in eating and drinking is very popular. And the excessive fat of food and thick taste exceeds the digestion and absorption capacity of spleen and stomach. Accumulation of food and wetness produces phlegm, within a long time, the evil of turbid toxin arises. As the saying goes, "Fat food bears inner heat, sweet food fills up stomach" (*Simple Conversation-Discussion on Special Diseases*), "More fat and thick food bears wet phlegm" (*Discussion On Medical Prescription-The Agent of Elimination*).

饮食失节，影响人体气血的运行。《素问·五脏生成》指出："多食咸，则脉凝泣而变色。"《张氏医通·诸血门》亦曰："人饮食起居，一失其节，皆能使血瘀滞不行也。"血瘀久则成毒，百病乃变化而生。这也是现代社会高脂血症、高血压、心脑血管疾病、糖尿病、肥胖症等发病率大大增高的主要原因之一。故《素问·通评虚实论》指出："消瘅仆击，偏枯痿厥，气满发逆，甘肥贵人，则膏粱之疾也。"

Diet out of control affects the operation of breath and blood. *Simple Conversation-Discussion on Various Relationships Concerning Five Storing Organs* points out: "Too much salty food makes the pulses blocked, blood coagulated and complexion gloomy." *Zhang's Medical Guide-Blood Division* also says: "Irregular diet and daily life, makes blood stasis." Long-term stasis of blood produces toxin evil which promotes the arising all diseases. This is also one of the main reasons for the greatly increased incidence of hyperlipidemia, hypertension, cardiovascular and cerebrovascular diseases, diabetes and obesity in modern society. Therefore, *Simple Conversation-General Discussion on Deficiency and Excess* points out: "To treat diabetes, apoplexy, paralysis, flaccidity, short of breath or reverse flow of breath of fat and noble people, (doctors should understand) the above (diseases) are diseases of rich and fat diet."

（三）情志不畅

1.3 Depression of mood

《素问·八正神明论》说："血气者，人之神，不可不谨养。"神态是内在气血的总体体现，因此所谓"清静"，指的是人体精神状态的安详，是一个人内在脏腑气血功能正常的外在表现。人体在精神上能够长期保持清静，营卫之气运行有序，肌肉腠理的功能状态正常，表现为致密而柔顺，邪气难以进犯机体，人体就不会得病。正所谓"正气存内，邪不可干"。喜、怒、忧、思、悲、恐、惊原本是人对外在环境各种刺激所产生的正常的生理反应。但当外来的刺激突然、强烈或持久不除，使情志激动过度，超过了人体生理活动的调节范围，则可使人体气机失调，进一步导致脏腑功能紊乱，气血运行失常，津液水湿不化，痰浊瘀血内停，浊毒由此而生。故《证治准绳·杂病·喘》谓："七情内伤，郁而生痰。"《医述·杂证汇参·血证》亦曰："或因忧思过度，而致营血瘀滞不行；或因怒伤血逆，上不得越，下不归经，而留积于胸膈之间者，此皆瘀血之因也。"情志因素与痰瘀的关系亦受到现代学者的重视。日本学者永田胜太郎认为慢性紧张是导致瘀血证的主要原因之一，瘀血状态就是低血清辅酶Q状态，它是一种慢性应激反应，即虽然交感神经释放儿茶酚胺，而其靶器官的心肌处于劳损状态，使全身的最小动脉收缩，末梢血液循环障碍，以致毛细血管系统、静脉系统瘀血。国内也有学者对冠心病瘀血证与A型性格、心理应激的关系进行调查分析，发现情志因素与瘀血的关系密切。《黄帝内经》说："喜则气下，悲则气消，消则脉虚空。因寒饮食，寒气熏满，则血泣气去，故曰虚矣。"大喜不止，削弱人体正气，正气一虚，病从内生；悲伤过度。人体"脉空虚"，正气不足，过食寒凉，寒气主凝滞，血凝之后，进一步加重气虚，为生理物质的"浊毒化"打下了基础。

Simple Conversation-Discussion on Mysterious Influences on the Eight Directions on Acupuncture says: "Vigor and vitality, the spirit of man, must be nourished carefully." The state of spirit is the over-all embodiment of the internal breath and blood, so the so-called "quiet" refers to the serenity of the human mind, and is the normal external expression of the energy and blood function of a person's internal organs. The man who can keep quiet in spirit for a long time, with good order of nourishing and defending mechanism, and normal function of muscle and striae performing densely and softly, can not be invaded by external evil, and will not fall ill at all. As the saying goes, "When positive energy is (abundantly) stored inside, evil can not work". Joy, anger, sorrow, thought, sadness, fear, surprise are originally the normal physiological reactions to various stimulation of the external environment, but when the external stimulation turns to be sudden, strong, lasting, or too exciting, beyond the adjustment range of human physiological activities, it can cause irregular work of energy mechanism of human body, further lead to disorder of the viscera function, abnormal operation of breath and blood, sweat and fluid clustered with water and wet failing to be vaporized, phlegm turbidity, stasis blood retaining inside, turbid toxin arises from this. Therefore, *Treatment Criterion-Miscellaneous Diseases-Asthma* says: "Depressing of seven emotions internally injured produces phlegm." *Doctor Statement-References of Miscellaneous disease-Blood Disease* also says: "Blood stasis is either because the excessive worry and thinking blocks the flow of nutrient-blood, or because the injury of anger makes blood reverse, failing to flow upward, failing to return to channels, retaining and accumulating between the chest and diaphragm, causing blood stasis." The relationship between emotional factors and phlegm stasis has also been valued by modern scholars. Japanese scholar Seitara Nagata thinks that chronic tension is one of the main causes of blood stasis disease, state of blood stasis is the state of low serum levels of coenzyme Q, it is a chronic stress reaction, although sympathetic nerve release catecholamine, but the target organ of myocardium in the strain state, makes the systemic artery contracted, obstruct peripheral blood circulation, resulting the stasis of blood capillary and venous blood. Domestic scholars also investigated and analyzed the relationship between blood stasis of patient with coronary heart disease and type A personality and psychological stress, and found that the relationship between emotional factors and blood stasis was close. *The Medical Classic of the Yellow Emperor* says: "Excessive joy sinks down the energy, excessive sorrow dissipates the energy, when the energy is dissipated, the pulses turns to be void. Using cold diet full of coldness, makes the blood flow obscure and heat energy dissipated, so it is called disease of deficiency." Excessive joy weaken the positive energy of human body, when the positive energy is weak or absent, disease arises; Excessive sadness makes the pulses "empty", positive energy insufficient. As cold induces stagnation, overtaken of cold food makes blood coagulation which further aggravates the energy deficiency, prepares the foundation for "turbid toxin change" of physiological substances.

《素问·举痛论》曰，"百病生于气也"。气不通畅，则毒邪内生。如气盛生毒，因气有余便是火热，火热之极即为毒；热毒、火毒的存在又可进一步伤害人体脏腑组织产生腑实、阴伤、血瘀等一系列病理后果；气郁生毒，情志变化刺激过于突然、持久，使脏腑功能紊乱，升降出入失常，影响气机的通调条达、津血的输布，可蓄郁而为毒，从而导致疾病。浊毒在体内蕴积日久，又可对人体脏腑经络造成严重损害，百病由此乃变化而生。这就是"郁生浊毒"。

Simple Conversation-Discussion On Pains says: "All diseases are born of abnormal work of energy mechanism." When energy mechanism does not work, toxin evil arises endogenously. For example, excessive energy produces toxin, because surplus energy is hot, ultra hot becomes toxin. Hot toxin and fire toxin further injures viscera tissues of human body, causing pathogenic result as solidity of transporting organs, injury of storing organs, blood stasis and so on. The depressed mood leads to disease. If the emotional stimulation is too sudden and lasting, which causes disorder of the viscera function, abnormal rise and fall, enter and withdraw, influences the regular work of energy mechanism, affects the spreading of sweat and blood, the stored depression turns to be toxin, resulting disease. Turbid toxin accumulated in human body for a long time, will cause serious damage to viscera meridians, arising all kinds of diseases. Therefore, accumulated depression bears turbidity.

（四）环境改变
1.4 Environmental changes

《素问·宝命全形论》指出："人以天地之气生，四时之法成。"人只有顺应自然气候的变化规律才能保持健康。随着各种现代化的生活设施不断地介入人类的生活，人们不必再"动作以避寒，阴居以避暑"，悠然地生活在人工营造的舒适环境之中。即使夏季室外酷暑炎热，室内也可以冷气习习；冬季户外冰雪凛冽，屋内也可以暖气融融。人们出入于这样乍热乍凉，或乍寒乍暖温度悬殊的环境，使机体腠理汗孔骤开骤闭，卫外功能难以适应，久而久之，闭阻体内的浊气即可化为浊毒而致病。

Simple Conversation-Discussion on Preserving Health and Life points out: "Man exists depending on the energy of heaven and earth, grows up in accordance with the rules of four seasons." People can only keep healthy by conforming to the changing rules of natural climate. With variety of modern living facilities constantly intervene in human life, people leisurely live in the artificial comfortable environment, no longer need to "do exercises to get away coldness, live in shade place to escape form the hotness of summer". Even in specially hot summer, we can keep cool indoors; in terribly cold winter, the house can be filled with warm air. People are involved in such an environment with temperature changing abruptly from cool to hot, and from warm to cold, making the striae and sweat holes of human body suddenly open and suddenly close, the defensive function can hardly be adapted, with time going, the turbidity within the body will be turned into turbid toxin and diseases.

环境的自然变化和人类对环境的干预使人类的生活环境发生了空前的变化，这种变化对人体的影响是巨大的、多层面的。从中医学的角度看，湿浊阻滞是一个不容忽视的方面。现代流行病学调查亦已证明了这一点。有人对石家庄市各行业共1005人进行整体随机抽样调查，结果表明：有湿阻症状者占10.55%，且与性别、年龄、职业无明显联系，主要病因为环境湿气过重、性格急躁或忧郁以及饮食不节，主要病位在脾。湿浊阻滞，气机不畅，进一步导致血行受阻，结滞成瘀，百病由此变化而生。

Natural evolution and artificial intervening greatly changed the environment of human living. The impact of these changes on the human body is huge and multifaceted. From the perspective of traditional Chinese medical science, wet and turbidity block is an aspect that cannot be ignored. This has also been proved by modern epidemiological investigations. Someone conducted a random sampling survey of 1005 people from various industries in Shijiazhuang city. The result showed that 1005 of them had wet resistance symptoms, and there was no obvious connection with gender, age or occupation. The main diseases were due to excessive environmental moisture, impatience or melancholy, and poor diet, and the main diseases were in the spleen. Block of wet turbidity, and abnormal work of energy mechanism, further lead to blood flow obstruction, stagnation develops to blood stasis, resulting various diseases.

（五）运动缺乏
1.5 Lack of exercises

《素问·宣明五气》云："久视伤血，久卧伤气，久坐伤肉。"若长年伏案，以车代步，室外活动减少，不仅可以导致气血亏虚，而且还可以使气机阻滞，津液运化、布散失常，从而浊毒之邪难免滋生。多食少动，对于浊毒体质的产生具有重要作用。颜元在《颜习斋言行录》中写道："习行、礼、乐、射、御之学，健人筋骨，和人气血，调人情绪，长人仁义……为其动生阴阳，下积痰郁气，安内抒外也。"这充分表明：体育运动既可强身健体，娱乐身心，磨炼意志，促进德智发展，又可防病治病，帮助身体早日康复。

Simple Conversation-Discussion on the Elucidation of Function of Five Storing Organs says: "Seeing for a long time impairs blood, lying for a long time impairs breath, sitting for a long time impairs flesh." If we sit at the desk year by year, tour by car instead of walking, with outdoor activities reduced, it will not only lead to deficiency of breath and blood, but also induce the obstruction of energy mechanism, disorder of fluid transmission and spreading, thus the evil of turbid toxin will inevitably breed. Eating more and moving less plays an important role in the production of turbid toxin constitution. Yan Yuan wrote in Words and Behavior Record of Yan Xi Zhai: "Learning and Practicing skills and art like ritual, music, archery, horse-riding will strengthen people's muscles and bones, harmonize human breath and blood, regulate people's mind, increase people's benevolence and righteousness... because exercises produce Yin and Yang, unload accumulated phlegm and depressed mood, make peace inside and defend evil-attacking from outside." This fully shows that sports can strengthen human body, entertain the body and mind, temper the will, promote moral and intellectual development, and can prevent and cure diseases, and help recovering the patient as early as possible.

（六）虚损劳倦

1.6 Deficiency and fatigue

人体是否发病，主要取决于人体的正气强弱。"正气存内，邪不可干""邪之所凑，其气必虚"，是中医药贡献给人民大众的养生智慧。《灵枢·百病始生》说："风雨寒热不得虚，邪不能独伤人。卒然逢疾风暴雨而不病者，盖无虚，故邪不能独伤人。此必因虚邪之风，与其身形，两虚相得，乃客其形。两实相逢，众人肉坚。其中于虚邪，也因于天时，与其身形，参以虚实，大病乃成。气有定舍，因处为名。"

Whether the person will be attacked by diseases mainly depends on the strength of positive energy in his body. "When (abundant) positive energy exists inside, evil can not do anything", "if evil can gather together in one's body, its positive energy must be deficient", of this is the health nourishing wisdom contributed by traditional Chinese medical science to the people. Spiritual Pivot-The Occurrences of all Diseases says: "If the human body is not deficient, the evil of wind, rain, cold and heat itself can not hurt people. People who do not fall ill when they were suddenly involved in abrupt wind and hard rain, are not deficient, so evil can not hurt people itself. This is because when the wind of deficient evil come across deficient human body, the wind evil wins the attack, and stays as the guest of the body. But the evil of wind will fail the attack, if the human body is strong enough. The occurrence of serious disease of deficient evil is because the abnormal weather further weaken the deficient human body. The pathogenic evils retain in different region of the body, and are named according to the region they stays."

虚易招邪，虚处留邪；邪碍气机，化生浊毒。这往往是一个连续的过程。《黄帝内经》说："有所劳倦，形气衰少，谷气不盛，上焦不行，下脘不通，胃气热，热气熏胸中，故内热。"由劳倦导致的形气衰少，还只是一个"纯虚无邪"的病理状态，一旦在这个基础上出现"上焦不行，下脘不通"，就不是纯虚无邪了，而是清浊相干，浊毒内生的一种现象，所以患者见到"内热"的各种证候表现。

Deficient person is easy to be attacked by evils, the evil which wins the attack will retain in deficient part of human body. Evils in human body obstruct the normal operation of energy mechanism, and produce turbid toxin. This is usually a continuous process. *The Medical Classic of the Yellow Emperor* says: "Fatigue reduces energy in human body, if the grain essence is not abundant, the upper energizer does not work well, the function of middle energizer is abnormal, people feel hot in stomach, the heat in stomach fumigate in chest, causes internal hot of human body." Reduction of energy in human body caused by fatigue is only a pathological state of "pure deficiency without evil affection". Once the phenomenon occurs that "the upper energizer does not work, the middle energizer is obstructed", it is no longer pure deficiency without evil affection, but a phenomenon of interaction of lucidity and turbidity, resulting internal turbid toxin. So patients see various manifestations of "internal heat".

（七）他邪转化

1.7 The evil transformed from other evils

浊毒之邪为与内生五邪、外感六淫密切相关，又有不同。浊毒兼具浊与毒的特性，可以由他邪转化，且为诸邪致病之甚者也。如食积，本为伤食，食积日久则生湿聚痰，湿与痰即具浊之性，湿痰蕴积日久则生毒，至此浊毒生焉。浊毒生则导致胃病渐重，甚至癌变。饮食若超过自身耐受量，则可转化成浊毒。如过饮久饮之酒浊毒；过食为病之食积化浊毒；大便干燥影响毒素排出，吸收毒素过多成粪毒；血糖、血脂过高形成糖浊毒、脂浊毒等。

The evil of turbid toxin is different from but closely related with endogenous five evil and external six evil. Turbid toxin with characteristics of both turbidity and toxin which can be transformed by other evils is more powerful to cause diseases than other evils. For example, food accumulation, originally is simply impairment of over-eating, but accumulation of food for a long time produces wet and phlegm with characteristic of turbidity, stagnation of wet and phlegm over a long time produces toxin, so far turbidity and toxin arises. The arising of turbid toxin makes stomach disease gradually become more and more severe, or even develop to cancer. If the diet exceeds the tolerance of stomach, it will be converted into turbid toxin. Other examples such as turbid toxin of over drunk or long-time drinking of wine, turbid toxin of accumulated food, turbid toxin of excrement (some dry excrement absorb in instead of discharging excessive toxin finally turn to be excrement toxin); sugar toxin transformed from high blood glucose, grease toxin transformed from high blood fat.

另外，水湿痰饮可转化为浊毒，汗液、二便不通，浊阴或水湿无以出路，内困日久而成"浊毒"；更多久病虚损，肺、脾、肾及三焦等脏腑气化功能失常，肾元衰败，导致浊毒内生。水、津、液本为体内的正常物质，若超出生理需要量，或停留于局部，或失其所，也成为一种毒。如水液代谢紊乱，水液过多为病之水毒、湿毒；机体在代谢过程中产生的各种代谢产物排出困难，蓄积日久，郁而化毒则为浊毒。瘀血亦可转化为浊毒之邪。瘀血是血液运行失常而化生的病理产物，常表现为瘀毒、出血、癥瘕。若瘀久不消，全身持久得不到气血的濡养，则出现面色黧黑、口唇紫暗、皮肤粗糙状如鳞甲，则成瘀毒；瘀血阻滞脉络，血液不循常道，溢出脉外，可见各种出血；体内肿块日久不化，质硬，固定不移，夜间痛甚，即癥瘕。血瘀则气滞，气血瘀滞则脉络阻塞、脏腑功用失常，从而导致浊毒内生。另外，所瘀之血，所溢之血，日久即聚浊毒之性，致人病生。

In addition, water, wet, phlegm, fluid retention can be converted into turbidity. Sweat, fluid, obstructed stool and urine, retained turbid evil or water wet, are transformed into "turbid toxin" after long-time accumulation; more deficiency of chronic disease, vaporization dysfunction of lung, spleen, kidney and triple energizer viscera, decay of renal essence, result in the arising internal turbid toxin. Water, sweat, fluid is the normal substances in human body, if they surpass the physiological needs, retain in local part of the body, or stay in uncertain part of the body, will become a kind of toxin. If water and liquid metabolism is disordered, excessive water and liquid will become water toxin and wet toxin; various metabolites produced in process of metabolism which is difficult to be discharged, will be transformed to turbid toxin after a long-time accumulation. Blood stasis can also be converted into the evil of turbid toxin. Blood stasis is the pathological product of abnormal blood operation, usually manifested as evil of stasis, bleeding and abdominal mass. If the blood stasis retains for a long time, the human body can not be nourished by sufficient energy and blood, the complexion will be dark black, lips will be purple, the skin will be rough and scaly, the stasis turns to be stasis toxin; blood stasis will block the pulses, blood will abnormally flow outside the veins, arising different kind of bleeding; the phyma in human body which does not dissipate in a long time, turns to be hard, fixed, terribly painful at night, is called abdominal mass. Blood stasis causes breath stagnation, blood stasis plus breath stagnation causes vein obstruction, viscera dysfunction, leading to the arising of endogenous turbid toxin. In addition, the accumulated stasis and overflow of blood, with the nature of turbid toxin, causes diseases.

二、浊毒病机特点
2. The characteristics of the pathogenesis mechanism of turbid toxin

（一）浊毒黏滞，病程缠绵
2.1 Sticky and stagnant turbid toxin, lingering disease course

"黏"，即黏腻；"滞"，即停滞。所谓黏滞是指浊毒致病具有黏腻停滞的特性。这种特性主要表现在两个方面：一是症状的黏滞性。浊病症状多黏滞而不爽，如大便黏腻不爽，小便涩滞不畅及分泌物黏浊和舌苔黏腻等。二是病程的缠绵性。因浊性黏滞，蕴蒸不化，胶着难解，故起病缓慢隐袭，病程较长，往往反复发作或缠绵难愈。如湿温，它是一种由湿浊热邪所引起的外感热病。由于浊毒性质的特异性，在疾病的传变过程中，表现出起病缓、传变慢、病程长、难速愈的明显特征。其他如湿疹、着痹等，亦因其浊而不易速愈。

"Sticky", means glutinous; "stagnation", means stubborn. The so-called sticky stagnation indicates that the turbid toxin disease has the characteristic of sticky stagnation. This characteristic is mainly manifested in two aspects: one is the stickiness of the symptoms. The symptoms of turbid toxin disease are sticky and unpleasant, such as sticky and greasy stool difficult to be discharged, dull urine, sticky and turbid secretions and sticky and greasy tongue coating. Another, the lingering course of disease. As the turbidity is sticky, it can neither be melted by accumulating steam, nor be resolved abruptly. So the beginning of the disease is slow and concealed, the course of the disease is longer, recurrent or lingering long but difficult to heal. Such as damp warm, it is an exogenous fever caused by damp turbidity and heat evil. Due to the nature of turbid toxin, it shows the characteristic of concealed occurrence, slow transmission, long course and difficult recovery in the process of disease transmission. Other diseases like eczema, damp arthralgia, are also difficult to recover quickly because of their turbidity nature.

浊毒之邪积聚体内，相互为用，日久必凝结气血，燔灼津液，致脏腑败伤，其病多深重难愈，病期冗长，病久入血入络，可致瘀血出血。许筱颖等认为：浊性黏滞，易结滞脉络，阻塞气机，缠绵耗气；毒邪性烈善变，易化热耗伤阴精，壅腐气血。"毒"之形成，与"浊"有密切的关系。若浊毒日久不解，深伏于内，耗劫脏腑经络之气血，而呈现虚实夹杂之证，在临床表现为缠绵难愈，变化多端。

Along with accumulating, gathering and interacting of turbid toxin evil in human body, breath and blood will be stagnated over time, sweat and fluid will be burnt, viscera will be attacked and damaged, the disease is internal, severe, and difficult to recover, will sustain for long time, then develops into blood and collateral, causing blood stasis and bleeding. Xu Xiaoying thinks: turbidity with the nature of sticky can easily stagnate the pulses, block the operation of energy mechanism, waste energy in lingering disease course; toxin evil with nature of fiery and fickle, will easily be transmitted into heat and consume and hurt the essence of storing organs, obstruct and erode energy and blood. The formation of "toxin" is closely related to "turbidity". If the turbid toxin can not be removed, it will retain deep inside human body for a long time, wear off the energy and blood of the viscera and meridians, cause the disease mixed with deficiency and solidity, with the clinical performance as lingering, changeable but difficult to heal.

（二）滞脾碍胃，阻滞气机

2.2 Turbidity obstructs the spleen, hinders the stomach, blocks the operation of energy mechanism

浊为阴邪，其性黏滞，最易困阻脾之清阳，阻塞气机，脾胃为人体气机升降运动的枢纽，脾不升清，胃不降浊，气机升降失常。如《灵枢·小针解》云："言寒温不适，饮食不节，而病生于肠胃，故命曰浊气在中也。"若湿邪阻中，脾胃受病，气机升降之枢纽失灵，人体之气机升降，权衡在于中气。三焦升降之气，由脾鼓动，中焦和，则上下顺。阳明为水谷之海，太阴为湿土之脏，胃主纳谷，脾主运化，脾升则健，胃降则和。所以中焦气和，脾胃升降皆得适度，则心肺在上，行营卫而光泽在外；肝肾在下，养筋骨而强壮于内；脾胃在中，传化精微以溉四旁，人体保持正常的气机升降运动，是为无病。脾为浊困，湿浊内聚，使脾胃纳运失职，升降失常。脾阳不振，湿浊停聚而胸闷脘痞、纳谷不香、不思饮食、肢体困重、呕恶泄泻等，以及分泌物和排泄物如泪、涕、痰、带下、二便等秽浊不清，舌苔白腻润滑而液多，脉沉濡而软，或沉缓而迟。

Turbidity is negative evil, with nature of sticky, can easily trap the lucid energy of spleen, block up the operation of energy mechanism. Spleen and stomach is the motion hub of the human air lifting movement, when spleen does not rise clear, stomach does not drop turbidity, air lift mechanism is abnormal. *Spiritual Pivot-Explanation of Small Needles* says: "If the patient feels unable to the weather change from cold of winter to the warmth of spring, with diet out of control, turbidity arises in middle energizer, disease will be born in the stomach and intestine." If the damp evil is blocked in middle energizer, spleen and stomach are involved in disease, the hub of the energy mechanism does not work. The key factor which influence the normal operation of rising and falling of energy mechanism of human body is function of spleen and stomach. Gases rising and falling in triple energizer, is encouraged by spleen. Harmony in middle energizer, ensures normal operation of upper and lower energizer. Yangming is the sea of water and grains, Taiyin is the storing organ of wet soil, stomach is responsible for accepting and digesting grains, spleen is responsible to transport and transform matured essence of water and grain, the up-transporting function of spleen ensures healthy, the down discharging of stomach function improves harmony of human body. If the middle energizer works well, the up-transporting function of spleen and the down discharging function of stomach is normal and moderate, heart and lung in upper energizer of the body perform their duties of nourishing and defensing, people look shining and bright; liver and kidney in lower energizer strengthen the inner body by nourishing muscles and bones; spleen and stomach in middle energizer transform essence to irrigation the whole body, people maintain normal operation of rising and falling energy mechanism, no disease occurs. When spleen is trapped with turbidity, wet turbidity gather together inside, which causes disorder of spleen transporting and stomach digesting performance, abnormal operation of rising and falling of energy mechanism. Therefore, the function of spleen is depressed, wet and turbidity retain and unite together, people will feel the chest distressed, stomach full and distention, with no desire to eat and no sense of taste, sick, vomiting and diarrhea, their legs blocked and difficult to move, their secretions and excrement such as tears, snivel, phlegm, menstruation, stool and urine turns to be turbid and filthy, their tongue coating look white greasy and lubricant, the pulse feels deep and soft, or deep and late.

（三）常相兼夹，耗气伤阴

2.3 Turbid toxin is often mixed with phlegm, wet, stasis and toxin, consumes energy and injures the organs

浊毒为病，常与痰、湿、瘀、毒并存。浊毒较之湿邪，更为黏腻滞涩，重浊稠厚。因此，病势更为缠绵难愈，多久久不能尽除。较之痰邪，浊毒变化多端，可侵及全身多个脏腑、四肢百骸，同时又会随体质及环境因素寒化、热化，从而出现种种变局。浊毒的存在可导致痰、瘀、毒等病理产物的产生，相兼为病，加重病情。浊毒困扰清阳，阻滞气机，可以导致津液停聚，加重痰浊；浊毒胶结，阻碍气血运行，更可加重气血瘀滞。浊毒伤人正气，蕴结成毒，或化热生毒，更可耗血动血，败坏脏腑。四者相兼，元气日衰，则病归难治。

Turbid toxin often coexists with phlegm, wet, stasis, toxin, causing diseases. Comparing with the wet evil, turbid toxin is more sticky and astringent, muddy and thick, therefore, causes disease more lingering and difficult to heal, most of them can not be removed thoroughly within a long time. Comparing with phlegm, turbid toxin is more changeable, can invade into multi viscera, limbs and various bones of the body at the same time. It can be transformed from coldness or heat due to different constitution and environment. The existence of turbid toxin can lead to the arising of phlegm, stasis, toxin and other pathological products, joining them to produce and aggravate diseases. Turbid toxin disturbs lucid essence and block the operation of energy mechanism, which can cause sweat and fluid stagnation, aggravate phlegm turbidity; cementation of turbidity and toxin obstruct the operation of breath and blood, and aggravate breath and blood stasis. Turbid toxin hurt the positive energy of human body, will be accumulated and transformed into toxin, or heat toxin, consume and hurt blood, corrupt viscera. Combining with other four pathogenic factors as phlegm, wet, stasis and toxin, turbid toxin make the vitality decay day by day, and the disease difficult to cure.

（四）阴阳相并，浊毒害清

2.4 Combining Yin and Yang, turbid toxin impairs the lucidity

浊性类水，水属于阴，故浊为阴邪。浊为阴邪，易阻气机，损伤阳气，"湿胜则阳微"。由湿浊之邪郁遏使阳气不伸者，当用化气利湿通利小便的方法，使气机通畅，水道通调，则浊毒可从小便而去，湿浊去则阳气自通。浊毒为阴邪，郁久化热生毒，兼具湿热毒性，此时多见湿热结聚，毒性昭彰之特点。故此说，浊毒为阴邪、阳邪相并，正如湿与热相并，如油入面，而浊毒为湿热之甚，阴阳更难分离，驱散消解更加困难。

Turbidity is similar to water, as water belongs to Yin, so turbidity is Yin evil which can easily obstruct the operation of qi mechanism, impairing Yang qi. "When dampness is excessive, Yang qi decays". When the damp evil depresses the extension of Yang qi, we should use the method of warming yang and eliminating water to unblock the urination and restore the operation of qi mechanism, regulate and dredge the water channel, so as to discharge the turbid toxin by way of urine, then positive energy is relieved when the wet turbidity is removed. Turbidity is Yin evil, which will be transformed into heat and toxin, with both wet and heat toxicity, at this time, the characteristic of aggregation of wet and heat with strong toxicity. Therefore, turbid toxin is a mixture of Yin and Yang evil, just as the mixture of wet and heat, like oil cemented with flour. Turbid toxin is the progress of wet and heat, it makes Yin and Yang evil more difficult to be separated, more difficult to be dissipated and removed.

湿浊之邪害人，阻遏清阳，蒙蔽神明、心窍、头部孔窍，出现头昏目眩，神昏谵语，甚或失聪。所以叶天士《温热论》有"浊毒害清"之说。《格致余论》云："湿者土浊之气……湿气熏蒸，清道不通，沉重而不爽利，似乎有物以蒙冒之。"慢性肾衰竭尿毒症脑病、肝衰竭肝性脑病都具有浊毒胶塞黏滞，蒙蔽清窍，神明失守的特点。

Wet and turbid evil impairs people by restraining lucid Yang, hoodwink brain, mind, and head orifice, generating dizziness, delirium, or even deaf. Therefore, Ye Tianshi has a saying in *Wen Re Lun (Discussion on Seasonal Febrile Diseases)* that "turbid toxin impairs lucidity". *Ge Zhi Yu Lun* says: "Dampness is soil turbid substance... moisture fumigation block the way of lucidity, patients feel heavy and uncomfortable, as if they are covered and coated with strange materials." Both uremia encephalopathy of chronic renal failure and hepatic encephalopathy of liver failure have the characteristics of cementing of turbid toxin, hoodwinks in lucid orifice, causes absence of spirit.

（五）易积成形，蕴久生变

2.5 Easy to form masses, make changes after long-time accumulation

浊毒之邪重浊、黏滞，易损脏腑，腐血肉，生恶疮癌肿。浊毒之邪表现有气味秽臭，或腥臭如败卵，肌肉组织多有腐烂，或易生赘疣；头昏蒙，甚则意识不清，身痛不可名状；骨蒸、恶寒、微热、自汗或盗汗，大便水样如注，或溏浊、黏滞不爽，或吐、呕或便冻血如烂肉样，或出流腐汁黄水，如妇女黄白带下、外阴瘙痒或刺痛、出浊水物等。如浊毒犯肾，开阖失司，可见通身浮肿，二便俱闭。浊毒日久不去，肾脏持续损害可致肾衰竭。王永炎强调毒邪在缺血性中风发病中的重要性，提出中风后常有瘀毒、痰毒、热毒互结，破坏形体，损伤脑络。周仲瑛认为乙肝慢性期，症状相对隐伏，病势缠绵，病程较长，"瘀毒"为其主要的病理环节，解毒化瘀为其基本治疗大法。我们所谈的浊毒要与一般的湿热之邪区别开来。这里的浊毒之邪是在原有病邪的基础上化生而又保留了原有病邪的特点，虽然与湿邪、热邪、瘀血等有联系，但已是完全不同的概念。

The evil of turbid toxin is heavy turbid and sticky, easy to damage viscera, corrupt flesh and blood, arise malignant sores and cancer. The evil of turbid toxin smells foul or stinking as rotten eggs, makes muscle tissue decay, or easy to generate wart; causes dizziness, or even unconsciousness, indescribable body pain; bone steaming, cold disliking, a little bit fever, sweating or night sweating, water, loose, or sticky stool, or vomiting, retching or passing frozen blood like rotten meat in one's stool, or passing yellow water like rotten juice, such as women's passing of yellowish leukorrhagia, vulva itching, or tingling, turbid water, etc. If turbid toxin attacks kidney, damage the switch for urine passing, it will cause visible edema in patient's body, both shit and piss cannot be discharged. Prolonged persistence of turbid toxin will sustainably damage kidney organ, causing kidney failure. Wang Yongyan emphasized the importance of toxic evil in the onset of ischemic stroke, proposed that after stroke patients often see interbinding of stasis, phlegm and heat toxin, destroy the body, impair the brain collateral. Zhou Zhongying thinks that in chronic stage of hepatitis B, the symptoms are relatively vague, the disease potential is lingering, the course of disease is longer, "stasis toxin" is its main pathological link, to remove toxin and resolve blood stasis is the basic treatment method. The turbid toxin which we are talking about should be distinguished from the general evil of dampness and heat. The evil of turbid toxin here is transformed from the original disease evil and retains the characteristics of the original disease evil. Although it is associated with dampness, heat evil, and blood stasis, but it is a completely different concept.

第三节　浊毒与脏腑关系
Section 3 The Relationship between Turbid Toxin and Viscera

一、脾胃与浊毒
1. The relationship of spleen, stomach, and turbid toxin

脾主运化、主升清，胃主受纳、腐熟水谷，主通降，以降为和。脾胃同属中焦，通过经脉相互络属构成表里关系。两者一纳一化，一升一降，脾为胃行其津液，共同完成饮食物的消化吸收及其精微的输布，从而滋养全身，因此脾胃被称为"后天之本"。脾主升，胃主降，两者相反相成。脾气升，则水谷之精微得以输布；胃气降，则水谷及其糟粕才得以下行。《临证指南医案》曰："脾宜升则健，胃宜降则和。"胃属燥土，脾属湿土，胃喜润恶燥，脾喜燥恶湿，燥湿相继，阴阳结合，才能完成饮食物的运化。《临证指南医案》曰："太阴湿土得阳始运，阳明燥土得阴自安。"脾运化失职，清气不升，即可影响胃的受纳与和降。反之，如饮食失节，食滞胃脘，胃失和降，亦可影响脾的升清与运化，脾失健运，水谷精微输布异常，湿聚成浊，郁而成毒，浊毒由内而生。

The spleen is mainly responsible for transporting and lucidity rising, the stomach is responsible for water and grain accepting and decomposing, the main task is opening up and discharging. To discharge the metabolites in time means harmony in stomach. Spleen and stomach belong to the same middle coke, forming the relationship of interior and exterior connected through channels and vessels, one accepts, one transports, one raises up the lucid essence to heart and lung, one discharge the metabolites into intestines, through transporting fluid for the stomach, spleen and stomach jointly complete the process of digestion and absorption of the diet and transporting and spreading of the essence, so as to nourish the whole body, therefore, spleen and stomach provide the material basis for "the acquired" constitution. The spleen, the stomach, the opposite. When temper rises, the essence of the valley is lost, and the valley and its dross are reduced. *Medical Case of Clinical Guide* says: "Spleen is healthy when it ascends, stomach is harmonious when it descends." Stomach belongs to dry soil, spleen belongs to wet soil, stomach likes moist, but dislikes dryness, spleen likes dryness but dislikes wetness. To combine dryness and wet, Yin and Yang, is a must to complete the transportation of diet. *Medical Case of Clinical Guide* says: "Wet Soil of Taiyin can transport when spleen get Yang, Dry Gold of Yangming is harmony when stomach get Yin." If the spleen transporting function does not work, lucid essence cannot rise, it will affect the accepting and declining performance of stomach, On the contrary, if diet is out of control, excessive food is stagnated in stomach, thus the stomach looses the function of declining and state of harmony, it can also affect the rising and transport performance of spleen, spleen looses the state of smooth transporting, the essence of water and grain cannot be transported and spread normally, wet is gathered into turbidity, depression of turbidity turns into toxin, turbid toxin arises internally.

二、肝胆与浊毒
2. Liver, gallbladder and turbid toxin

肝主疏泄，胆主决断，共同助脾主运化。中医的整体观认为，人体脏腑气血是一个有机的整体，靠相互协调和制约来保证其生理功能的完成，五脏六腑的功能多赖肝之疏泄。肝的疏泄周转功能有助于脾胃气机的升降、饮食的消化和吸收、肺气的宣发和敷布、胆汁的排泄及气血的周转，它们是一个生命活动的有机整体，共同协调，维持脏腑气血的平衡。肝的疏泄功能正常，脾气能升，胃气能降，则既能纳，又能化，从而保持正常的消化吸收功能。若肝失疏泄，无以助脾之升散，可见"木不疏土"，即"肝脾不和""肝郁气滞"。肝失疏泄，肝气郁结，三焦气机不畅，则横逆而克脾，脾失健运，肝失疏泄，气机不畅，水液代谢功能失常，湿邪内蓄，继而积湿成浊，并可引起血行受阻，气滞血瘀，或为气血逆乱，可致浊毒内生。

The liver governs catharsis, the gallbladder governs decision. Liver and gallbladder work together to help the spleen implementing transportation. According to the holistic view of traditional Chinese medical science, the viscera, breath and blood of human body form an organic constitution to ensure the completion of physiological functions through coordination and co-restriction. The function of the viscera depends more on the catharsis of the liver. The catharsis and turnover function of liver contributes to the lifting of spleen power and declining of stomach power, the digestion and absorption of diet, the promotion and spreading of lung power, the excretion of bile and the turnover of breath and blood. They are an organic whole of life activities and are coordinated together to maintain the balance of qi and blood in the zang and fu organs. When the catharsis function of the liver is normal, the spleen power can rise, the stomach power can fall. Normal operation of accepting and transporting maintains the normal performance of digestion and absorption function. If the liver looses its catharsis function, failing to assist the rise of the spleen power, we will see "wood does not soften soil", "liver and spleen are not in harmony". When liver looses the function of dispersing, liver qi will be depressed and stagnated, the qi mechanism of triple energizer does not work, liver qi transverses and restrains the spleen, the function of water fluid metabolism is abnormal, wet evil is stored internally, then accumulated into turbidity, which will cause blood obstruction, breath stagnation and blood stasis, or turmoil of breath and blood, resulting the arising of turbid toxin endogenously.

三、肾、膀胱与浊毒
3. Kidney, bladder and turbid toxin

肾与膀胱相表里，肾司二便，专主开阖，所谓开阖，即二便之排泄机关也。膀胱主储存和排泄尿液。肾与膀胱功能正常，则二便通利。二便不利，则浊物内蕴，此为化生浊毒之源也。肾者主水，肾与膀胱的疾病均可见水液代谢异常。水液代谢异常也是浊毒内生的主要病机。脾为后天之本，肾为先天之本。脾之健运，化生精微，须借助于肾阳的推动，因此有"脾阳根于肾阳"之说。若肾阳不足，可致脾阳亏虚，运化失职，必易导致浊毒内蕴。

The relationship between Kidney and bladder is the relationship of interior and exterior organ. Kidney controls passing of stool and urine, masters opening and closing of the kidney switch, which is the switch to control the excretion of two feces. The bladder stores and excretes urine. When the function of kidney and bladder is normal, the defecation is fluent. If the defecation does not work well, there must be the accumulation of the turbid substances, which is the source of turbid toxin. Kidney governs water. Abnormal water metabolism often occurs in kidney and bladder disease. Abnormal water and liquid metabolism is also the main pathogenesis of turbid toxin. The spleen provides the material basis for the acquired constitution, the kidney is the origin of the congenital constitution. The normal function of spleen and the transportation of essence, should be assisted by the promotion of kidney Yang, so there is a saying that "the kidney Yang is the root of spleen yang". If the kidney Yang is insufficient, it can cause the deficiency of spleen Yang, absence of spleen transportation, which will easily lead to the internal accumulation of turbid toxin.

四、肺、大肠与浊毒
4. Lung, large intestine and turbid toxin

肺与大肠相表里，大肠为传导之官，传导失职，则浊物排出不畅最易郁而生毒，日久致生他变。肺主宣发肃降，通调水道。所谓宣发，含有宣布发散之意。肺主宣发是指肺把宗气、血液、津液输布散发到全身各处的功能。所谓肃降，含有清肃下降之意；肺主肃降是指肺居上焦，它的气机以下降为顺。只有肺气肃降，才能使呼吸均匀平稳，不咳不喘。若肺失宣降，肺气上逆或壅滞郁闭，则气机不畅，浊毒中生。所谓通调水道，是指肺气有调节和维持水液代谢平衡的功能。水道指水液排泄的途径，如呼吸、汗液的蒸发、尿液的排泄等。这一功能主要是由肺气的宣发和肃降来完成的。因为肺的宣发肃降能促进和调节水液代谢，所以称"肺为水之上源"。《素问·经脉别论》说"饮入于胃，游溢精气，上输于脾，脾气散精，上归于肺，通调水道，下输膀胱"，这就是对这一代谢过程的概括。若宣发肃降功能失调，则可出现水液代谢异常，从而蕴生浊毒。

The relationship between the lung and the large intestine is the relationship between exterior and interior organ. Large intestine is the conduction officer, absence of conduction causes abnormal discharging of turbidity, stagnation of turbidity arises toxin and other changes over time. Lung governs vaporizing and spreading, elimination and declining, regulates the water diversional channel. The so-called vaporizing and spreading refers to the function of lung power to vaporize and spread initial energy, blood, body fluid to everywhere of the body. The so-called elimination and declining indicates that as lungs are located in upper energizer of human body, declining means normal performance. Only elimination and declining makes breathing even and stable, without cough and asthma. If the lung looses the function of elimination and declining, the lung power will ascend or be stagnated, the energy mechanism could not work smoothly, turbid toxin arises. The so-called regulation of water diversion channel refers that the lung power has the function of regulating and maintaining the balance of water and liquid metabolism. Water channel refers to the way of water excretion, such as breathing, evaporation of sweat, urine excretion, etc. The above regulation is mainly completed by vaporizing and spreading, elimination and declining of lung power. Because the promotion of the lung can promote and regulate the metabolism of water, so called "the lung as the source of water". *Simple Conversation-Special Discussion on Channels and Vessels* says: "Drink accepted by stomach produces essence, which is transported and spread up to lung by spleen, can be used to regulate water diversion, and discharged through the bladder." This is a generalization of this metabolic process. If the dysfunction, water metabolism can be abnormal, thus containing turbid toxin.

五、心、小肠与浊毒
5. The heart, the small intestine and turbid toxin

心与小肠相表里。小肠主泌别清浊，因此说小肠功能正常则清浊分明，各归其道，若泌别不清，则浊郁毒生。心为神之居、血之主、脉之宗，心主血脉，血液与津液同源互化，血液中的水液渗出脉外则为津液，津液是汗液化生之源。心又藏神，汗液的生成与排泄又受心神的主宰与调节。心神清明，对体内外各种信息反应灵敏，汗液的生成与排泄就会随体内生理情况和外界气候的变化而有相应的调节，所以情绪紧张、激动、劳动、运动及气候炎热时均可见汗出现象。故《素问·经脉别论》说："惊而夺精，汗出于心。"由此可见，心以其主血脉和藏神功能为基础，主司汗液的生成与排泄，从而维持了人体内外环境的协调平衡。若心失所主，血脉代谢紊乱，则浊毒中生。

The relation between heart and small intestine is the relation between interior and exterior organ. The small intestine governs the separation of lucidity and turbidity. When the function of the small intestine is normal, lucidity and turbidity is separated clearly and transported in their own way. If the separation is not clear, turbidity is stagnated and toxin arises. The heart is the house of mind, the governor of blood, the source of the pulse, blood and body fluid are born homologously and mutual-transformable. The water in blood oozed out of the pulse is fluid, body fluid is the source to transform sweat. The mind is hidden in heart, and the generation and excretion of sweat are governed and regulated by mind. When the mind and is smart, sensitive to all kinds of information inside and outside the body, the generation and excretion of sweat, will be properly adjusted to fit the physiological situation of the body and the changes of the external climate, therefore, sweating phenomenon usually occurs in the circumstances of emotional tension, excitement, laboring, exercising and hot climate. Therefore, *Simple Conversation-Special Discussion on Channels and Vessels* says: "Essence is exhausted by frightening, sweat is generated from the heart." Thus it can be seen that the heart with the power of governing blood and pulses, with the function of hiding the mind and controlling the generation and excretion of body sweat, maintains the coordinated balance of the internal and external environment of the human body. If the heart doesn't work, the metabolic disorder of blood and pulses occurs, turbid toxin arises.

第四节　浊毒体质
Section 4　Turbid Toxin Constitution

中医学认为人体是一个以脏腑经络为内在联络的有机整体。自然界存在着人类赖以生存的必要条件，同时自然界以及包括社会环境、工作环境等环境因素的变化又常常直接或间接地影响着人体，而人体受外界的影响也必然相应地发生生理或病理上的反应。早在《黄帝内经》中就认识到人的健康和疾病与自然环境、精神因素有着密切的关系，天人合一、形神合一、阴阳平衡是最佳的生理状态，明确提出"六淫""七情"等是引起疾病发生的重要致病因素。

Traditional Chinese Medicine believes that the human body is an organic integration of internal viscera and meridians. Nature provides the necessary conditions for human survival, at the same time, natural and social, and working environment often directly or indirectly affect the health of human body, inducing corresponding physiological or pathological reaction of human body. Early in the time of *The Medical Classic of The Yellow Emperor*, it was realized that human health and disease are closely related to the natural environment and spiritual factors, the unity of nature and man, the unity of body and mind, and the balance of positive and negative energy are the best physiological state. It is clearly put forward that "six excessive evil" and "seven emotions" are important pathogenic factors causing the occurrence of diseases.

浊毒体质的形成，有先天禀赋、后天失调、药物作用等因素所导致。而大多数人是由于外感之邪，大量饮酒，或过食肥甘厚味，或过度思虑，脾虚不运，而致水液不化，聚湿生痰，浊毒内蕴。《灵枢·寿夭刚柔》认为："人之生也，有刚有柔，有弱有强，有短有长，有阴有阳……"说明体质与先天禀赋关系密切，体质差异与生俱来。有资料表明，肥胖者通常有明确的家族史，父亲或母亲肥胖，其子女约有40%～50%出现肥胖；如父母均肥胖，则其子女肥胖的机会可以达70%～80%。

The formation of turbid toxin constitution is caused by congenital (kidney essence) deficiency, acquired function (of spleen) disorder, improper using of medicine and other factors. but most probably it is caused by evil of exogenous, large quantity of alcohol, or too much eating of fat and sweet food, or excessive thinking. As the deficient spleen does not transport, water fluid cannot be vaporized, wet is accumulated into phlegm, turbid toxin arises inside. *Spiritual Pivot-Discussion On Long and Short Life, Sturdiness and Softness* thinks: "The constitution of people is classified as sturdy, soft, weak, strong, short-life and long-life, and active and passive." It shows that constitution is closely related to innate endowment, and constitution differs from the very beginning of life. Data shows that obese people usually have a clear family history, if the father or mother is obese, about 40% to 50% of their children are obese, if the parents are obese; the obese chance of their children can be up to 70% to 80%.

浊毒体质包括痰浊与热毒体质两种。痰浊体质是目前比较常见的一种体质类型，当人体脏腑、阴阳失调、气血津液运行失常，易形成痰浊时，便可认作痰浊体质。痰浊体质多见于肥胖人，或素瘦今肥之人。该体质的人常表现有体形肥胖，腹部肥满松软，面部皮肤油脂较多，多汗且黏、胸闷、痰多，面色秽浊，眼胞微浮，容易困倦，舌体胖大，舌苔白腻或黄腻，身重不爽，喜食肥甘甜黏，大便不实或不爽，小便不多或微混，性格偏温和、稳重，多善于忍耐。此种体质类型有易患高血压、糖尿病、肥胖症、高脂血症、哮喘、痛风、冠心病、代谢综合征、脑血管疾病等疾病的倾向。而热毒体质，则常见面垢油光，易生痤疮，口苦口干，身重困倦，大便黏滞不畅或燥结，小便短黄，阴囊潮湿，或带下增多，质偏红，苔黄腻，脉滑数，容易心烦急躁，易患疮疖、黄疸、热淋等病，对夏末秋初湿热气候，湿浊重或气温偏高环境较难适应。

Turbid toxin constitution includes phlegm turbidity constitution and hot toxin constitution. Phlegm turbidity constitution is a more common constitution type at present. When the viscera, balance of positive and negative energy of human body are irregular, the operation of breath, blood, liquid and fluid is abnormal, it will be easy to form phlegm turbidity, thus the constitution can be recognized as phlegm turbidity constitution. Sputum turbidity constitution is more common in obese people, or people thin in past but fat at present. People with the above constitution often look fat, with full and soft belly, more fat in facial skin, more sticky sweat and phlegm, chest tightness, filth face, floating eyes, easy to drowsiness, fat and enlarged tongue body with white greasy or yellow greasy tongue coating, heavy body, preferring fat, sweet and sticky food, stool is not solid but a little bit difficult, little urine or slightly muddy, with mild, stable personality, and more patience. People of this constitution type is prone to hypertension, diabetes, obesity, hyperlipidemia, asthma, gout, coronary heart disease, metabolic syndrome, cerebrovascular diseases and other diseases. People of hot toxic constitution, usually see dirt but greasy face, easy to acne, dry and bitter mouth, lazy and sleepy, stool is sticky or dry, urine is short and yellow, damp scrotal, or more leukorrhea, red tongue, yellow and greasy tongue coating, slippery and rapid pulse, easy to upset, easy to suffer from boils, jaundice, fever and other diseases. They are difficult to adapt to the wet and hot climate, with more wet turbidity or high temperature in late summer and early autumn.

浊毒体质观在中医病因学上与现代以西方医学为主体的生物–心理–社会医学模式有着共同的思维方式。体质健康是人的生命活动和劳动工作能力（包括运动能力）的物质基础。在形势和发展过程中，人的体质具有明显的差异性和阶段性。不同人的体质差异表现在形态发育、生理功能、心理状态、身体素质和运动能力，对环境的适应以及对疾病的抵抗力等方面，包括从最佳功能状态到严重疾病和功能障碍等各种不同的体质水平。体质的稳定性由相似的遗传背景形成，年龄、性别等因素也可使体质表现出一定的稳定性。然而，体质的稳定性是相对的.每一个体在生长壮老的生命过程中，因受环境、精神、营养、锻炼、疾病等内外环境中诸多因素的影响，而使体质会发生变化，从而使得体质只具有相对的稳定性，同时具有动态可变性。这种特征是体质可调的理论基础，也可有效地指导浊毒证的临床诊断与用药。

Constitution view of turbid toxin theory in TCM etiology shares the same mindset with the modern bio-psychological-society model of medical science. Physical health is the material basis of human life activities and ability of labor and work (including exercising ability). In the process of situation and development, it has obvious differences and stage. The constitution differences of different people are shown in morphological development, physical function, mental state, physical quality and exercise ability, and ability to adapt to the environment and resistance to disease, etc. Besides, the constitution differences of people are related to different phase or state of life development process, including the phase of best functional state of body, the phase of serious disease and dysfunction of body and other phase of physical level. The stability of the constitution depends on similar genetic background, and other factors such as age and sex. However, the stability of the constitution is relative. During the life process of birth, growing up, prime and ageing, the constitution will changes due to the affection of many factors, such as factor of internal and external environment, factor of spirit, factor of nutrition, factor of exercise and diseases, therefore the stability of constitution is relative, the dynamic variability of constitution is constant. This characteristic is the theoretical basis for the possibility of constitution adjustment, and can also effectively guide the clinical diagnosis and medication of turbid toxin diseases.

第五节　浊毒辨证
Section 5　The Syndrome Differentiation of Turbid Toxin

浊毒既是一种对人体脏腑经络及气血阴阳均能造成严重损害的致病因素，同时也是指多种原因导致脏腑功能紊乱、气血运行失常，机体内产生的代谢产物不能及时正常排出蕴积体内而化生的病理产物。浊毒证是指以浊毒为病因使机体处于浊毒状态从而产生特有临床表现的一组或几组症候群。浊有浊质，毒有毒性。浊质黏腻导致浊邪为病，多易结滞脉络，阻塞气机，缠绵耗气，胶着不去而易酿毒性；而毒邪伤人，其性烈善变，损害气血营卫。两者相合则因毒借浊质，浊夹毒性，多直伤脏腑经络。浊毒可侵犯上、中、下三焦，但以中焦最为常见，在中焦中以脾胃最为常见。

Turbid toxin is not only a pathogenic factor which can cause serious damage to the viscera, breath, blood, Yin and Yang, but also a pathological product transformed from the accumulated metabolites failing to be discharged from human body in time caused by the dysfunction of viscera and the abnormal operation of breath and blood. Turbid toxin syndrome refers to a group or groups of symptoms that make the body in the state of turbid toxin and produce unique clinical manifestations.

Turbidity has turbid nature, toxin has toxic character. Sticky and greasy nature promotes the turbid evil to cause disease, easier to knot veins, block energy operation mechanism, lingering and energy wasting, gluey and easy to be transformed into toxin; when toxin hurt people, it will abruptly and seriously damage breath and blood, nourishing and defensive energy. The combination of turbidity and toxin will directly damage viscera, invading triple energizers of the body, especially the middle energizer i.e. spleen and stomach, because toxin is assisted by turbid nature, turbidity carries toxic character.

一、浊毒证候的主症与兼次症
1. The main and co-time disease of turbid toxin syndrome

以浊毒为病因病机使机体产生特有临床表现的一组或几组症候群称为浊毒证候，包括主症、兼次症及舌脉等。在前期研究基础上，进一步建立、健全浊毒证诊断标准，逐步在全国范围内形成高度共识，是完善浊毒理论体系的重要举措。根据历代医家对"浊""毒"的记载，结合我们对浊毒的认识，将浊毒证概括为：浊毒主症：①疾病所在系统、器官等病位的主要症状；②大便黏腻不爽，臭秽难闻，小便或浅黄或深黄或浓茶样改变，汗液秽浊有味。浊毒兼次症：颜面色黄、晦浊、粗糙，褐斑，痤疮，头重如裹，皮肤油腻，眼睑红肿糜烂，鼻头红肿溃烂，咽部红肿，咳吐黏稠涎沫，口苦，口中黏腻，渴而不欲饮，肌表湿疹等。舌脉：舌质或红或红绛或紫，苔色或黄或白或黄白相间；脉或弦滑或细滑或弦细滑。因浊毒侵犯部位、疾病性质、疾病所处阶段、患者体质及既有的干预措施不同，临证之际，当详细审之。

A group or several groups of symptom with the etiology of turbid toxin are called turbid toxin syndrome, including the main symptom, secondary symptom, and manifestation of tongue and pulses. It is an important measure to improve the theoretical system of turbid toxin to further establish and improve the diagnostic standard of turbid toxin syndrome and gradually form a high consensus across the country on the basis of the preliminary research. Combining the records of "turbidity" and "toxin" by physicians in different dynasties with our understanding of turbid toxin, the turbid toxin syndrome is summarized as: the main symptoms of turbid toxin: a. the main symptoms of the disease in certain system, organ and other location; b. sticky stool, smelly, light yellow or deep yellow or thick tea like urine, turbid smell sweat. Secondary and complex symptoms of turbid toxin syndrome: dark, rough and yellow face with moth patch and acne in it, head as heavy as being wrapped, greasy skin, swollen eyelids with erosion, swollen apex nasi with ulceration, swollen throat, sticky and thick saliva, bitter and sticky mouth, thirsty but with no want to drink, muscle surface eczema, etc. Manifestation of tongue and pulses: red, deep red or purple tongue with tongue coating of tongue and pulses: red, deep red or purple tongue with tongue coating of yellow or white or alternation of yellow and white; string slippery pulse or thin slippery pulse or string thin slippery pulse. Clinical examination should be carefully made due to the different site of turbid toxin invasion, the nature of and phase of the disease, the patient's constitution and the medical intervention measures which have been implemented towards the patient.

浊毒存在于人体内部的时候，阻滞气机，影响气血升降，阻碍妨碍水液代谢，不利于水谷精微的传化与吸收。这样的病理机制可以发生在人体的很多部位，可以说从上到下，从里到外，都存在着浊毒停着的可能。浊毒停于头部，影响气机升降，可以出现大头瘟等传染病症，除了发热、口渴、脉搏洪大等全身症状之外，还会出现头痛、呕吐、眼目肿胀、耳肿、口疮、鼻塞、喉肿、咽痛等症状。内伤杂病的浊毒上涌头部，则可以出现突然昏厥、痰声辘辘、双目失明、暴聋失音等症状。浊毒见于胸部，则既影响肺气出入升降，也妨碍心血的输布运行，可见胸闷气短、咳嗽喘息、痰涎壅盛、心慌心悸、心痛彻背、神志异常等症。浊毒见于胃脘，影响胃之受纳，也影响脾之运化，因此可以见到恶心呕吐、脘腹胀满、心下疼痛、饮食难进、痞块积聚等症状。浊毒停于两胁，就会出现胁痛胀满、癥瘕积聚、口苦目眩等证候。浊毒流注经络骨节，致肢体疼痛，甚则痰瘀浊毒附骨，出现痛风结节；内则流注脏腑，加重脾运失司，升降失常，穷则及肾，脾肾阳虚，发为石淋、关格。浊毒停于下焦，就会出现小腹胀满、痞块硬肿、尿闭便坚、神识如狂、妇女月经适来适断、带下秽浊、便泻不畅、男女不育不孕、下肢浮肿等证。

When turbid toxin exists in the human body, it blocks the energy mechanism operation, affects the rise and fall of breath and blood, hinders the metabolism of water and liquid, and is not conducive to the transmission and absorption of water and grain essence. Such pathological mechanism can occur in many parts of the human body. That is to say turbid toxin may stay in any part of the body, from top to bottom, from inside to outside. When it stays in the head, it affects the rise and fall of energy mechanism, causes serious head fever and other infectious disease with main symptom as fever, thirst, full pulse and other systemic symptoms as headache, vomiting, swollen eye and ear, mouth sores, stuffy nose, swollen throat, sore throat. When turbid toxin attacks the head of the patients with viscera injuries and miscellaneous diseases, it will cause sudden fainting, noisy phlegm, blindness, sudden deafness and aphonia and other symptoms. When turbid toxin invades chest, it will not only affect the ascending, descending, entering and exiting of lung energy operation, but also hinder the spreading and transmission of heart blood, causing symptoms as chest distress, short of breath, cough and wheezing, congestion of phlegm and saliva, epigastric oppression and palpitation, cardiac pain hurting back, abnormal mind and other diseases. When turbid toxin is seen in the epigastric stomach, it will affect the acceptance function of stomach and the transporting function of spleen causing nausea and vomiting, abdominal distension, stomachache, difficult diet, ruffian block accumulation and other symptoms.When turbid toxin stays on the two lateral sides of thorax, there will be hypochondrium distending pain and fullness, gathering and accumulation of movable and unmovable masses, bitter mouth and dizziness. When turbid toxin retains in the meridians and bone joints, it will cause pain of limbs, even gout nodules produced by phlegm stasis and turbid toxin of lumbar vertebra; further more, turbid toxin will stays in storing and transforming organs, aggravating the dysfunction of spleen transporting, abnormal operation of energy ascending and descending, or even directly attacks kidney, causing function deficiency of spleen and kidney, inducing stone lymph, frequent vomiting and dysuria. When turbid toxin stays at the lower energizer, there will be abdominal distension, hard and swollen mass, urine closure and hard stool, mental crazy, women irregular menstruation with filthy leukorrhagia, sterility of woman and infertility of man, edema of lower limbs and other symptoms.

二、常见浊毒脏腑辨证
2. Common turbid toxin viscera syndrome differentiation

（一）浊毒在胃
2.1 The turbid toxin is in the stomach

1.主症　胃脘疼痛，脘腹胀满，纳呆，嗳气，恶心呕吐，烧心反酸。

2.1.1 Main symptoms　Epigastric pain, abdominal distension, anorexia, belching, nausea and vomiting, heartburn and acid regurgitation.

2.兼次症　口干口苦，气短懒言，周身乏力，心烦易怒，小便短赤，面色晦浊，泄泻不爽，或大便秘结等。

2.1.2 Secondary symptoms　Dry and bitter mouth, short of breath and lazy to speak, body fatigue, irritability, short and red urine, cloudy complexion, diarrhea, or constipation, etc.

3.舌象　舌红，苔黄腻。

2.1.3 Tongue image　Red tongue with yellow greasy tongue coating.

4.脉象　脉滑数。

2.1.4 Pulse image　Slippery and rapid pulse.

5.证候分析　饮食内伤，情志不舒，胃之通降失职，浊邪内停；日久脾失健运，水湿不化，湿浊中阻，郁而不解，蕴积成热，热壅血瘀成毒。浊毒之邪影响气机升降，气机阻滞，则胃脘疼痛，脘腹胀满，嗳气；胃失和降，脾失健运则纳呆。浊毒壅盛积滞中焦，胆气上逆，故烧心反酸，口干口苦；浊毒困脾，脾胃受损，肠道功能失司，清浊不分则泄泻。浊毒日久，津伤液耗，肠失濡润，则大便秘结，小便短赤。浊毒犯胃，致胃气痞塞，升降失调，则恶心呕吐。肝藏魂，心藏神，毒热之邪内扰魂则心神不宁，魂不守舍，而见心烦易怒。脾失健运，化源乏力，脏腑功能减退，故见气短懒言，周身乏力。浊毒蕴结，郁蒸体内，上蒸于头面，则面色晦浊。浊毒中阻则见舌红苔黄腻，脉滑数。

2.1.5 Analysis of syndrome　Internal injury, discomfort in emotion, dysfunction of stomach energy descending, retaining of turbidity evil; after a long time, spleen fails to transport water and grain essence, wet water cannot be vaporized, damp turbidity is depressed and confused, then accumulated into heat, heat congestion and blood stasis are transformed into toxin. The evil of turbid toxin affects the ascending and descending of energy mechanism, the obstruction of energy mechanism causes epigastric pain, abdominal distension, belching; when stomach looses the function of harmonious descending, spleen looses the function of smooth transporting, anorexia occurs. Accumulation of excessive turbid toxin in middle energizer causes adverse flow of bile energy, resulting heartburn and acid reflux, dry and bitter mouth; When turbid toxin traps spleen, it affects the normal work of spleen and stomach, causes the dysfunction of intestine to separate lucidity and turbidity, thus diarrhea occurs. If turbid toxin stays in human body for a long time, it will consume and waste body fluid and liquid, make the intestines loss of lubrication, stool constipation, urine short and red. When turbid toxin attacks stomach, it causes gastric qi ruffian, disorder of ascending and descending operation, nausea and vomiting occurs. Liver hides the soul, heart hides the mind. When the evil of toxin and heat interrupts the mind and soul, the mind cannot not be quiet, soul is difficult to be held, therefore upset irritation occurs. When spleen lost the function of healthy transporting, it lacks the motivation to transport, viscera function declines, resulting shortness of breath, lazy to speak, and overall fatigue. When turbid toxin is accumulated and stagnated, it will be steamed in body. When head and faces are steamed, the face is cloudy. In case of turbid toxin resistance, the tongue is red with yellow greasy tongue coating, and the pulses are slippery and rapid.

（二）浊毒在肝

2.2 The turbid toxin is in the liver

1.主症　胁肋部胀满疼痛，遇烦恼郁怒则痛作或痛甚，口干口苦，嗳气则舒，善太息，急躁易怒，头痛眩晕。

2.2.1 Main symptoms　Hypochondrium distending pain and fullness, pain occurs or turns to be more serious in case of worries and depression rages, dry and bitter mouth, belching, feel better to sigh, irritability, headache and dizziness.

2.兼次症　或胃脘胀痛，胃痛连胁，或胸膈胀闷，上气喘急，不思饮食，或精神抑郁，寐差，或心烦纳呆，或后背疼痛，沉紧不适，小便短赤，大便秘结，妇女见乳房胀痛，月经不调，痛经。

2.2.2 Secondary symptoms　Epigastric distension and pain, pain of stomach and lateral sides of thorax, or sealed and distended chest diaphragm, asthma, anorexia, or mental depression, poor sleep, or upset and anorexia, or backache and pain, tightness and discomfort, short and red urine, stool constipation, breast distension and pain, irregular menstruation, dysmenorrhea of female patients.

3.舌象　舌红紫或红绛，苔黄腻或黄燥。

2.2.3 Tongue image　The tongue is red purple or crimson, with yellow greasy or yellow dry tongue coating.

4.脉象　脉弦数或弦滑。

2.2.4 Pulse image　String rapid or string slippery pulse.

5.证候分析　感受湿热之邪或脾失健运，积湿化浊，郁久蕴热成毒，浊毒内伏肝络，肝气郁滞，则胁肋胀满疼痛，情志抑郁。肝气不条达，影响气机升降则善太息或嗳气则舒，遇烦恼郁怒则痛作或痛甚。肝气受损，浊毒痰火内盛，不得宣泄而熏蒸，蒙蔽脑神则头痛眩晕。浊毒内蕴，夹胆气上逆则口干口苦。浊毒内蕴助肝阳上亢则急躁易怒，失眠多梦。浊毒日久入络，波及背部，阻遏经络则出现背痛，沉紧不适。邪毒热盛灼津则小便短赤，大便秘结。女子以肝为用，浊毒阻碍气机，气血失和，冲任失调则妇女乳房胀痛，月经不调，痛经。舌红紫或红绛，苔黄腻或黄燥，脉弦滑数均为浊毒中阻内伏于肝之象。

2.2.5 Syndrome analysis　Attacked by the evil of dampness and heat or affected by spleen disorder in smooth transporting, accumulated dampness is transformed into turbidity, constant depression is transformed into heat and then toxin, turbid toxin retains in liver collateral, causes stagnation of liver energy, hypochondrium distending pain and fullness, depression in emotion.

Dysfunction of liver affects the ascending and descending of energy mechanism, thus patients feel better to sigh, and feel comfortable after belching, pain occurs or turns to be more serious in case of worry and depressed anger. When liver function is damaged, phlegm fire of turbid toxin is excessively abundant and fumigated as it can not be discharged in time, headache and vertigo arises when the fumigated phlegm fire hoodwink the brain and mind. Accumulation of turbid toxin plus reverse flow of gallbladder qi causes dry and bitter mouth. Accumulation of turbid toxin promotes hyperhepatic of liver function, resulting irritable rages and insomnia with more dreams. For time being, turbid toxin will enter the collateral, affect the back, inhibit the meridians, cause back pain, heavy, tight and discomfort. Toxin evil is terribly hot to burn fluid, making the urine short and red, stool constipated. Health of women depends on liver, turbid toxin hinders the operation of energy mechanism, causes disharmony of breath and blood, abnormal work of thoroughfare and conception vessel, causing distention and pain of breast, irregular menstruation, dysmenorrhea. The tongue is red purple or crimson, with yellow greasy or yellow dry tongue coating, the pulses are string, slippery and rapid, forming the image of obstruction of turbid toxin retaining in liver.

（三）浊毒在肺
2.3 The turbid toxin is in the lung

1.主症　咳嗽痰多，质稠色黄，胸闷，气喘息粗，心烦口渴，大便秘结，小便短赤。

2.3.1 Main symptoms　Cough with more thick and yellow phlegm, chest distress, asthma with thick breathing, upset and thirsty, constipated stool, short and red urine.

2.兼次症　或咳吐脓血腥臭痰；或骤起发热，咳嗽气喘，甚则鼻翼翕动；或壮热口渴，烦躁不安。

2.3.2 Secondary symptoms　Vomiting smelly phlegm with pus and blood; or sudden fever, cough with asthma, or even nostrils fluttered; or extreme fever, thirsty and restlessness.

3.舌象　舌红苔黄腻。

2.3.3 Tongue image　Red tongue with yellow greasy tongue coating.

4.脉象　脉弦滑数。

2.3.4 Pulse image　String slippery and rapid pulse.

5.证候分析　外伤湿热之邪，久郁不化则发为浊毒。浊毒蕴肺，肺气失司则发为咳嗽；浊邪壅滞则痰多质稠，毒邪害清则咳痰色黄，甚则咳吐脓血腥臭痰；肺气不降，浊毒阻肺则胸闷气喘。浊毒瘀滞以致肺不布津，并导致肠道津液缺乏，故心烦口渴，大便秘结，小便短赤，甚则壮热口渴，烦躁不安。风热浊毒犯肺，热壅肺气，故骤起发热。热盛伤津则壮热口渴。舌红苔黄腻，脉弦滑数则为浊毒内蕴脏腑之象。

2.3.5 Syndrome analysis　Attacked by external evil of dampness and heat, which is transformed into turbid toxin from long-time accumulation. When turbid toxin retains in lungs, cough occurs in case of disorder of lung function; when turbidity evil is abundantly stagnated, phlegm turns to be more and thicker, when evil of toxin affect the lucidity, phlegm turns to be yellow, or even smelly phlegm with pus and blood; if the lung energy does not descend, it is because lung energy is blocked by turbid toxin, thus chest distress and asthma occurs. Stagnation of turbid toxin causes dysfunction of fluid spreading of lungs, makes the intestine short of fluid and fluid, patient feels thirsty, stool constipated, urine short and red, or extreme fever and thirsty, restlessness. When lungs are attacked by turbid toxin of wind and heat evil, heat obstructs the lung energy, thus sudden fever occurs. When excessive fever consumes the fluid, patient feels thirsty, and restless. Red tongue with yellow greasy tongue coating, string, slippery and rapid pulse, forms the image of turbid toxin accumulated in viscera.

（四）浊毒在心
2.4 Turbid toxin is in the heart

1.主症　心胸憋闷疼痛，心悸怔忡，气短，烦躁易怒，多梦易惊，口舌生疮，谵语烦渴。

2.4.1 Main symptoms　Chest distress, heart pain, severe palpitation, short of breath, irritability, easy to be shocked by more dreams, sores in mouth and tongue, delirium and thirsty.

2.兼次症　或昏蒙眩晕；或发热，面红目赤，呼吸气粗；或面色晦暗；或小便短赤，大便秘结。

2.4.2 Secondary symptoms　Dizziness; or fever, red eyes and faces, thick breathing; or dark complexion; or short and red urine, constipation.

3.舌象　舌红苔黄腻。

2.4.3 Tongue image　Red tongue with yellow greasy tongue coating.

4.脉象　脉弦数。

2.4.4 Pulse image　String rapid pulse.

5.证候分析　浊毒之邪盘踞于心，胸阳失展则胸闷心痛，久而导致心之功能下降，血亏气虚，故心悸怔忡。浊毒蕴结，内扰心神，则心烦失眠，面红目赤。邪陷心包则意识模糊或狂躁谵语。毒蕴日久则心火旺盛故口舌生疮。外感毒邪或浊毒内蕴里热蒸腾上炎则发热，面红目赤，呼吸气粗。浊毒内阻，清阳不升，浊气上泛，气血不畅则面色晦暗。热移小肠则小便短赤。火热津伤则大便秘结。舌红苔黄腻，脉弦数则为浊毒在心之象。

2.4.5 Analysis of syndrome　When evil of turbid toxin stays in heart, heart function declines, chest distress and heart pain occurs, blood and breath turns to be deficient, palpitation occurs; stagnation of turbid toxin disturbs heart and mind, causing irritability and insomnia, red faces and eyes. When evil sunk in pericardium, confusion of consciousness occurs, patient becomes crazy with constant delirium. Long-time accumulation of toxin e burns the heart fire, and causes sores in mouth and tongue. External toxin evil and internal accumulated turbid toxin transpiring, causes fever, red face and eyes, thick breathing. Obstructed by turbid toxin, energy of lucidity cannot rise, energy of turbidity works, circulation of breath and blood is not smooth, thus the complexion is dark. When heat enters small intestine, urine turns to be short and red. Extreme fever consumes fluid, causes constipation. Red tongue with yellow greasy tongue coating, string and rapid pulse are the image of turbid toxin in the heart.

（五）浊毒在肾

2.5 The turbid toxin is in the kidney

1.主症　腰膝酸软，少腹胀闷疼痛，下肢甚或周身浮肿，尿道灼痛，尿频尿急，尿黄短赤。

2.5.1 Main symptoms　Soft waist and acid knee, abdominal distension and stuffy pain, lower limbs or even peripheral body swollen, urethra burning urinary pain, frequent and abrupt urination, yellow or short red urine.

2.兼次症　或血尿，血淋，或女子不孕，男子不育。

2.5.2 Secondary symptoms　Hematuria, bloody, or sterility of woman and infertility of man.

3.舌象　舌红，苔薄黄或黄腻。

2.5.3 Tongue image　Red tongue with thin yellow or yellow greasy tongue coating.

4.脉象　弦或滑数。

2.5.4 Pulse image　String pulse or slippery and rapid pulse.

5.证候分析　外感湿热之邪久而加重化为浊毒，或久居湿地等感受寒湿之邪蕴积日久化为浊毒，浊毒入肾，导致肾之经络受邪而气血壅滞，故腰膝酸软、少腹胀满疼痛；浊毒影响肾之主水功能可出现水肿；肾与膀胱相表里，浊毒害肾必连及膀胱，膀胱功能失司，则出现尿频、尿急、尿痛等症；浊毒之邪灼伤肾与膀胱之脉络，则出现血尿、血淋等症；浊毒郁久影响肾主生殖之功则发为女子不孕，男子不育等症；舌红苔黄腻或薄黄，脉弦滑或数为浊毒内蕴脏腑之象。

2.5.5 Syndrome analysis　The long-time accumulation of evil of external dampness and heat, or accumulation of cold and wet evil arisen from long-time living in wetland, are gradually aggravated and transformed into turbid toxin. When turbid toxin invades kidney, it will attack the kidney meridians leading to breath and blood stagnation, therefore, lassitude of loin and knees occurs, and the lower abdominal is distended, full and painful. When turbid toxin affects the water controlling function of kidney, it may possibly cause edema. As the relationship between kidney and bladder is the couple relation between exterior and interior organs, bladder will be affected when kidney is attacked by turbid toxin. Once bladder function is abnormal, frequent urination, urgent urination and painful urination occurs. When the evil of turbid toxin burns the pulses of the kidney and bladder, hematuria, blood dribbling occurs. Long- time accumulation of turbid toxin will influence the reproduction controlling function of the kidney causing sterility of woman and infertility of man. Red tongue with yellow greasy or thin yellow tongue coating, string slippery pulse or rapid pulse is the image of turbid toxin in kidney.

（六）浊毒在脑

2.6 The turbid toxin is in the brain

1.主症　头痛，眩晕，记忆力下降，口舌㖞斜，舌强语謇，半身不遂，甚或至昏迷，肢体强急。

2.6.1 Main symptoms　Headache, vertigo, decline of memory ability, oblique mouth and tongue, stiff tongue and speechless, hemiplegia, or even coma, stiff and tight body.

2.兼次症　耳鸣或精神异常，或思维障碍，或烦躁谵妄，神识昏蒙，不省人事，循衣摸床；或口吐白沫，四肢抽搐；或面赤身热，躁扰不宁；或言行呆傻，睁眼若视，貌似清醒的植物人状态等。

2.6.2 Secondary symptoms　Tinnitus or spiritual abnormal, or thinking obstruction, or irritably delirium, unconscious dizzy, insensibility or foaming at mouth, limbs convulsions; or red face and hot body, restless disturbance; or silly words and deeds, eyes opening as if watching, as awake as in vegetative state.

3.舌象　舌红苔黄腻。

2.6.3 Tongue image　Red tongue with yellow greasy tongue coating.

4.脉象　弦数。

2.6.4 Pulse image　String rapid pulse.

5.证候分析　浊毒作为一种病理产物，可以上蒙清窍，或者阻碍气血上行，脑窍失养，产生头痛眩晕。脑之玄府通利失和则滞气停津，积水成浊，浊蕴为毒，浊毒泛淫玄府，碍神害脑，变生中风诸症可出现舌歪语謇，半身不遂，甚则昏迷肢强。脑为元神之府，浊毒郁脑影响脑的功能则记忆力下降。毒淫脑髓，浊气上扰，内伤神明，蒙闭清窍，气血逆乱，轻则精神异常，或思维障碍，或烦躁谵妄，重则脑髓受损，神识昏蒙，不省人事，循衣摸床。浊毒蒙蔽清窍，扰乱神明则口吐白沫，四肢抽搐。情志不遂，生湿化痰，痰浊郁而化热久酿浊毒，浊毒上扰清窍，逆扰神明则面赤身热，躁扰不宁，浊毒阻滞脑络，脑失所养则言行呆傻。若神明失用，经久不愈，则发为睁眼若视、貌似清醒的植物人状态。舌红苔黄脉弦数是为浊毒内蕴脏腑之象。

2.6.5 Syndrome analysis　Turbid toxin as a pathological product, can block the orifices, hinder the upward moving of breath and blood, make the brain short of nourishment, causing headache and vertigo. Disharmony of the brain stagnate the breath and fluid, accumulation of water becomes turbidity, turbidity is then transformed into toxin. Turbid toxin attacks and occupies the brain, disturbs the mind and mental work, causing allogenic stroke with symptoms as oblique tongue and speechlessness, hemiplegia, or even coma and limb stiffness. When brain, as the house of mentality, is functionally affected by accumulation of turbid toxin, memory ability declines. When toxin attacks the brain pulp, evil of turbidity rises upward, disturbs the mentality, hoodwinks the orifices, makes breath and blood move reversely, causing spiritual abnormal, thinking obstruction, or irritably delirium, more severely, it damages the brain marrow, causing unconscious dizzy, insensibility, floccitation. When turbid toxin hoodwinks the orifices, disturbs the mental work, it causes foaming at the mouth, tic of limbs. Emotional discomfort produces dampness and phlegm, accumulation of phlegm turbidity will be transformed into heat, then into turbid toxin after a long time. Turbid toxin disturbs the orifices, disorders the mental peace, patients see red face and hot in whole body, irritable restlessness. When turbid toxin obstruct the brain collateral, foolish words and deeds occurs as the brain is short of nourishment. If dysfunction of mind fails to recover for a long time, the patient will become vegetative.

Red tongue with yellow tongue coating, string and rapid pulse is the image of turbid toxin retaining in the brain.

（七）浊毒在皮、脉、筋、骨

2.7 The turbid toxin is in the skin, veins, muscles and bones

1.主症　皮肤晦暗如烟熏色，甚则皮肤起斑；或皮肤起群集小疱，瘙痒，红肿灼痛，脱屑，粗糙；关节灼热红肿疼痛，屈伸不利，身体重着，肢倦神疲。

2.7.1 Main symptoms　The skin is as dark as fumigated, or even skin spots occur; or skin cluster of vesicles arises, itching, reddish swollen, burning pain, skin desquamation, rough; joints become reddish swollen, burning painful, difficult to flex and extend, body is heavy, fatigue in limbs and tired in spirit.

2.兼次症　或发热恶风，口渴烦闷；或心烦易怒，失眠多梦，心悸怔忡；或肌肤麻木不仁，阴雨天加重；或关节肿大畸形。

2.7.2 Secondary symptoms　Fever with aversion to wind, thirsty, boredom; or irritability, insomnia with more dreams, severe palpitation; or numb skin, more severe in rainy days; or joint enlargement and deformity.

3.舌象　舌红苔黄腻。

2.7.3 Tongue image　Red tongue with yellow greasy tongue coating.

4.脉象　弦滑数。

2.7.4 Pulse image　String, slippery and rapid pulse.

5.证候分析　外感风热或脾胃内热蕴生浊毒，蕴于皮肤则皮肤晦暗如烟熏，甚则皮肤斑疹。浊毒壅滞皮肤则皮肤起群集小疱，灼热刺痒。肝脾湿热，助浊毒之邪循经蕴肤，则瘙痒，红肿灼痛。浊毒阻滞气血运行，肤失濡养则皮肤脱屑，粗糙。如若浊毒之邪深陷皮肤之络，可发为肌肤麻木不仁，不知痛痒。浊毒蕴于筋骨，损伤脉络，筋骨失养，则出现关节灼热肿胀疼痛，屈伸不利。浊为湿之甚，浊性重着，故会出现身体重着，肢倦神疲；浊毒泛于肌表，营卫失和，可表现为发热恶风，口渴烦闷。热扰心神则心烦易怒，失眠多梦，心悸怔忡。舌红、苔黄腻、脉弦滑数为浊毒侵袭筋脉皮骨之象。

2.7.5 Syndrome analysis　Accumulation of external wind heat or heat in the spleen and stomach produces turbid toxin, when turbid toxin attacks skin, the skin will be as dark as fumigated, or even skin rash arises. When turbid toxin retains in the skin, clusters of skin vesicles arise, patients will feel burning hot and irritable itching. Dampness and heat in the liver and spleen helps turbid toxin evil invading the skin along with the meridian, causing itching and, reddish swelling and burning pain. Turbid toxin blocks the operation of breath and blood, make the skin loss of nourishment, skin turns to be rough with desquamation. If the evil of turbid toxin sinks deep in the skin, it can cause skin numbness, insensitivity to pain and itch. If the turbid toxin lies in muscles and bones, it will injure pulses. When muscles and bones are short of nourishment, the joints will be burning hot, swollen, distended and painful, difficult to flex and extend. Turbidity is transformed from wetness, when turbidity is of dampness, patients will see body damp and heavy, fatigue in limbs and tired in spirit.

When turbid toxin is found in muscle surface, disharmony of nourishing and defensive energy occurs, patients will have fever, fear of wind, thirsty, and restlessness. When mind is affected by heat evil, patients will have restless anger, insomnia with more dreams, palpitations. When turbid toxin invades skin, muscles, bones and pulses, the tongue image is red tongue with yellow greasy tongue coating, the image of pulse is string, slippery and rapid.

三、浊毒三焦辨证
3. Triple energizer differentiation of turbid toxin syndrome

（一）浊毒在上焦
3.1 The turbid toxin is in upper energizer

1.主症　胸闷咳喘，身热口渴，头晕，面红目赤，心烦失眠，甚则心悸怔忡。

3.1.1 Main symptoms　Chest distress, cough and asthma, fever and thirsty, dizziness, red eyes and faces, upset, insomnia, and even severe palpitation.

2.兼次症　或恶寒发热，身热不扬，午后热甚；甚或神昏谵语，言语謇涩；或胸痛，咳吐黄稠脓痰，心烦肢厥。

3.1.2 Secondary symptoms　Fever with aversion to cold, the patient feels hot in body, even more severe in afternoon; even dizzy and delirium, faint and astringent language; or chest pain, vomiting yellow thick pus phlegm, upset and cold limbs.

3.舌象　舌暗红或紫暗，苔黄腻或厚腻，或薄黄。

3.1.3 Tongue image　Tongue dark red or purple dark with yellow greasy, thick greasy, or thin yellow tongue coating.

4.脉象　弦滑数。

3.1.4 Pulse image　String slippery rapid pulse.

5.证候分析　浊毒盘踞上焦，影响心肺功能则出现胸闷咳喘，咳吐黄稠痰，心悸怔忡之症。浊毒上扰清窍则头晕，蕴于颜面则面红目赤。浊毒影响津液输布则身热口渴，心烦失眠。邪陷心包则神昏语謇，甚或心烦肢厥。浊毒夹湿困阻肌表，肺气不宣，卫外失司，故恶寒。正气抗邪，正邪相争则发热。湿遏热伏，热不得宣扬，故身虽热而不扬。午后阳明经气主令，阳明乃多气多血之经，当其主令之时则正气充盛，抗邪有力，正邪相争，故午后热甚。舌暗红苔黄腻或薄黄，脉弦滑数则为浊毒盘踞上焦之象。

3.1.5 Syndrome analysis　When turbid toxin occupies upper energizer, it affects cardiopulmonary function, causes chest distress, cough and asthma with yellow thick phlegm, palpitation and severe palpitation. When turbid toxin disturbs the sense organs of the head, dizziness occurs. When turbid toxin retains in the face, faces and eyes turn to be red. When turbid toxin affects the spreading of body fluid, patient will feel general fever and thirsty, dysphoria and insomnia. When evil sinks in pericardium, it causes unconsciousness, dysphoria and cold limbs. When turbid toxin and dampness perplexes muscle surface, pulmonary energy cannot be released to defend against the external evil, therefore, the patient will feel fever with aversion to cold, while positive energy is fighting with the negative evil. Dampness obstructs the embedded heat, thus general fever cannot be dispersed. Afternoon is the time dominated by Yangming meridian which contains more breath and blood, when it governs, positive energy is abundant to fight against the pathogenic factor, so fever seems more severe in the afternoon. Dark red tongue with yellow greasy or thin yellow tongue coating, and string slippery pulse is the image of tongue and pulses when turbid toxin occupies the upper energizer.

（二）浊毒在中焦

3.2 The turbid toxin is in middle energizer

1.主症　胃脘连及胁肋胀满疼痛，烧心反酸，不思饮食，急躁易怒，嗳气频数，情志抑郁不舒，大便或溏滞不爽，色黄味臭或秘结不通，小便不利。

3.2.1 Main symptoms　Full, distension and painful in epigastric and flank, heart-burn and acid reflux, anorexia, irritability, frequent belching, depression, sluggish stool or loose stool, yellow, smelly or secret knot, adverse urine.

2.兼次症　或头晕目眩，胁有痞块，恶心腹胀，或寒热往来，身目发黄，或面色晦暗，口苦口干，身重肢倦，或恶心干呕，入食则吐。

3.2.2 Secondary symptoms　Dizziness, ruffian in two lateral sides of thorax, nausea and abdominal distension, alternative cold and pyretic malaria, yellow eyes and body, or dark face, bitter and dry mouth, heavy body and fatigue in limbs, or nausea and retching, vomiting.

3.舌象　舌质红或暗红，苔黄厚腻或薄黄。

3.2.3 Tongue image　Red or dark red tongue with yellow thick and greasy tongue coating or thin and yellow tongue coating.

4.脉象　弦数或弦滑。

3.2.4 Pulse image　String rapid or string slippery pulse.

5.证候分析　浊毒内蕴于肝胃，肝胃不和，浊毒郁阻气机，故胃脘连及胁肋胀痛。胃气壅滞，胃失和降，胃气上逆则嗳气。浊毒壅盛，积滞中焦，则烧心反酸。浊毒影响中焦脾胃运化功能，出现不思饮食、纳呆等症。肝气不舒则急躁易怒，情志抑郁。浊毒不去，饮食不化，浊气不降，清气不升，故头晕目眩，胁有痞块，腹胀，恶心呕吐。浊毒蕴于肌肤则身目发黄，或面色晦暗。湿热浊毒下注大肠，则大便溏滞不爽，若热势较重则色黄味臭，或秘结不通。气机阻滞，膀胱气化障碍，故小便不利。舌红，苔黄腻，脉弦滑或数为浊毒内蕴中焦之象。

3.2.5 Syndrome analysis　Turbid toxin retains in liver and stomach, causes liver-stomach disharmony, obstruction of energy mechanism operation, in result, distension and pain of epigastric and flank occurs. Block of gastric qi affects the harmony and descending function of stomach, when gastric qi moves upward reversely, belching occurs. When the turbid toxin is abundantly accumulated in middle energizer, heartburn and acid regurgitation occurs. When turbid toxin affects the transport function of spleen and stomach of middle energizer, patients will have no desire to eat, anorexia occurs. When liver is abnormal in function, people will feel irritable, and depressed emotion. If the turbid toxin cannot be removed, diet cannot be thoroughly consumed. Therefore dizziness, ruffian in two lateral sides of thorax, nausea and abdominal distension will occur. Red tongue with yellow greasy tongue, and string slippery or rapid pulse is the image of tongue and pulses when turbid toxin stays in middle energizer.

（三）浊毒在下焦

3.3 The turbid toxin is scorched in lower energizer

1.主症　小腹胀满，痞块硬肿，尿闭便坚或尿频而急，溺时热痛，淋漓不畅，尿中带血，便泻不畅或下痢腹痛、便下脓血、里急后重、肛门灼热，妇女月经时来时断，带下秽浊。

3.3.1 Main symptoms　Lower abdominal distension with hard and swollen mass, urine closure and dry stool, or frequent and acute urination, patient feels hot and painful when urine is discharged, drainage urine, or urine with blood, difficult discharging of stool, diarrhea, or dysentery abdominal pain, stool with pus and blood, tenesmus, anal burning hot, women irregular menstruation, foul leukorrhea.

2.兼次症　身热呕恶，脘痞腹胀，头晕而胀，神识昏蒙，或神识如狂，口干不欲饮，男女不育不孕，下肢浮肿等证候。

3.3.2 Secondary symptoms　Body heat, nausea, gastric pain and abdominal distension, dizziness and head distension, consciousness confusion or mania, dry mouth but with no want to drink, sterility of woman and infertility of man, swollen lower limbs.

3.舌象　舌红，苔黄腻。

3.3.3 Tongue image　Red tongue with yellow greasy tongue coating.

4.脉象　滑数。

3.3.4 Pulse image　Slippery rapid pulse.

5.证候分析　浊毒内蕴，下迫膀胱，故尿频而急，溺时尿道热痛。浊毒黏滞于膀胱，下窍阻塞，水道不利，故溺时淋漓不畅。浊毒煎熬而津液耗伤，故尿液浑浊黄赤。热邪灼伤血络，血溢于尿中，则尿中带血。浊毒滞于大肠，大肠传导失职，则下利频繁。浊毒阻滞气机，腑气不通，则腹中作痛。浊毒郁蒸，血肉壅滞腐败，化而为脓，故便下脓血。里急及肛门灼热，是热毒之邪逼迫所致，后重乃浊滞大肠，黏着难下之征。浊毒内蕴，正邪相争，故身热。浊毒阻滞气机，脾胃升降失司，故恶心呕吐，脘痞腹胀。火性炎上，浊毒上涌则头晕而胀。气滞食阻则少腹硬满。浊阻气机，气化不利，津不上承，故口干而不欲饮。浊毒内蕴，壅阻于经络、筋脉，则气血不能畅达而致筋脉失养，引动肝风，则神识昏蒙或神识如狂。舌红，苔黄腻，脉滑数为浊毒在下焦之象。

3.3.5 Syndrome analysis　Accumulated turbid toxin bears pressure to bladder, so urination becomes frequent and acute, hot and painful. When turbid toxin is sticky in the bladder, the lower orifices are obstructed, the waterway is blocked, so dribbling urine occurs. Suffering from turbid toxin torments and consumption of fluid and liquid, urine turn to be turbid and yellow red. When heat evil burns blood collateral, blood overflow in the urine, thus blood is found in urine. When turbid toxin is stagnated in the large intestine, the conduction function of large intestine does not work, frequent dysentery and diarrhea occurs. When turbid toxin obstructs energy mechanism operation, the transporting organ cannot function, patient feels painful in the abdomen. When turbid toxin is fumigated, flesh and blood is obstructed and corrupted into pus, so pus and blood is found in stool. Contraction of genital organ and burning hot in anus is caused by pressure of heat toxin evil, tenesmus is the symptom caused by stagnated turbidity in large intestine, which can hardly be discharged. When turbid toxin retains inside, positive energy and disease evil contends against each other, fever occurs as a result. When turbid toxin obstructs the energy mechanism operation, spleen and stomach looses their function of ascending and descending, so nausea and vomiting, abdominal distension occurs. On fire inflammation, turbid toxin moves upwards, thus dizzy and distension in head occurs. Breath stagnation and food resistance causes hard and fullness of lower abdomen. When turbidity resisted the smooth operation of energy mechanism, the gasification is adverse, fluid cannot be transported upward, so patient feels dry in mouth, but with no want to drink. When turbid toxin is stagnated inside human body, it obstructs the meridians and pulses, breath and blood can not reach freely, meridians and pulses are short of nourishment, the liver wind is promoted which causes unconsciousness or crazy. Red tongue with yellow greasy tongue coating, slippery rapid pulse is the image of tongue and pulses when turbid toxin invades the lower energy.

第二章 慢性胃炎浊毒论
Chapter 2 On Turbid Toxin Of Chronic Gastritis

第一节 病因病机
Section 1 Etiology and Pathogenesis

一、古代中医名家对慢性胃炎的认识
1. The understanding of ancient traditional Chinese medicine masters on chronic gastritis

慢性胃炎在中医学中无系统论述。根据其临床症状表现，该病可归入"胃脘痛""痞满""嘈杂""反酸"等范畴。有关本病的记载，始见于《黄帝内经》。《素问·六元正纪大论》曰："木郁之发……民病胃脘当心而痛，上支两胁，膈咽不通，食饮不下。"隋代巢元方《诸病源候论·诸痞候》提出"八痞"之名，说明引起痞的原因非止一端，究其病机却不外乎营卫不和、阴阳隔绝、血气窒塞不得宣通。痞满病名首见于《伤寒论》。《黄帝内经》认为其病因是饮食不节、起居不适和寒气为患等，如《素问·太阴阳明论》说："食饮不节，起居不时者，阴受之……阴受之则入五脏……入五脏则膜满闭塞。"张仲景在《伤寒论》中明确指出："满而不痛者，此为痞。"明清时期，张介宾在《景岳全书·痞满》中更是明确地指出："痞者，痞塞不开之谓；满者，胀满不行之谓。盖满则近胀，而痞则不必胀也。"并指出："凡有邪有滞而痞者，实痞也；无物无滞而痞者，虚痞也。有胀有痛而满者，实满也；无胀无痛而满者，虚满也。实痞实满者，可消可散；虚痞虚满者，非大加温补不可。"金元时期李东垣的《兰室秘藏》立"胃脘痛"专病、专方，对治疗慢性胃炎起到了指导作用。清代叶天士《临证指南医案·胃脘痛》对于本病的辨证治疗有许多独到之处，提出"胃痛久而屡发必有凝痰""久痛入络"。

Chronic gastritis is not systematically discussed in traditional Chinese medical works. According to clinical symptoms, the disease was classified into the "epigastric pain", "thoracic fullness", "abdominal noisy", "acid reflux" and other categories. The earliest records of this disease is found in the *The Medical Classic of the Yellow Emperor. Simple Conversation-Major Discussion on the Progress of the Six Climatic Changes* says "When liver depression occurs... people will feel painful under the heart for stomach disease with hypochondrium pain, food and drink cannot be discharged because of the obstruction of diaphragm and pharynx". Chao Yuanfang of Sui dynasty put forward eight symptoms of abdominal mass in *Discussion on Causes of Different Diseases-Abdominal Mass*, indicating that the cause of abdominal mass is not only one, but the pathogenesis is nothing more than disharmony of nourishment and defensive energy, isolation of Yin and Yang, obstruction of blood and breath. Abdominal mass as the name of disease is first seen in *Treatise on Febrille and Miscellaneous Diseases*. *The Medical Classic of The Yellow Emperor* thinks that its cause is uncontrolled diet, irregular daily life, and cold-attacking, such as *Simple Conversation-Discussion on Taiyin and Yangming* says: "Uncontrolled diet and irregular daily life will first affect Yin Channels, then the five storing organs which suffer from abdominal mass due to obstruction of energy mechanism operation." Zhang Zhongjing clearly pointed out in *Treatise on Febrille and Miscellaneous Diseases*: "Full but not painful, this is abdominal mass." In the Ming and Qing dynasties, Zhang Jiebin pointed out more clearly in *Complete Works of Jingyue- Distention and fullness*: "Abdominal mass, means obstructional closure; abdominal fullness, means abdominal distentional block. Fullness is similar to distention, but abdominal mass is not necessarily distentional." And pointed out: "Abdominal mass with evil and stagnation is excess abdominal mass, abdominal mass with no substance and stagnation is deficient abdominal mass. Fullness with distention and pain is excess fullness; fullness without distention and pain is deficient fullness. Excess abdominal mass and fullness can be dissipated, deficient abdominal mass and fullness must be treated by pyretic tonification" In the Jin and Yuan dynasties, Li Dongyuan's *Lan Shi Mi Cang (Secret Book of Orchid Chamber)* establishes special prescriptions to treat the disease of "epigastric pain", which played a guiding role in the clinical treatment of chronic gastritis. Ye Tianshi of Qing dynasty put forward in *Clinical Guide Medical Case of-Medical Case of Epigastric Pain* that "Frequent repeat of stomach pain for a long time must be caused by stagnation of phlegm", "long-time stomach pain will enter the collateral", made many unique contributions to the syndrome differentiation and treatment of this disease.

其病因病机为外感表邪误用攻里泻下，脾胃受损，外邪乘虚内陷入里，阻塞中焦气机，升降失司，遂成痞满。胃气壅塞，而成痞满。饮食不节制，嗜好食生冷粗硬，或偏嗜肥甘厚味，或嗜浓茶烈酒及辛辣过烫饮食，损伤脾胃，脾胃失健，水液输布失司，酿生痰浊，痰气交阻于胃脘，则升降失司，以致食谷不化，阻滞胃脘，升降失司，胃气壅塞，而成痞满。七情失和，肝失疏泄，横逆犯胃致胃气阻滞而成之痞满为多见，即如《景岳全书·痞满》所谓："怒气暴伤，肝气未平而痞。"久病体虚，脾胃虚弱纳运失职，升降失调，胃气壅塞，而生痞满。

The cause and pathogenesis of the disease is misusing endopurgation and tuina method to treat external surface evil, which affects the function of spleen and stomach, presses the external evil to enter the internal body, blocks the energy operation mechanism of middle energizer, causes dysfunction of ascending and descending system, then abdominal mass and fullness occurs. Obstruction of stomach qi causes abdominal mass and fullness. Uncontrolled diet, favor of raw, cold, rough and hard food, or favor of fat, sweet and thick tastes, or favor of thick tea and strong liquor, or too spicy and too hot diet, will damage spleen and stomach. When spleen and stomach is disordered, water liquid which cannot be transported and irrigated breeds phlegm turbidity. When phlegm and qi are resisted in stomach, the ascending and descending cannot be implemented, so the grains which cannot be consumed in stomach blocks epigastric qi become abdominal mass and fullness. Commonly, disharmony of seven emotion makes liver loose releasing function, transverse arrest the stomach to cause gastric qi block and then become abdominal mass and fullness. Just as *Complete Works of Jingyue- Distention and Fullness* says: "Unexpected injure of anger, discomfort in liver leads to abdominal mass." Long-time disease makes body deficient, spleen and stomach weak and unable for consuming and transporting, abnormal in ascending and descending, causing gastric qi obstruction, and then abdominal mass and fullness.

慢性胃炎病机错综复杂，病程较长，发病认识主要与饮食不节、进食粗糙或刺激性食物、嗜好烟酒、情志不遂、素体虚弱、劳倦内伤、用药不当、久病体虚等因素有关。其病在胃，与肝脾有关，病机为虚实夹杂。

Chronic gastritis has complicated pathogenisis and long course of disease, and the incidence of chronic gastritis is mainly related to uncontrolled diet, rough or stimulating food, tobacco and alcohol, depression, weakness, fatigue, improper medication, chronic body deficiency and other factors. The disease is in the stomach in relation with liver and spleen, the pathogenesis is a mixture of deficiency and excess.

二、基于浊毒理论对慢性胃炎病因病机的认识
2. The etiology of chronic gastritis based on the theory of turbidity toxicity

慢性胃炎病位在胃，细究之应在胃膜（胃络），而与肝之疏泄、脾之升清、胃之降浊均有密切关系。胃主受纳，为水谷之海，以通为用，以降为顺；脾主运化，以升为常。两者共为后天之本，气血生化之源。肝属木，为刚脏，喜条达，主疏泄，胃之功用依赖于脾之运化、肝之疏泄，若情志不调、脾胃虚弱，或感受邪气，致肝郁气滞，横犯中土，克脾伐胃，中土既虚，水湿停聚，继而积湿成浊，浊郁化热，热蕴成毒，浊毒之邪深伏胃络血分，最终导致本病的发生。

Although the location of chronic gastritis disease is in the stomach, specifically in the gastric membrane (gastric collateral), the chronic gastritis is in close relation with the liver releasing function, the lucidity ascending function of the spleen, the turbidity descending function of the stomach. The stomach is the sea of water and grain, responsible for receiving and accepting, ensuring normal metabolism and smooth descending of stomach qi. Spleen is mainly responsible for transporting and transmission, ensuring normal ascending of spleen qi. The energy of stomach and spleen are acquired from grain and water, which is also the source of breath and blood. The nature of the liver is similar to wood, responsible for releasing, favor of harmony. The function of the stomach depends on the transporting function of the spleen, releasing function of liver, if the patient is not in good mood, feels weak in spleen and stomach, or attacked by evil qi, it will cause liver depression and qi stagnation, aggression to middle soil, the spleen and stomach will be attacked. Excessive water retains and gathers in deficient middle-soil, then accumulated into turbidity, turbidity transmitted into heat, heat turned to be toxin, the evil of turbid toxin are deeply hidden in collateral of stomach, and blood, finally causes the occurrence of the disease.

（一）病因
2.1 Cause of disease

1.脾胃虚弱　脾胃虚弱多由于劳倦伤脾，素体虚弱，久病损伤脾胃，或者先天肾阳不足，胃失于温煦或年高体衰，脾虚胃缓均可引起脾胃虚弱或虚寒，使脾失运化，胃失温养，升降失常，出现胃痛、胀满等症，久之形成慢性胃炎。

2.1.1 Weak spleen and stomach　　Spleen and stomach weakness are most probably due to fatigue, body deficiency, damage of long-term of disease. Besides, congenital deficiency of kidney Yang, cold in stomach or debility because of elder age, spleen deficiency or stomach slowness can also cause spleen and stomach weakness and coldness, which will make the spleen loose the function of transporting and transmission, stomach loose the function of warm and cultivation, causing disorder of ascending and descending of energy mechanism, stomachache, full in stomach, etc, and with time passes, chronic gastritis as a result.

2.饮食因素　　暴饮暴食，饥饿失常；过食生冷，寒积胃脘；恣食肥甘、辛辣，过饮烈酒，致饮食停滞，损伤脾胃。寒凝阻络则气滞血瘀，湿热中阻则脾胃受困，日久损伤脾胃，形成胃炎。《兰室秘藏·中满腹胀》云："或多食寒凉，及脾胃久虚之人，胃中寒则胀满，或脏寒生满病"，"也有膏粱之人，湿热郁于内而成胀满者"。

2.1.2 Dietary factors　　Overeating and drinking, abnormal hunger; over-eating of raw and cold food, accumulated coldness in stomach; overtaken of sweet, spicy or spirits, will cause diet stagnation and make damage to spleen and stomach. Cold coagulated in collateral will cause qi stagnation and blood stasis, dampness and heat blocked in middle energizer will trap the spleen and stomach, with time passes will damage the spleen and stomach, forming gastritis. *Secret Works in Orchid Room-Full bloating* says: "People who over-take cold and cool diet, or long-time deficiency in spleen and stomach, feel full in stomach, or we say cold in storing organs cause full disease", "Besides, there are also people in favor of thick and fat tastes, feel full inside because of depression of heat and dampness".

3.情志因素　　肝主疏泄，性喜条达，忧思恼怒，情志不畅，肝郁气滞，疏泄失职，横逆犯胃，郁滞不行，不通则痛。故《沈氏尊生书》谓："胃痛，邪干胃脘病也。唯肝气相乘为尤甚，以木性暴，且正克也。"肝气久郁，化而为火，五脏之火又以肝火最为横暴，火性炎上，迫灼肝胃之痛往往经久不愈。忧思伤脾，脾气郁结，运化失常，水谷不化，也可见胃脘胀满之症。

2.1.3 Emotional factors　　Liver is mainly responsible for dispersing, in favor of harmony. Worry, thinking, anger and rage, will make the mood unhealthy, liver depressed and qi stagnated. The function of liver dispersing does not work. The depression and stagnation transverse stomach, pain occurs because of blockage. Therefore, *Shen's Life Cultivation Book* says: "Stomachache is the disease which indicates that stomach is attacked by evil. The disease will become more serious when liver qi joins in, as the character of wood is violent, and it restrains the soil." Long-time depressed liver qi will turn to be fire. And the fire of liver is the most violent one among the fire of all the five storing organs. The pain of liver and stomach burnt by fire inflammation will keep for a long time and difficult to recover. Worry and thinking will hurt the spleen, with the spleen qi depressed, the transporting function will be abnormal, water and grain which cannot be digested, will also cause the disease of epigastric distension.

（二）病机

2.2 Pathogenesis

1.病机特点　　脾胃虚弱为本，邪气干胃为标。慢性胃炎临床表现多种多样，如胃脘部疼痛、胀满、痞满、痞塞、嗳气、嘈杂等，属中医"痞满""嘈杂"等范畴。引起本病的病因非常复杂，有外感六淫也有内伤七情及不节饮食等，根据中医"正气存内，邪不可干""邪之所凑，其气必虚"及《金匮要略》中"若五脏元真通畅，人即安和""四季脾旺不受邪"等理论，可以认为慢性胃炎的病机特点是虚实夹杂，脾虚为本，邪气干胃为标，脾胃虚弱，多为脾胃气虚，部分可伴阴血不足。邪气包括六淫、饮食、痰浊、瘀血等。邪气犯胃致脾胃运化失职，水湿不化，日久蕴生浊毒，浊毒中阻，气机不畅，中焦痞塞不通而发本病。

2.2.1 Characteristics of pathogenesis　Weakness of the spleen and stomach is the root, evil attacks the stomach is the leaf. The clinical manifestations of chronic gastritis are various, such as epigastric pain, distension, ruffian full, ruffian plug, belching, upset, etc. It belongs to "ruffian full", "upset" and other categories of TCM. The cause of the disease is very complex, including the attacking of six external evilness, injury of seven internal emotions and uncontrolled diet. According to the TCM discipline "when healthy energy is sufficient, evil cannot attack", "wherever evil invades, the healthy energy must be deficient" and the theory "if the circulation of the vital energy is unobstructed, people is safe and harmonious", "if the spleen is flourishing in four seasons, people will not be invaded by evil" in *Synopsis of Golden Chamber*, it can be considered that chronic gastritis pathogenesis is mixed with deficiency and excess, spleen deficiency is the root, stomach attacked by evil is the leaf, the weakness in spleen and stomach is mainly due to qi deficiency of spleen and stomach, part of them is accompanied with Yin blood deficiency. The evil includes six external evils, diet, phlegm turbidity, blood stasis, etc. Evil invades the stomach and causes dysfunction of the spleen and stomach transporting, excess of water and dampness retains and is accumulated into turbid toxin, when turbid toxin is obstructed, energy mechanism is not smooth, the ruffian plug in middle energizer promotes the occurrence of this disease.

2.主要病机

2.2.2 The main pathogenesis

（1）胃气壅滞：腑气以通为用，胃气主降，脾胃功能受损，胃气不降，阻滞于中焦，则胃胀满疼痛，气或聚或散，故胀痛走窜不定。胃气失降而上逆，则嗳气、欲吐。胃肠气滞则肠鸣、矢气频作，矢气或嗳气之后，阻塞之气机暂得通畅，故胀痛减轻。若气急阻塞严重，上不得嗳气，下不得矢气，气聚不散，则脘腹胀痛加剧。胃肠之气不降则大便秘结。苔黄，脉弦，为浊气内停，气机阻滞之象。

2.2.2.1 Stomach qi stagnation: the function of qi of transporting organs is to transport, when the function of the spleen and stomach is affected, the stomach qi does not descend, and is obstructed in middle energizer, the epigastric distension and pain occurs, the qi will gather or separate, thus the pain of distension keeps moving uncertainly. When the stomach qi moves upward, belching occurs accompanied with vomiting. Qi stagnation in stomach and intestine causes frequent occurrence of gurgling and farting. Distension pain will be less serious when the obstruction of energy mechanism is dredged after farting and belching. If the energy mechanism is seriously obstructed, the qi gather tightly without separation, patient can neither belch, nor break wind, the distension pain will be more serious. When the stomach and intestine qi does not descend, constipation occurs. Yellow tongue coating, string pulse is the image of turbidity stagnation and energy mechanism obstruction.

（2）湿浊中阻：脾喜燥恶湿，湿浊中阻，湿困脾阳，运化失职，水湿内停，脾气郁滞，则脘腹痞胀或痛，食少。脾失健运，湿滞气机，则口中黏腻无味。水湿下渗则见大便稀溏，湿性重浊，也可见到大便黏腻不爽。湿性重浊，泛溢肌肤，则见头身困重，肢体肿胀等。舌红，苔腻，脉濡或滑，同为湿浊中阻之象。

2.2.2.2 Wet and dampness resistance: spleen likes dry, dislikes dampness, when damp turbidity affects spleen Yang, spleen transporting is dysfunction, water dampness retains, spleen qi is stagnated, patient eats less than usual, and feels abdominal distension or pain. When spleen does not transport normally, wet stagnation affects the energy mechanism, patient feels sticky and tasteless in mouth. When water wet infiltrates, the patient's stool will be loose; when the dampness is heavy and turbid, the patient's stool will be sticky. when wet and heavy turbidity spread over through the skin, patient will have head and body trapped, limb swelling, etc. Red tongue with greasy moss, lingering or slippery pulse, is also the characteristic of wet turbidity obstruction.

（3）浊犯肝胃：情志不遂，肝失疏泄，气不通畅，则浊邪内生，浊气横逆犯胃，胃气郁滞，则胃脘、胸胁胀满疼痛，走窜不定。胃气上逆而见呃逆、嗳气。肝失条达，情志失调，则见精神抑郁，善太息。木郁作酸，肝气犯胃，则吞酸嘈杂。胃不主受纳，则不思饮食。肝气郁滞，则可见大便不爽。舌红，苔薄黄，脉弦滑，为肝气郁滞，浊犯肝胃之象。

2.2.2.3 Turbidity invades liver and stomach: when liver and stomach are invaded by turbidity, patient will feel depressed in emotions, liver looses the function of dredging, qi obstruction promotes the production of internal turbidity evils. When turbidity invades stomach, stomach qi is stagnated, patient feels distension and walking pain in stomach and chest. When stomach qi moves upwards, patient will hiccup or belch. When liver function is abnormal, patient will be disorder and depressed in mood, sigh frequently. Depressed liver produces sour, when liver qi invades stomach, patient feels upset and swallow sour liquid. When stomach fails to receive, patient will have poor appetite. Liver qi stagnation makes patient difficult to discharge feces. Red tongue with thin and yellow moss, string and slippery pulse, is the image of turbidity invading liver and stomach.

（4）浊毒内蕴：胃病日久，湿浊之气留滞于中焦，郁久化热，则见胃脘胀满，胀痛灼热。湿热浊毒之气耗伤气阴，则见口干口苦。浊气犯胃，胃失和降，胃气上逆，则见恶心呕吐。胃气受浊影响，不主受纳，则见纳呆。中焦气机阻滞，浊毒内蕴，阳气不能输布于体表四肢，则见怕冷。浊毒之气内蕴于中焦脏腑，气机不通，可见到大便不爽或便溏。舌红或紫红，苔黄腻，脉滑或滑数，为浊毒内蕴，湿热中阻之象。

2.2.2.4 Turbid toxin accumulation: when stomach disease keeps for a long time, pathogenic dampness remains in middle energizer, stagnation and heat, patient feels abdominal distension, distention pain and burning. Turbid toxin with dampness and heat consumes and injures qi Yin, patient feels dry and bitter in mouth. When turbidity invades stomach, the stomach looses the function of harmony and descending, the stomach qi rises adversely, patient will have nausea and vomiting. When the stomach qi is affected by turbidity, the stomach fails to receive and accept, patient will have a poor appetite. When the connotation of turbid toxin obstructs the normal operation of energy mechanism in middle energizer, the positive energy fails to be spread through limbs and body surfaces, patient will fear coldness. When turbid toxin is accumulated in spleen and stomach, the energy mechanism cannot work normally, patient will feel difficult to discharge feces or discharge loose feces. Red or purple red tongue with greasy and yellow coating, slippery or slippery and rapid pulse is image of accumulation of turbid toxin causing obstruction of dampness and heat.

（5）浊毒壅盛：湿浊之气郁滞于中焦，日久郁而化热，蕴热为毒，灼伤真阴，阴液不能上蒸于口，故见口干口苦。中焦气机郁滞，故见脐腹胀满疼痛。浊毒壅盛，上扰清窍，故见心烦躁扰，头晕胀痛，寐差。浊毒壅盛，中焦气机不通，湿浊之气壅滞，故见大便秘结不通，小便短赤或黄。舌紫红，苔黄厚腻，脉滑数或弦滑数，均为湿热中阻，浊毒壅盛之象。

2.2.2.5 Abundant turbid toxin: long time depression and stagnation of damp turbidity in the middle energizer will be transmitted into heat, then accumulated heat into toxin, the vital Yin is burnt and affected, Yin liquid cannot be steamed out through mouth, so patient feels dry and bitter in mouth. Energy mechanism in middle energizer is depressed and stagnated, therefore, umbilical abdominal pain occurs. Abundant and excess turbid toxin interrupts the clear orifices, thus patient feels irritable dizziness, distention pain and insomnia. When damp turbidity stagnation are transmitted into excessive abundant turbid toxin, the energy mechanism is obstructed in meddle energizer, so constipation and short red urine or yellow urine occurs. Purple red tongue with yellow and thick greasy moss, slippery and rapid pulse or string slippery and rapid pulse is the image of damp and heat obstruction in middle energizer with excessive and abundant turbid toxin.

（6）瘀血内结：脾胃病日久常见瘀血内结之象。瘀血阻滞，则可见胃脘部刺痛，痛有定处，以夜间为甚。血瘀日久伤阴，阴伤则胸满口燥，面色暗滞也较为常见。舌质紫或紫暗，或有瘀点、瘀斑，脉弦涩，均为瘀血内结之象。

2.2.2.6 stagnation of blood stasis: stagnation of blood stasis occurs when spleen and stomach disease keeps for a long time. The patient feels stabbing epigastric pain in certain position, usually more serious at night. Blood stasis hurts Yin with time passes, patient feels dry in mouth and full in chest when Yin is injured, dark complexion is more common. Purple or purple dark tongue with petechial, stasis spots, weak string pulse, is the image of stagnation of blood stasis.

（7）毒热伤阴：胃病日久，毒热盛，耗伤阴液，常出现阴伤之象。胃阴不足，虚热内生，热郁于胃，气失和降，则见胃脘胀满、灼痛，嘈杂不舒，痞满不适。胃失阴滋，纳化迟滞，则饥不欲食或食少。胃阴亏耗，阴津不能上滋，则口燥咽干；不能下润，则大便秘结，小便短少。舌红少津，苔少或花剥，脉弦细或细数，是毒热内结，耗伤胃阴之象。

2.2.2.7 Toxic heat injures Yin: when stomach disease keeps for a long time, abundant toxic heat consumes and damages Yin liquid. When Stomach Yin is insufficient, deficient heat is born endogenously, as heat is depressed in the stomach, stomach qi looses harmony and descending function, thus patient feels stomach distension, burning pain, upset, ruffian discomfort. Without nourishing of Yin, the digestion turns to be slow and late, patient does not want to eat or has a poor appetite even at the time when he is hungry. When stomach Yin is poor, body fluid fails to be sent upwardly, patient feels dry mouth and throat; meanwhile, the body fluid cannot lubricate the intestine, phenomenon of constipation and short urine occurs. Red tongue with less fluid, less or exfoliative moss, string and thready pulse or thready and rapid pulse is the image indicating stagnation of toxic heat consumes and damages the stomach Yin.

（8）脾胃虚弱：素体虚弱或浊毒日久伤脾，导致脾胃功能虚弱者在临床上也较为常见。脾胃功能虚弱，脾失健运，胃失和降，脾胃气机壅滞于中焦，则见胃脘部胀满或隐痛，胃部喜按喜暖。脾胃虚弱，其受纳腐熟水谷及运化功能失司，则见食少。气血生化乏源，机体失于濡养，则见气短、懒言、口淡、乏力、大便稀溏等；舌质淡，边有齿痕，脉细弱，均为浊毒伤脾，脾胃虚弱之象。

2.2.2.8 Weak spleen and stomach: for time being, weak body or turbid toxin hurts the spleen, even causes the weakness of spleen and stomach function in clinical practice. Thus, spleen looses the function of healthy transporting, stomach looses the function of harmony and descending. The energy of spleen and stomach is stagnated in middle energizer, patient feels stomach distension or hidden pain, the stomach likes to be pressed and warmed. Weak spleen and stomach affects the function of the stomach to digest water and grain, and the spleen to transport and transmit, patient has a poor appetite. As the source of breath and blood turns to be poor, patient feels short of breath, lazy to speak, tasteless in mouth, hypodynamic, discharges loose stool, weak and teeth-printed tongue, weak and thready pulse is the image indicating that turbid toxin damages spleen, the spleen and stomach turns to be weak.

第二节　辨证要点
Section 2　Key Points of Syndrome Differentiation

一、辨主证
1. Distinguish the principal syndrome

慢性胃炎的主症变化多样，有以胃痛为主，则按胃脘痛辨证，有以痞胀为主，则按痞满辨证，还有以纳呆、便溏、嗳气、泛酸等症为主，有时数症同兼并见，则要根据具体症状分别辨证。

The principal syndromes of chronic gastritis are changeable variously. If the principal is stomach pain, it should be treated as epigastric pain. If the principal syndrome is ruffian distension, it should be treated as ruffian full. If the principal syndrome is anorexia, loose stool, belching, pantothenic acid, or sometimes a few symptoms occur simultaneously, we should differentiate according to the specific symptoms.

二、辨缓急
2. Distinguish slow and abrupt syndrome

凡胃痛暴作，起病急者，多因外受寒邪，或恣食生冷，或暴饮暴食，以致寒伤中阳，或积滞不化，胃失和降，不通则痛。胃胀突发者，多因暴怒伤肝，肝气失于疏泄，胃络失和，或饮食失宜，食滞胃脘，胃失和降所致。凡胃痛胃胀渐发，起病缓者，多因脾胃虚，胃络失其气血温煦或土壅木郁，而致肝胃不和，气滞血阻。

All the abrupt occurrences of stomach pain, are mostly due to invading of external cold evil, taking-in of cold food and drink, or over-taken of drink and food, therefore coldness injures the middle Yang, then stagnated inside, causes stomach loose the function of harmony and descending, obstruction produces the pain. Abrupt occurrences of stomach distension, are mostly because severe rage injures liver, liver qi fails to be dispersed, stomach collateral looses the state of harmony, or improper diet causes food stagnation in stomach, so stomach looses the function of harmony and descending. All gradual and slow occurrences of stomach pain and distension, are mostly because the spleen and stomach are so deficient that stomach collateral looses breath and blood warming, or obstruction of spleen and depression of liver causes disharmony of liver and stomach, stagnation of qi and resistance of blood.

三、辨虚实
3. To distinguish excess and deficiency

胃痛而胀，大便闭结不通者多实，痛而不胀，大便不秘结者多虚；喜凉者多实，喜温者多虚；拒按者多实，喜按者多虚；食后痛胀甚者多实，饥则腹痛胀满者多虚；脉实气逆者多实，脉细弱者多虚；痛胀起病徐缓，按之濡软而不坚者多虚；新病体壮者多实，久病体衰者多虚。

The disease of stomach pain and distension with the symptom of constipation, is most probably sthenia; stomach pain and distension without constipation is mostly deficient. If the patients of stomach pain and distension like cool food or drink, their disease is mostly sthenia. If the patients of stomach pain and distension like warmer food and drink, their disease is mostly deficient. If the patients refuse to be pressed, their disease is mostly sthenia. If the patients like to be pressed, their disease is mostly deficient. If the patients with pain and distension feel more serious after meals, their disease is mostly sthenia. If the patients with pain and distension feel more serious before meals, their disease is mostly deficient. Patients with sthenia pulse and adverse flow of stomach qi, their disease is mostly sthenia. Patients with thready and weak pulse, their disease is mostly deficient. If the Patients with gradual and slow occurrences of pain and distension feel soft when they are pressed, their disease is mostly asthenia. Fresh patients with strong body, their disease is mostly sthenia. Weak patients with long course of disease, their disease is mostly deficient.

四、诊法

4. Diagnosis method

（一）望诊

4.1 Inspection

1.整体望诊

4.1.1 Overall observation

（1）望神

4.1.1.1 Spirit observation

1）浊毒轻证表现：神清语利，面色晦暗不洁，面部表情抑郁；目光无神，反应慢，动作缓慢；呼吸平稳，肌肉不消瘦。

4.1.1.1.1 Spirit of patients with light turbid toxin syndrome: calm clarity and fluent speaking, dark face, depressed facial expression, dull eyes, slow reaction, slow movement; smooth breathing, not emaciated.

2）浊毒重证表现：神昏嗜睡，语言艰涩，面色秽浊，面无表情；目光呆滞，反应迟钝，动作艰难，体态笨拙；呼吸浅快，肌肉消瘦。

4.1.1.1.2 Spirit of patients with heavy turbid toxin syndrome: drowsiness, difficult to speak, turbid face, depression in facial expression; dull eyes, slow reaction, difficult movements, clumsy posture; shallow and rapid breathing, emaciated muscles.

3）浊重毒轻者多表现为神情淡漠，浊毒并重者多表现为神志如蒙，毒重浊轻者多表现为神昏谵语。

4.1.1.1.3 Patients with heavy turbidity and light toxin syndrome are mostly indifferent in facial expression, those patients with same degree of turbidity and toxin are mostly confused in facial expression, and those patients with heavier toxin and lighter turbidity syndrome are mostly confused in mind but delirium in speaking.

（2）望色：浊毒在胃者临床多表现为面色萎黄，暗淡无光。

4.1.1.2 Complexion observation: patients with turbid toxin syndrome in the stomach, their clinical manifestations are yellow complexion, dull and gloomy.

（3）望形体：若浊轻毒重者，患者形体多肥胖；若毒重浊轻尤其浊毒伤阴者，患者形体多消瘦。

4.1.1.3 Body observation: if the patient is with syndrome of lighter turbidity and heavier toxin, the patient is more obese; if the patient with syndrome of heavier toxin and lighter turbidity, especially those who are injured in Yin, by turbid toxin, will be thinner in body.

2.望舌象　临床上浊毒证患者以黄腻苔多见，但因感受浊毒的轻重不同而有所差别。以湿浊之邪为主者，舌苔腻、薄腻、厚腻，或黄或白或黄白相间；浊毒并重者，舌苔多为黄厚而腻；以热毒为主者，舌苔黄而微腻，或黑或中根部黄腻。脾胃感受浊毒之邪，舌苔腻微黄；胃肠感受浊毒之邪，苔腻；肝胆感受浊毒之邪，舌苔黄腻。初感浊毒，津液未伤时苔黄腻而滑；浊毒伤津时苔黄而燥。

4.1.2 Observation of tongue image Most of the patients with turbid toxin syndrome see yellow and greasy moss in clinical manifestation. But there might be some differences due to the degree of turbid toxin in body. Patients with syndrome of wet turbidity evil mostly have tongue coating of greasy, thin greasy, thick greasy, either yellow, white, or yellow-white. Patients with the syndrome of same degree of turbidity and toxin will mostly have yellow thick and greasy tongue coating. Patients with syndrome of heat toxin have tongue coating of yellow and mild greasy, or black, or yellow greasy in middle and the root part. When the spleen and stomach feel the evil of turbid toxin, the tongue coating will be greasy and slightly yellow. When the stomach and intestine feel the evil of turbid toxin, the tongue coating will be greasy. When the liver and gallbladder feel the evil of turbid toxin, the tongue coating will be yellow and greasy. Patients of fresh occurrence of turbid toxin syndrome, have tongue coating of yellow greasy and slippery when the body fluid has not been hurt, and the tongue coating will be yellow and dry when the body fluid is hurt by turbid toxin. First feeling of toxin, yellow and greasy and smooth, yellow and dry.

3.望排出物

4.1.3 Observation of the discharge

（1）望痰涎：浊重毒轻者，痰多，色白黏腻或呈泡沫，咳吐不爽；浊毒并重者，痰色黄或白，黏浊稠厚，排吐不利；毒重浊轻者，痰黄，黏稠难咳。

4.1.3.1 Observation of the sputum saliva: patients with the syndrome of heavier turbidity and lighter toxin have more phlegm of white sticky and greasy or in the state of foam, and feel difficult to cough and vomit. Patients with the syndrome of same degree of turbidity and toxin, have sticky and thick phlegm of yellow and white color, feel difficult to discharge. Patients with syndrome of heavier toxin and lighter turbidity have yellow, sticky and thick phlegm which is difficult to be discharged.

（2）望呕吐物：浊重毒轻者，呕吐物多为清水痰涎；浊毒并重者，呕吐物多为酸腐不化之谷物；毒重浊轻者，多为干呕。

4.1.3.2 Observation of the vomit: patients with syndrome of heavier turbidity and lighter toxin usually vomit cloudy and light sputum and saliva. Patients with syndrome of same degree of turbidity and toxin usually vomit sour grains which is not digested. Patients with syndrome of heavier toxin and lighter turbidity usually retch without vomit.

（3）望二便：若浊重毒轻，大便溏滞不爽，溲浑浊；若浊毒并重，溲黄赤；若毒重浊轻，溲涩赤。

4.1.3.3 Observation of shit and urinate: patients with syndrome of heavier turbidity and lighter toxin, usually discharge loose and stagnated stool and turbid urine. Patients with syndrome of the same degree of turbidity and toxin usually discharge yellow red urine. Patients with syndrome of heavier toxin and lighter turbidity usually discharge astringent red urine.

（二）闻诊

4.2 Listening and smelling diagnosis

闻诊包括听声音和嗅气味两个方面的内容。医者通过听觉和嗅觉了解由病体发出的各种异常声音和气味，以诊察病情。

Listening and smelling diagnosis includes listening to the sound and smelling the smell. Doctors detect the disease condition by listening to the various abnormal sounds and smelling odors issued by the patient.

1.听声音　呕吐有声有物称为呕；有物无声称为吐，如吐酸水、吐苦水等；干呕是指欲吐而无物有声，或仅呕出少量涎沫。其临床统称为呕吐。浊毒之邪侵袭胃部，导致胃失和降，胃气上逆，临床上可表现为呕吐。若浊重毒轻，吐势较缓，声音较弱；若浊毒并重，吐势较急，声音响亮；若毒重浊轻，临床上多闻及干呕之声。

4.2.1 Listen to sound　Vomiting with sound and discharge is called vomit; spitting something without sound is called spitting, such as spitting sour water, spitting bitter water; retching refers to vomit soundly with nothing, or only vomit a small amount of saliva foam. Clinically, it is collectively referred to as vomiting. The evil of turbid toxin attacks the stomach, leading to stomach dysfunction of harmony and descending. Gastric qi moves adversely, clinically causes vomiting. If the toxin is more severe, the turbidity is lighter, the tendency of vomiting will be slow, the sound of vomiting will be weak. If the turbidity is as severe as toxin, the tendency of vomiting will be rapid, the sound of vomiting will be louder. If toxin is more severe than turbidity, retching is usually heard clinically.

2.嗅气味　浊毒之邪侵袭胃肠，患者口中发出臭秽之气。

4.2.2 Smelling the smell　When the evil of turbid toxin attacks the stomach and intestines, patient's mouth emits foul breath.

3.排出物气味　浊毒之邪袭胃，呕吐物气味臭秽。

4.2.3 Smell the smelling of the discharge　When the evil of turbid toxin attacks stomach, smell of the vomit will be foul.

（三）问诊

4.3 Consultation

浊毒轻重程度辨证：若患者表现为身热不扬，汗少，口黏不渴或渴不欲饮，多诊断为浊重毒轻。若患者表现为发热汗出热不解，口苦腻，渴不多饮，多诊断为浊毒并重。若患者表现为壮热汗多，口苦烦渴，多诊断为毒重浊轻。

Differentiation of the severity of turbidity and toxin: if the patients feel hot with less sweat, sticky mouth but not thirsty, or thirsty with no want to drink, their syndromes are most probably more severe in turbidity but lighter in toxin. If the patient feels fever with sweat, but difficult to expel, with bitter and greasy mouth, thirsty but do not want to drink more, they will mostly be diagnosed as same degree of turbidity and toxin. If the patient feels high fever with much more sweat, bitter and polydipsia in mouth, they may be diagnosed as heavier turbidity and lighter turbidity.

若患者主要表现为身热不扬、胸脘痞闷、头胀身重、烦恶者，多诊断为浊毒之邪侵犯中焦。

If the patient mainly feels uncomfortably hot, with ruffian and stuffy chest, distension head and heavy body, restlessness, he may be diagnosed as the evil of turbid toxin invades the middle energizer.

若患者表现为身热不扬，脘腹痞胀，呕恶，口苦口腻，多诊断为浊毒之邪侵犯脾胃；若身体重着，脘痞不饥，口淡不渴，大便溏滞不爽，多诊断为浊重毒轻；若身热心烦，脘痞腹胀，恶心呕吐，大便溏薄，色黄气臭，汗出热不解，多诊断为浊毒并重；若高热，心烦口渴，脘闷身重，多诊断为毒重浊轻。

If the patient is uncomfortably hot, abdominal ruffian and distension, vicious, bitter and greasy mouth, he will usually diagnosed as turbid toxin evil invades spleen and stomach. If the patient feels heavy and damp, the stomach is weak, but the appetite is poor, tasteless but not thirsty, the stool is loose, stagnated and difficult, he will usually be diagnosed as heavier in turbidity, lighter in toxin. If the patient feels hot and restless, with stomach ruffian and abdominal distension, nausea and vomiting, loose, thready, yellow and foul stool, sweating but sustainable fever, he will usually be diagnosed as same degree of turbidity and toxin. If the patient feels high fever, restless and thirsty, with stuffy stomach and heavy body, he will usually diagnosed as heavier toxin and lighter turbidity.

（四）切诊

4.4 Feeling diagnosis

1.脉诊

4.4.1 Pulse feeling and palpation

（1）浊毒之邪侵犯脾胃，脉象多濡滑。

4.4.1.1 When the evil of turbid toxin invades the spleen and stomach, the pulse feels sluggish and sllppery.

（2）浊重毒轻者，脉多濡缓；浊毒并重者，脉多濡数；毒重浊轻，脉多滑数。

4.4.1.2 Patients with syndrome of heavier turbidity and lighter toxin, their pulses feel sluggish and slow. Patients with syndrome of same degree of turbidity and toxin, their pulses feel sluggish and rapid. Patients with syndrome of heavier toxin and lighter turbidity, their pulses feel slippery and rapid.

2.按诊

4.4.2 Palpation

（1）辨凉热：浊毒之邪侵袭胃脘，浊重毒轻，导致阳气郁于内而不达于外，按胃脘多表现为寒凉；毒重浊轻，按胃脘多表现为灼热。

4.4.2.1 To differentiate cool and heat: if the evil of turbid toxin attacks the epigastric, and turbidity is heavier and toxin is lighter, Yang energy stagnated inside, cannot be transported outside, when the stomach is pressed, patient will feel cold and cool; if toxin is heavier, turbidity is lighter, patient will feel burning hot when the stomach is pressed.

（2）辨疼痛：若胃脘部按之疼痛，多为浊毒之邪侵袭胃。

4.4.2.2 To differentiate pain: if the patient feels epigastric pain when the stomach is pressed, it indicates that the evil of turbidity toxin invades the stomach.

（3）辨腹胀：腹部胀满，按之有充实感觉，有压痛，叩之声音重浊的，为实满。

4.4.2.3 To differentiate abdominal distension: if the patient feels abdominal full and solid and pressing pain when he is pressed in abdomen, and percussion sound is heard when he is knocked in abdomen, he is solidly full in abdomen.

（4）辨痞满：痞满是自觉心下或胃脘部痞塞不适和胀满的一种症状。脘部按之有形而胀痛，推之辘辘有声者，多为浊毒之邪作为致病产物，导致水停胃中。

4.4.2.4 To differentiate ruffian full: ruffian full is an uncomfortable ruffian plug and distension full symptom under heart or in stomach felt by patients. If patients feel tangible and swelling pain in stomach when being pressed, the stomach makes rumbling sound when being pushed, mostly because evil of turbid toxin as a pathogenic product causes water stopping in stomach.

（5）辨肿块：肿块的按诊要注意其大小、形态、硬度、压痛等情况。若胃脘部按之有肿物，压之不痛，按之不移，多考虑为浊毒之邪停滞胃脘，发生癌变。

4.4.2.5 To differentiate masses: masses pressing diagnosis should should be made according to the size, shape, hardness, tenderness and other conditions of the mass. If we feel a mass in the epigastric part of the patient, which is not painful when being pressed, unmovable when being pushed, it should most probably be considered as canceration occurs due to turbid toxin stagnated in stomach.

第三节 治疗原则
Section 3 Principles of Treatment

根据浊毒致病特点，化浊解毒为其治疗原则。化浊解毒可使浊化毒除，从而气行血畅，痰消火散，积除郁解，恢复脾升胃降之特性。而化浊解毒之法可随证灵活辨用，或给邪以出路，使浊毒从大便而出，从小便而去，从汗液而排，或从根本截断浊毒生成，阻断湿、浊、痰、热、毒胶结成浊毒之势。

According to the pathogenic characteristics of turbid toxin, to resolve turbidity and remove toxin is its therapeutic principle. To resolve turbidity and remove toxin can reduce and terminate the injury and damage from turbidity and toxin, thus normalizing the circulation of breath and blood, diminish phlegm and cease the fever, solve the accumulation and depression, restore the characteristics of the spleen ascending the stomach descending. Method of turbidity resolving and toxin removing can be flexibly used according to syndrome, either to leave a way out for evil, let it be discharged with stool, urinate, sweat. Or to fundamentally stop the production of turbid toxin, resist the turbid-toxin change tendency of wet, turbidity, phlegm, heat, toxin.

一、给邪以出路化浊解毒
1. Leave a way out for evil to resolve turbidity and remove toxin

（一）通腑泄浊解毒——从大便而出
1.1 To unblock the Fu-organs to resolve turbidity and remove toxin—to discharge it with the stool

六腑以通为用，以降为和，浊毒内停日久，可致腑气不通，邪滞壅盛，《金匮要略》中就指出："谷气不消，胃中苦浊……"可通过通腑泄浊将浊毒排出体外。

The six Fu-organs are normal when there are nothing obstructed, harmony when the discharging is regular. Accumulation of turbid toxin for a long time can cause abnormal operation of qi mechanism of Fu-organs, evil excessive stagnation of evils, *Synopsis Of Golden Chamber* points out: "If the grain qi cannot not be dispersed, the stomach feels bitter and turbid..." Turbid toxin can be removed form the body through unblocking the Fu-organs and discharge the turbidity.

（二）渗湿利浊解毒——从小便而去
1.2 To diminish the turbidity and remove the toxin by draining the dampness—to discharge with urinate

湿浊同源，湿久凝浊，久则浊毒内蕴。《丹溪心法·赤白浊》指出："胃中浊气下流，为赤白浊……胃中浊气下流，渗入膀胱。"可见浊毒之邪可下注膀胱。苏东坡在《养身杂记》中说"要长生，小便清"。只有小便通利，人体水液代谢正常，才可以使浊毒从小便排出；也有利于稀释血液，预防血浊。

Wet and turbidity share the same resource, turbidity is stagnated by long-time wet, turbid toxin will be accumulated internally with time passes. *Danxi's principle of Medical Method-Red and white turbidity* points out: "Turbid substance in the stomach flows downward produces red and white turbidity...The substance flows downward and seeps into the bladder." It can be seen that the evil of turbid toxin can flow downward into the bladder. Su Dongpo said in *Collected Works of Life Nourishing*, "To live a long life, urine should be discharged regularly". Only urine discharging is unblocked and fluent, water metabolism in human body is normal, the turbid toxin can be discharged with urine; this is also conducive to dilute blood and prevent blood turbidity.

（三）达表透浊解毒——从汗液而排
1.3 To resolve turbidity and remove toxin by promoting sweating—to discharge with sweat

浊毒蕴结肌表，保持汗出可以疏通腠理、宣通肺卫，有利于体内浊毒通过汗液透达于体外，从而排出浊毒。本法属中医学汗法范畴，达表透浊解毒以汗出邪去为目的，中病即止，不可过汗。如发汗太过，易损伤津液，甚则大汗不止，导致虚脱。此外可配合使用蒸浴、针灸等疗法达到出汗的目的。张从正《儒门事亲·汗下吐三法该尽治病诠》曰："灸、蒸、熏、渫、洗、熨、烙、针刺、砭射、导引、按摩，凡解表者，皆汗法也。"

When turbid toxin is accumulated in muscle surfaces, to promote sweating can dredge striae, diffuse lung and defensive gases, to discharge turbid toxin out of the body together with sweat. This method belongs to the sweating method of Chinese medical science. The purpose of resolving the turbidity and removing the toxin by promoting sweating is to remove the evil through sweating, sweating should be controlled when the purpose is realized. If sweat is excessive, it will affect the body fluid. Furthermore, sustainable sweating will cause collapse. In addition, steaming bath, acupuncture may be used to assist sweating. Zhang Congzheng said in *Confucian Physician -Sweating, Constipation and Vomiting Three Methods Cure All Diseases*: "Moxibustion, steaming, fumigation, dispersing, bathing, ironing, flipping, needling, ulceration puncturing, directing, massage, all solutions to release the external belongs to sweating method."

二、截断浊毒的生成
2. Truncate the generation of turbid toxin

（一）健脾除湿解毒
2.1 To resolve the dampness and remove the toxin by reinforcing the spleen

湿为浊毒之源，脾虚运化失职，湿邪内生，湿凝成浊，日久蕴热，热极成毒，呈浊毒内蕴之势，脾健则湿不内生，正气存内，外湿则不可干，而脾胃为后天正气之本，故健脾除湿为化浊解毒的治本之法。

As dampness is the source of turbid toxin, spleen deficiency and dereliction of transporting and transmission function causes the generation of internal dampness evil, dampness will be stagnated into turbidity, then turbidity is accumulated into heat for a long time, extreme heat is transmitted into toxin, turbid toxin is internally generated gradually. Spleen health will block the generation of internal dampness, when positive energy is sufficient inside, external dampness cannot invade. Spleen and stomach is the root of acquired positive energy. Therefore, to reinforce the spleen and resolve the dampness is the fundamental way to resolve the turbidity and remove the toxin.

（二）芳香辟浊解毒
2.2 To repel the turbidity and remove the toxin with aroma

"脾主升清，胃主降浊"，无论是内因还是外因，脾胃失司，湿浊之邪阻于中焦，日久化生浊毒，单纯祛湿难获良效，需以芳香辟浊类药物"解郁散结，除陈腐，濯垢腻"（《本草便读》）。

"Spleen promotes the ascending of lucidity, stomach promotes the descending of turbidity", regardless of internal or external causes, if spleen and stomach are dysfunctional, the evil of dampness will be blocked in middle energizer, and transmitted into turbid toxin with time passes. Simple diminishing of dampness is difficult to obtain good results, it needs aroma to "release stagnation and dissipate binds, to remove the old and decayed,and eliminate the external interference". *Ben Cao Bian Du (Reference to Materia Medica)*.

（三）祛痰涤浊解毒

2.3 To cleanse turbidity and remove toxin by dispelling phlegm

因痰性流连黏结，积着胶固，需加以荡涤才能祛除。痰郁而不解，蕴积成热，热壅血瘀，热极则生毒，形成浊毒内壅之势，本法可从发病之来源，祛痰涤浊解毒，临床用于胃脘堵闷，肢体困重，纳呆，口中黏腻无味，大便溏或大便不爽等症。

Because phlegm usually lingers on agglutination, easy to accumulate like glue, it needs to be removed by cleansing. If sputum stagnation is resolved in time, it will be accumulated into heat, heat obstruction causes blood stasis, extreme heat turns to be toxin, forming the tendency of internal obstruction of turbid toxin. This method can dispel phlegm, cleanse turbidity and remove toxin from the source of the disease, is clinically used for epigastric congestion, limb sleepiness, dull, sticky tasteless in mouth, loose or bad stool and other syndromes.

（四）清热化浊解毒

2.4 To resolve turbidity and remove toxin by heat clearing

因湿凝成浊，痰浊内阻，致血瘀气滞，气郁而化热，热极则生毒，浊毒蕴结，缠绵难愈，故化浊解毒的最后关键在于清热化浊解毒。本法可从发病的来源上遏制浊毒的产生和传变。

Because wet will be coagulated into turbidity, phlegm turbidity generates internal resistance and causes blood stasis and qi stagnation, qi stagnation will turns to be heat, extreme heat generates toxin. When accumulation of turbid toxin lingers and difficult to recover, so the last key to resolve turbidity and remove toxin is to clear heat. This method can curb the generation and transmission of turbid toxin from the source of the disease.

（五）攻毒散浊解毒

2.5 To disperse turbidity and remove toxin by eliminating toxin

浊毒已成，久居体内，毒陷邪深，胶结固涩，非攻不克，需以毒攻毒，活血通络，故常用有毒之品，借其性峻力猛以攻邪，才能将聚集在一起的浊毒攻散，使浊毒流动起来，或排出体外，或归于清气。但应用此法需注意，有毒性的药物多性峻力猛，故在正气尚未衰竭而能耐攻的情况下，可借其毒性以攻毒。若患者正气多已受损，其治不耐一味猛烈攻伐，因此，以毒攻毒之应用，应适可而止，衰其大半而止，要根据患者的体质状况和耐攻承受能力，把握用量、用法及用药时间，方能收到预期的效果。

When turbid toxin has been living in the body for a long time, the toxin evil is bogged deep inside, cemented and astringent, it cannot be removed without elimination. It is necessary to treat the virulent pathogen with toxic agents, to promote blood circulation so as to unblock the collateral. The powerful characteristic and strong force of the toxic drugs are utilized to eliminate the evil, so as to break through the stagnated turbid toxin, make the turbid toxin flow, or discharge it out of body, or restore it to lucidity. However, attention should be paid that the above method should be used when the healthy qi of the patient is not exhausted and can withstand attacking. When the patient's healthy qi has been damaged, he cannot bear the blindly attacking, therefore, the application of poisonous agents should be stopped. The method of treating the virulent pathogen with toxic agents should be stopped when most of the evil is eliminated. At the same time, to realize the expected medical effect, the dosage, usage and medication time should be decided according to the patient's physical condition and the ability to bear the attacking.

临床上浊毒证的表现千差万别，十分复杂。浊邪秽浊不清，故治以芳香化浊、渗湿化浊、健脾化浊、通腑泄浊、行气降浊等。毒由热生，变由毒起，毒不除，变必生，故治以清热解毒、通络解毒等。浊毒病邪有轻、中、重相对量化的划分，治疗上也要根据浊毒病邪之轻重分而治之。治疗浊毒应根据邪之浅深，病之新久，在气、在血，是否入络成积等情况分层选药。浊毒的治疗不能拘泥于一方一药，而应辨证论治，灵活用药，这样才能取得较好疗效。

The clinical performance of turbid toxin is varied and complicated. As turbidity evil is not clear, so we treat it by using aroma, by draining the dampness, reinforcing the spleen, unblocking the Fu-organs, smoothing the qi mechanism to discharge it etc. Toxin is generated from heat, changes are made from toxin, if toxin is not removed, changes will certainly be made, so we remove toxin by clearing heat, unblocking collateral. and etc. There is a quantitative degree division of turbid toxin evil including light, medium and heavy, and the treatment should also be made according to the severeness of turbid toxin disease. The prescription to treat turbid toxin should be decided according to the depth of evil, the course of disease, either in breath or blood, whether accumulated or not and other conditions. The treatment of turbid toxin can not be confined to one prescription or one drug, but by syndrome differentiation and flexible medication, so as to achieve better curative effect.

第四节　辨证治疗
Section 4　Treatment with Syndrome Differentiation

一、胃气壅滞型
1. Gastric qi obstruction type

（一）主要症状
1.1 Main symptoms

脘腹痞胀疼痛，痛而欲吐，或腹胀痛剧，肠鸣走窜不定，矢气频作，矢气后胀痛减轻，或胀痛剧而无肠鸣矢气，大便秘结，舌红，苔厚，脉弦。

Abdominal distension and pain, painful with eager to vomit, or abdominal distension with severe pain, gurgling sound and uncertain position, frequent breaking of wind, distension pain reduced after wind-breaking, or severe distension pain without gurgling sound and wind-breaking, constipation, red tongue with thick moss, pulse string.

（二）病机

1.2 Pathogenesis

浊蕴胃肠，气机阻滞。

Turbidity is accumulated in stomach and intestines, and qi mechanism is blocked.

（三）治则

1.3 Treating principle

理气和胃，降逆消痞。

Regulate qi and harmonize stomach, reduce the counterflow and resolve stuffiness.

（四）方药

1.4 Prescription

木香9g，枳实15g，厚朴15g，槟榔15g，炒莱菔子20g。

Mu xiang (Radix Aucklandiae) 9g, zhi shi (Fructus Aurantii Immaturus) 15g, hou po (Cortex Magnoliae Officinalis) 15g, bing lang (Semen Arecae) 15g, chao lai fu zi (fried Semen Raphani) 20g.

（五）加减运用

1.5 Addition and reduction principle

胃气上逆，食入则吐，加大黄、甘草；胃脘疼痛，加延胡索、白芷；嗳气，加石菖蒲、郁金、紫苏叶、黄连；食积滞气，嗳腐吞酸，加鸡内金、焦三仙；呃逆，加丁香、柿蒂。

Adversing of stomach qi, vomiting while eating, add da huang (Radix et Rhizoma Rhei), gan cao (Radix Glycyrrhizae); epigastric pain, add yan hu suo (Rhizoma Corydalis), bai zhi (Radix Angelicae Dahuricae); belching, add shi chang pu (Rhizoma Acori Graminei), yu jin (Radix Curcumae), zi su ye (Folium Perillae), huang lian (Rhizoma Coptidis); food accumulation and qi stagnation, fetid eructation and acid regurgitation, add ji nei jin (Endothlium Corneum Gigeriae Galli), jiao san xian (fried Hordei Fructus Germinatus, fried Massa Medicata Fermentata, fried Crataegi Fructus); hiccups, add ding xiang (Clove), shi di (Calyx Kaki).

二、湿浊中阻型
2. Dampness and turbidity obstructed in middle energizer

（一）主要症状

2.1 Main symptoms

胃脘堵闷，肢体困重，纳呆，口中黏腻无味，大便溏或不爽，舌红，苔腻，脉濡或滑。

Epigastric congestion, limb heavy with sleepiness, poor appetite, sticky and tasteless mouth, loose or difficult stool, red tongue with greasy moss, weak or slippery pulse.

（二）病机

2.2 Pathogenesis

湿浊内生，阻滞气机。

Dampness and turbidity generated internally blocks the energy mechanism.

（三）治则

2.3 Treating principle

除湿化浊，和胃消痞。

To remove dampness and resolve turbidity, harmonize stomach and eliminate ruffian.

（四）方药

2.4 Prescription

石菖蒲15g，郁金12g，茯苓15g，白术9g，茵陈15g，砂仁15g，肉豆蔻15g，苍术15g。

Shi chang pu (Rhizoma Acori Graminei) 15g, yu jin(Radix Curcumae) 12g, fu ling (Poria) 15g, bai zhu (Rhizoma Atractylodis Macrocephalae) 9g, yin chen (Herba Artemisiae Sccopariae) 15g, sha ren (Fructus Amomi) 15g, rou dou kou (Semen Myristicae) 15g, cang zhu (Rhizoma Atractylodis) 15g.

（五）加减运用

2.5 Addition and reduction principle

胸骨后隐痛，痰多，恶心加半夏、旋覆花、代赭石；胃灼热反酸，加乌贼骨、瓦楞子粉、煅龙骨、煅牡蛎；呕吐，加半夏、降香。

Substernal pain, more phlegm, nausea, add ban xia (Rhizoma Pinelliae), xuan fu hua (Flos Inulae), dai zhe shi (Hematitum Seu Ochra); gastropyrexia and acid regurgitation, add wu zei gu (Os Sepiellae seu Sepiae), wa leng zi fen (Concha Arcae), duan long gu (Charring Os Draconis), duan mu li (Charring Choncha Ostreae); vomiting, add ban xia (Rhizoma Pinelliae), jiang xiang (Legnum Dalbergiae Odorrifrae).

三、浊犯肝胃型
3. Turbidity invades liver and stomach

（一）主要症状

3.1 Main symptoms

胃脘胀满或胀痛，胁肋胀满，嗳气，泛酸，善太息，遇烦恼郁怒则症状加重，精神抑郁，寐差，大便不爽，舌红，苔薄黄，脉弦滑。

Epigastric distension or pain, flank distension, belching, pantothenic acid, frequent sighing, the disease becomes more severe in case of anger, mental depression, poor sleep, difficult stool, red tongue with thin yellow moss, string and slippery pulse.

（二）病机

3.2 Pathogenesis

肝气不舒，肝胃不和。

Abnormal flow of liver qi, disharmony of liver and stomach.

（三）治则

3.3 Treatment principle

疏肝理气，和胃消痞。

To disperse liver and regulate the liver qi, and harmonize the stomach to eliminate ruffian.

（四）方药

3.4 Prescription

柴胡15g，香附12g，青皮9g，荔枝核15g，佛手15g，预知子15g，香橼15g。

Chai hu (Radix Bulpleuri) 15g, xiang fu (Rhizoma Cyperi) 12g, qing pi (Pericarpium Citri Reticcuta-tae Viride) 9g, li zhi he (Semen Litchi)15g, fo shou (Fructus Citri Sarcodactylis) 15g, yu zhi zi (Fructus Akebiae) 15g, xiang yuan (Fructus Citron) 15g.

（五）加减运用

3.5 Addition and reduction principle

腹胀满，加焦槟榔、炒莱菔子、大腹皮；浊阻气机，脘痞苔腻，加茯苓、泽泻、石菖蒲；气郁化火，胃中灼热，加黄芩、黄连、生石膏；寐差，加合欢皮、夜交藤。

In case of abdominal distension, add jiao bing lang (burnt Semen Arecae), chao lai fu zi (fried Semen Raphani), da fu pi (Pericarpium Arecae). In case of turbidity blocking the energy mechanism, gastric mass with greasy tongue moss, add fu ling (Poria), ze xie (Rhizoma Alismatis), shi chang pu (Rhizoma Acori Graminei). In case of qi depression transmitted into fire, stomach feels burning hot, add huang qin (Radix Scutellariae), huang lian (Rhizoma Coptidis), sheng shi gao (Crude Gypsum Fibrosum); in case of sleepless, add he huan pi (Cortex Albiziae) and ye jiao teng (Caulis Polygoni Multiflori).

四、浊毒内蕴型
4. Turbid toxin inherent type

（一）主要症状

4.1 Main symptoms

胃脘胀满，胀痛灼热，口干口苦，恶心呕吐，纳呆，怕冷，小便黄，大便不爽或便溏，舌红或紫红，苔黄腻，脉滑或滑数。

Epigastric distension, distension, pain and burning hot, dry and bitter in mouth, nausea and vomiting, poor appetite, fear of cold, yellow urine, difficult or loose stool, red or purple red tongue with yellow and greasy moss, slippery or slippery rapid pulse.

（二）病机

4.2 Pathogenesis

湿热中阻，浊毒内蕴。

Dampness and heat resistance in middle energizer, turbid toxin connotation.

（三）治则

4.3 Treatment principle

化浊解毒，和胃消痞。

Resolve turbidity and remove toxin, harmonize stomach and eliminate masses.

（四）方药

4.4 Prescription

黄芩12g，黄连12g，黄柏12g，蒲公英12g，生石膏30g，茵陈15g，藿香15g，佩兰12g。

Huang qin (Radix Scutellariae) 12g, huang lian (Rhizoma Coptidis) 12g, huang bo (Cortex Phellodendri) 12g, pu gong ying (Herba Taraxaci cum Radice) 12g, sheng shi gao (Crude Gypsum Fibrosum) 30g, yin chen (Herba Artemisiae Scopariae) 15g, huo xiang (Herba Agastaches seu Pogostemonis) 15g, and pei lan (Herba Eupatorii) 12g.

（五）加减运用

4.5 Addition and reduction principle

伴恶心，加紫苏叶、黄连；大便不干、不溏，排便不爽，便次频数者，加葛根、白芍、地榆、秦皮、白头翁；伴肠化，加半枝莲、半边莲、绞股蓝、薏苡仁、白英；伴不典型增生，加三棱、莪术；伴幽门螺杆菌（HP）感染，加蒲公英、虎杖、连翘、黄连；心下痞，加瓜蒌、黄连、半夏；胃黏膜充血水肿，常加川芎、延胡索、三七。

In case of nausea, add zi su ye (Folium Perillae), huang lian (Rhizoma Coptidis); in case of frequent, difficult but not dry, not loose stool, add ge gen (Radix Puerarae), bai shao (Radix Paeoniae Alba), di yu (Radix et Rhizoma Sanguisorbae), qin pi (Cortex Fraxini Caulis), bai tou weng (Caulis et Folium Pulsatillae); if accompanied by intestinal metaplasia, add ban zhi lian (Herba Scutellariae Barbatae), ban bian lian (Herba Lobeliae Ciliatae), jiao gu lan (Herba Gynostemmatis Pentaphylli), yi yi ren (Semen Coisis), bai ying (Herba Solani Lyrati); if accompanied by atypical hyperplasia, add san leng (Rhizoma Sparganii), e zhu (Rhizoma Curcumae); if accompanied by HP infection, add pu gong ying (Herba Taraxaci cum Radice), hu zhang (Rhizoma Polygoni, lian qiao (Fructus Forsythiae), huang lian (Rhizoma Coptidis); in case of egastric mass, add gua lou (Fructus Trichosanthis), huang lian (Rhizoma Coptidis), ban xia (Rhizoma Pinelliae); in case of gastric mucosa and congestion edema, add chuan xiong (Rhizoma Chuanxiong), yan hu suo (Rhizoma Corydalis), san qi (Radix Notoginseng).

五、浊毒壅盛型
5. Obstruction of abundant turbid toxin

（一）主要症状
5.1 The main symptoms

口干口苦，脐腹胀满疼痛，心烦躁扰，头晕胀痛，寐差，大便秘结不通，小便短赤或黄，舌紫红，苔黄厚腻，脉滑数或弦滑数。

Dry and bitter mouth, umbilical abdominal distension and pain, heart irritability, dizziness and distension and pain, poor sleep, constipation, short, red or yellow urine, purple tongue with yellow thick and greasy moss, slippery rapid or string slippery rapid pulse.

（二）病机
5.2 Pathogenesis

湿热中阻，浊毒壅盛。

Dampness and heat resisted in middle energizer, obstruction of abundant turbid toxin.

（三）治则
5.3 Treatment principle

泄浊攻毒。

To discharge turbidity and eliminate toxin.

（四）方药
5.4 Prescription

半边莲15g，半枝莲15g，白花蛇舌草15g，苦参9g，板蓝根15g，鸡骨草12g。

Ban bian lian (Herba Lobeliae Ciliatae) 15g, ban zhi lian (Herba Scutellariae Barbatae)15g, bai hua she she cao (Herba Oldenlandiae Diffusae)15g, ku shen (Radix Sophorae Flavescentis) 9g, ban lan gen (Radix Isatidis) 15g, ji gu cao (Herba Abri) 12g.

（五）加减运用
5.5 Addition and reduction principle

口苦，纳呆，加龙胆草；心烦，加栀子、淡豆豉；便秘，加芦荟、番泻叶。对毒重浊轻者应以解毒为主，但对热毒治疗又常据毒之轻重而用药。毒轻用绞股蓝、黄芩、黄连、黄柏、蒲公英、连翘，毒中用半边莲、半枝莲、白花蛇舌草，毒重用白英、黄药子。伴肠化，加白花蛇舌草、薏苡仁、白英；伴不典型增生，加水红花子、穿山甲（现用替代品，下同）、全蝎、蜈蚣、水蛭。

In case of bitter mouth, poor appetite, add long dan cao (Gentianae Radix et Rhizoma); in case of dysphoria, add zhi zi (Fructus Gardeniae), dan dou chi (Sojae Semen Praeparatum); in case of constipation, add lu hui (Aloe)and fan xie ye (Sennae Folium). Patients with syndrome of heavier toxin and lighter turbidity should be treated mainly to remove toxin. But the prescription of heat toxin should be decided according to the severity of toxin. For lighter toxin, we choose jiao gu lan (Rhizoma seu Herba Gynostemmatis Pentaphylli), huang qin (Radix Scutellariae), huang lian (Rhizoma Coptidis), huang bo(Cortex Phellodendri), pu gong ying (Herba Taraxaci cum Radice), lian qiao (Forsythiae Fructus); for mid-degree of toxin, we use ban bian lian (Herba Lobeliae Ciliatae), ban zhi lian (Herba Scutellariae Barbatae), bai hua she she cao (Herba Oldenlandiae Diffusae); for severe toxin, we use bai ying (Herba Solani Lyrati), huang yao zi (Rhizoma Dioscoreae Bulbiferiae). If accompanied by intestinal metaplasia, add bai hua she she cao (Herba Oldenlandiae Diffusae), yi yi ren (Semen Coisis), bai ying (Herba Solani Lyrati); if accompanied by atypical hyperplasia, add shui hong hua zi (Fructus Polygoni Orientalis), chuan shan jia (Squanma Manitis)(substitute as priority), quan xie (Scorpio), wu gong (Scolopendra), shui zhi (Hirudo).

六、瘀血内结型
6. Blood stasis stagnated internally

（一）主要症状
6.1 Main symptoms

胃脘胀满，刺痛，痛有定处，夜间加重，胸满口燥，面色暗滞，舌质紫或紫暗，或有瘀点、瘀斑，脉弦涩。

Epigastric distension, tingling and fixed pain, aggravated at night, with full chest, dry mouth, dull complexion, purple or purple dark tongue with petechia or ecchymosis, string and astringent pulse.

（二）病机
6.2 Pathogenesis

浊毒中阻，瘀血内结。

Turbid toxin obstructed in middle energizer, blood stasis stagnated internally.

（三）治则
6.3 Treatment principle

理气活血，化瘀消痞。

Regulate qi and promote blood circulation, resolve blood stasis and eliminate ruffians.

（四）方药
6.4 Prescription

当归15g，川芎12g，延胡索15g，三七2g，蒲黄15g，五灵脂15g，姜黄9g，白芷15g，丹参15g，鸡血藤15g。

Dang gui (Radix Angelicae Sinensis) 15g, chuan xiong (Rhizoma Chuanxiong) 12g, yan hu suo (Rhizoma Corydalis) 15g, san qi (Radix Notoginseng) 15g, pu huang (Pollen Typhae) 15g, wu ling zhi (Faeces Trogopterorum) 15g, jiang huang (Rhizoma Curcumae Longae) 9g, bai zhi (Radix Angelicae Dahuricae)15g, dan shen (Salviae Miltiorrhizae) 15g, ji xue teng (Caulis Spatholobi) 15g.

（五）加减运用
6.5 Addition and reduction principle

伴胃脘胀满气滞，加柴胡、香附、木香；心血暗耗，虚火内浮所致眠差，加酸枣仁；伴异型增生，加三棱、莪术。

With epigastric distension full and qi stagnation, add chai hu (Radix Bulpleuri), xiang fu (Rhizoma Cyperi) , mu xiang (Radix Aucklandiae); for insomnia caused by internal consumption of blood and deficient fire floating, add suan zao ren (Semen Ziziphi Jujubae); with dysplasia, add san leng (Rhizoma Sparganii) and e zhu (Rhizoma Curcumae).

七、毒热伤阴型
7. Toxic heat injures Yin

（一）主要症状
7.1 Main symptoms

胃脘胀满，灼痛，胃中嘈杂，饥不思食或食少，口干，五心烦热，大便干结，舌红少津，苔少或花剥，脉弦细或细。

Epigastric distension, burning pain, upset in stomach, hungry with no want to eat or poor appetite, dry mouth, upset heat of five centres, dry stool, red tongue with less liquid, less or peeling moss, string thready or thready pulse.

（二）病机
7.2 Pathogenesis

毒热内结，耗伤胃阴。
Toxic heat knotted internally damages the stomach Yin.

（三）治则
7.3 Treatment principle

滋养胃阴，和胃消痞。
To nourish the stomach Yin, harmonize the stomach and eliminate ruffian.

（四）方药
7.4 Prescription

百合15g，乌药12g，沙参15g，麦冬15g，五味子15g，山茱萸15g，乌梅15g，玄参

15g，玉竹15g，黄精15g。

Bai he (Bulbus Lilii) 15g, wu yao (Radix Linderae) 15g, sha shen (Radix Adennophorae Strictae) 12g, mai dong (Radix Ophiopogonis) 15g, wu wei zi (Fructus Schisandalis) 15g, shan zhu yu (Arillus Corni) 15g, wu mei (Fructus Mume) 15g, xuan shen (Radix Scrophulariae) 15g, yu zhu (Rhizoma Polygonati Odorati) 15g, huang jing (Rhizoma Rolygonati) 15g.

（五）加减运用
7.5 Addition and reduction principle

伴胃中烧灼，加生石膏、黄连；胃痛兼背痛，加沙参、威灵仙；伴胃酸缺乏，加石斛；伴口干，加天花粉；伴咽堵，加射干、桔梗、板蓝根。

Accompanied by gastric burning heat, add sheng shi gao (Crude Gypsum Fibrosum), huang lian (Rhizoma Coptidis); stomach pain involving back, add sha shen (Radix Adennophorae Strictae), wei ling xian (Radix Clematidis); lack of gastric acid, add shi hu (Dendrobii Caulis); with dry mouth, add tian hua fen (Radix Trichosanthis); in case of throat blockage, add she gan (Rhizoma Belamcandae), jie geng (Platycodonis Radix), ban lan gen (Radix Isatidis).

八、脾胃虚弱型
8. Weak spleen and stomach

（一）主要症状
8.1 Main symptoms

胃脘胀满或隐痛，胃部喜按喜暖，食少，气短，懒言，呕吐清水，口淡，乏力，大便稀溏，舌质淡，边有齿痕，脉细弱。

Epigastric distension or dull pain, the stomach likes to be pressed and warmed, less food, short of breath, lazy to speak, vomiting water, light mouth, fatigue, loose stool, light tongue with teeth marks, tready and weak pulse.

（二）病机
8.2 Pathogenesis

浊毒伤脾，脾胃虚弱。

Turbid toxin hurts the spleen, and the spleen and stomach are weak.

（三）治则
8.3 Treatment principle

补气健脾，和胃消痞。

To tonify qi and reinforce spleen, harmonize stomach and eliminate ruffian.

（四）方药

8.4 Prescription

党参15g，茯苓15g，白术9g，陈皮15g，白扁豆15g，山药15g。

Dang shen (Radix Codonopsitis Pilosulae) 15g, fu ling (Poria) 15g, bai zhu (Rhizoma Atractylodis Macrocephalae)9g, chen pi (Pericarpium Citri Reticulatae) 15g, bai bian dou (Semen Dolichoris Album) 15g, shan yao (Tuber Dioscoreae) 15g.

（五）加减运用

8.5 Addition and reduction principle

脾阳不振，手足不温，加附子、炮姜；气虚失运，满闷较重，加木香、枳实、厚朴；气血两亏，心悸气短，神疲乏力，面色无华，加太子参、五味子；脾胃虚寒，加高良姜、荜茇。

When spleen Yang is sluggish, hands and feet are not warm, add fu zi (Radix Aconiti), pao jiang (prepared Ginger); in case of abnormal operation of energy mechanism because of qi deficiency, patient feels full and heavy, add mu xiang (Radix Aucklandiae), zhi shi (Fructus Aurantii Immaturus), hou po (Cortex Magnoliae Officinalis); when breath and blood are deficient, palpitation, short of breath, fatigue, ill complexion, add tai zi shen (Radix Pseudostellariae), wu wei zi (Fructus Schisandalis); For cold and deficient spleen and stomach, add gao liang jiang (Rhizoma Alphiniae Officinari)and bi bo (Radix Piperis Longi).

第三章 消化性溃疡浊毒论
Chapter 3 On Turbid Toxin of Peptic Ulcer

第一节 病因病机
Section 1 Etiology and Pathogenesis

一、古代中医名家对消化性溃疡的认识
1. The understanding of ancient TCM masters on peptic ulcer

消化性溃疡基本属于中医学"胃脘痛"的范畴，又与"痞满""吞酸""嘈杂"等有密切联系，现代临床上大多按胃脘痛进行辨证治疗。

Digestive ulcer basically belongs to the category of "epigastric pain" in TCM, and is closely related to "ruffian full", "swallowing acid" and "stomach upset". In modern clinical practice, it is mostly treated according to epigastric pain.

胃脘痛的病名，最早记载于我国的第一部古典医籍《黄帝内经》。如《灵枢·邪气脏腑病形》曰："胃病者，腹䐜胀，胃脘当心而痛，上支两胁，膈咽不通，饮食不下，取之足三里也。"《素问·痹论》云："饮食自倍，肠胃乃伤。"《素问·举痛论》云："寒气客于肠胃，厥逆上出，故痛而呕也。""寒气客于肠胃之间，膜原之下，血不得散，小络急引故痛。"《素问·六元正纪大论》云："木郁之发……民病胃脘当心而痛。"《灵枢·五邪》云："邪在脾胃……阳气不足，阴气有余，则寒中肠鸣腹痛。"以上论述说明饮食失常、寒邪、风邪、热邪、肝气犯胃（即情志失调，肝郁克土）及脾胃虚寒皆可引起胃脘痛。汉代张仲景《金匮要略·腹满寒疝宿食脉证》篇也有关于胃脘痛的类似记载，认为"按之不痛为虚，痛者为实"，其中的大建中汤、小建中汤、黄芪建中汤、四逆散、泻心汤、芍药甘草汤、吴茱萸汤、小柴胡汤皆为后世治疗胃脘痛的有效方。《金匮要略》为后世医家对胃脘痛的辨证、立法、处方奠定了基础。唐代孙思邈《备急千金要方》有九种心痛之说，实际上多指胃痛而言，但从此古代文献多把属于胃脘痛的心痛和属于心经本身病变的心痛混为一谈。宋代严用和《济生方》进一步分析《备急千金要方》提出的九种心痛的病因是外感六淫，七情内伤，饮食所伤。金元时期，医学家们的学术争鸣拓宽了本病的治疗门径。李东垣在《兰室秘藏》一书立"胃脘痛"一门，以脾虚寒凝立论，拟草豆蔻丸、神圣复气汤等方治疗本病，体现了补脾温中的治疗思想。朱丹溪首次为胃脘痛正名，指出前人所谓"心痛"，实指胃脘痛，澄清了心痛与胃脘痛的混淆，使胃脘痛成为独立的

病证。明代李中梓强调虚实的辨证施治，告诫人们治疗本病不可囿于"通则不痛"之说而不分虚实，应重视补虚止痛一法的应用。清代医家尤其重视医疗经验的积累，同时将治法理论向前推进了一步。如叶天士治疗本病立足肝胃，始终贯穿"以通为主"的原则，强调分辨气血阴阳及在经在络，认为病初"气结在经"，治宜苦辛通降或疏泄气机；久病"血伤在络"，治宜辛柔和络或搜剔缓攻为主。活血化瘀一法经过王清任、唐容川在医疗实践中的发展也更加完备。综上所述，中医学早在数千年前对消化性溃疡就有比较系统的认识。随着历代医家的不断完善、补充，消化性溃疡的病因、病机、辨证治疗更加丰富和完善。

The medical name of epigastric pain was first recorded in China's first classical medical book, *The Medical Classic of the Yellow Emperor*. For example *Spiritual Pivot-Symptoms of Viscera due to attack of Evil Qi* says: "The stomach disease chacterized by abdominal distension starts from epgastric pain, involving the hypochondria, obstruction of the diaphragm and throat and inability to take food, (can be treated by) needling Zusanli." *Simple Conversation-On Spasm* says: "Over-taken of diet hurts the intestines and the stomach". *Simple Conversation-Discussion on pains*: "Cold evil stays in the intestines and stomach, thus chronic headache occurs which leads to pain and vomiting.""Cold evil stays between the intestines and the stomach below the membrane, causes blood stagnation and contraction of small collateral, resulting pain." *Simple Conversation-Major Discussion on the Progress of the Six Climatic Changes* say: "Affected by wood (liver) depression... epgastric disease occurs acting as stomach pain."*Spiritual Pivot-Five Evil* says: "As evil stays in spleen and stomach...Yang qi is deficient, Yin qi is excessive, therefore when cold evil attacks, intestine gurgling and abdominal pain occurs." The above discussion shows that dietary disorder, cold evil, wind evil, heat evil, liver qi attacks stomach (i. e., emotional disorders, liver depression restrains soil) and the deficiency and coldness of spleen and stomach can cause epigastric pain. Zhang Zhongjing of Han dynasty in his *Synopsis of Gold Chamber-Discussion on disease, pulse and syndrome differentiation treatment of Abdominal Full, Cold Hernia, Dyspepsia* also had similar records about epigastric pain, he thought "If the patient does not feel pain when being pressed in stomach, the disease is deficient; if the patient feels painful when being pressed in stomach, the disease is excessive." The prescriptions as Dajianzhong Decoction, Xiaojianzhong Decoction, Huangqi Jianzhong Decoction, Sini Powder, Xiexin Decoction, Shaoyao Gancao Decoction, Wuzhuyu Decoction, Xiaochaihu Decoction are all effective solutions for treatment of epigastric pain. *The Synopsis of the Golden Chamber* laid a solid foundation for the syndrome differentiation, legislation and prescription of epigastric pain in later generations. There are nine kinds of heartache listed in *Qianjin Prescriptions* of Sun Simiao, in fact, it mostly refers to stomach pain. But since then, the ancient literature mostly confused the epigastric pain with the heartache of the heart meridian itself. Yan Yonghe of Song dynasty further analyzed in his *Jisheng Fang Prescriptions* that the causes of nine kinds of heartache listed in *Qianjin Prescriptions* include attacks of six excessive external evils, injuries of seven internal emotions, and injury of improper diet. In the Jin and Yuan era, the academic contention of medical scientists widened the treatment path of this disease. Li Dongyuan set up the independent division of "epigastric pain", in his book *Medical Secrets in Orchid Room*, creating Caodoukou Pill, Shensheng Fuqi Decoction and other prescriptions to treat the disease according to the differentiation of spleen deficiency and cold coagulation, reflecting the treatment principle to tonify the middle energizer by warming the spleen. Zhu Danxi for the first time clarified the name of epigastric pain, pointed out that the so-called "heartache" of predecessors, actually refers to epigastric pain, clarified the confusion between heartache and epigastric pain, and made epigastric pain become an independent disease certificate. Li Zhongzi of Ming dynasty emphasized the syndrome differentiation principle according to deficiency and excess of the disease, and warned that the treatment of this disease should not be confined to the principle of "no obstruction, no pains" regardless of deficiency and excess, and should pay attention to the application of the method of tonifying deficiency to relieve pains. Doctors in the Qing dynasty paid special attention to the accumulation of medical experiences and further pushed forward the theory and treatment principle of epigastric pain. Doctor Ye Tianshi treated this disease on the basis of liver and stomach, always implement the principle that "unobstruction is preferred", emphasizing the differentiation of location of the disease, either in breath, or in blood, either in Yin or in Yang, either in the meridians or in the collateral, he thinks that at the beginning of the disease, "qi is knotted in the meridians", the appropriate way of treatment is to resolve the knotting and descend the qi by using bitter and acrid medicines; long- courage- disease is because "blood has been injured in collateral", appropriate way of treatment is to harmonize the laterals by soft acrid medicines or to slowly attack and pick out the evil by using medicines of insects. The treatment method of promoting blood circulation to remove blood stasis is further developed and perfected by Wang Qingren and Tang Rongchuan in medical practice. To sum up, Chinese medical science had a relatively systematic understanding of peptic ulcer thousands of years ago. The continuous improvement and reinforcement of doctors in all dynasties enriched and perfected the treatment theory and practice of peptic ulcer disease in cause, pathogenesis and syndrome differentiation.

二、基于浊毒理论对消化性溃疡病因病机的认识
2. The understanding of peptic ulcer disease based on the theory of turbid toxin

我们提出消化性溃疡浊毒致病论，认为浊毒内蕴既是一种病理产物也是一种致病因素。因情志不畅、饮食不节、先天禀赋不足，脾胃虚弱；或因外感六淫，均可使脾失健运，水湿内生。湿邪郁久则化热，热煎津液成痰，痰凝生浊，浊聚日久成毒，浊毒壅盛于胃腑，进而脾胃气机升降失调，气机阻滞，不通则痛，故见胃脘疼痛。本病病位在脾胃，而与肝肾关系密切，为本虚标实之证。源于脾虚，以浊毒为标，多虚实并见，日久可伤阴耗液，阴损及阳，形成危急重症。消化性溃疡活动期浊毒壅盛，愈合期邪（浊毒）正（正气）相持或正虚邪恋，疾病反复发作，缠绵难愈。

We propose the turbid toxin pathogenesis of peptic ulcer disease and believe that the connotation of turbid toxin is both a pathological product and a pathogenic factor. Unhealthy mood, undesciplined diet, insufficient innate endowment, weak spleen and stomach, or six external evils, can make the spleen lose healthy operation, water wet is generated endogenously. Long-time depression of wet evil will be transmitted into heat, heat fries fluid and liquid into phlegm, phlegm coagulation will turn to be turbidity, unitation of turbidity for a long time will turn to be toxin, turbid toxin congests abundantly in the stomach, will then cause irregular operation of ascending and descending qi mechanism of the spleen and stomach, blocking of qi mechanism leads to pains, thus peptic ulcer occurs. Although the disease is usually located in spleen and stomach, it is closely related to liver and kidney, characterized by root deficiency and branch excess. Originated from spleen deficiency, with turbid toxin as the tip, peptic ulcer can usually see both deficiency and excess, with time passes, it can hurt Yin and consumes fluid, When Yin damages Yang, abrupt and critical illness occurs. Turbid toxin is abundantly obstructed in active period of peptic ulcer, stalemate with healthy qi or lingering with deficient healthy qi in healing period. The disease will repeat again and again, lingering and difficult to heal.

（一）病因
2.1 The etiology

1.脾胃虚弱　若先天禀赋不足，素体脾胃虚弱，或久病不愈，延及于脾或者先天肾阳不足，胃失于温煦或年高体衰，均可引起脾胃虚弱。脾失健运，胃中产生痰浊、水湿、积滞、浊毒等病理产物；土弱则肝木乘虚犯胃，造成胃病。脾胃虚弱是消化性溃疡发病的基础。

2.1.1 Weakness of the spleen and stomach　If the congenital endowment of the patient is deficient, spleen and stomach is usually weak, or with long-time disease lingering, which affects the spleen, or deficient in congenital kidney Yang, stomach looses warmth, or physical failure due to ages, can all cause weakness of the spleen and stomach. When the spleen looses the healthy operation, phlegm, moisture, stagnation, turbid toxin and other pathological products will be generated in the stomach; when the soil (spleen) is weak, liver attacks the stomach, causing different stomach disease. Therefore, weak spleen and stomach is the basis of peptic ulcer.

2.饮食因素　饮食不节造成的溃疡病主要有四种情况：一是暴饮暴食，饮食过量，脾运不及，导致宿食停滞，胃失和降，气机郁滞而发病；二是由于过食生冷，致使寒积胃脘，使胃寒而痛；三是由于过食肥甘，或偏嗜辛辣或烈酒，致使热郁于胃，使胃热而痛；四是由于长期的饥饱无常，进食没有规律，导致胃失和降，脾失健运，损伤脾胃而发病。

2.1.2 Dietary factors　There are mainly four causes of ulcer disease caused by irregular diet. Firstly, fulminant eating and drinking, over-taken of diet, dyspepsia stagnation due to delay of spleen transporting, obstruction of qi mechanism because of dysfunction stomach harmonizing and descending. Second, over-taken of rough and cold diet causes cold stagnation in stomach, leading to pains in case of cold of stomach. Third, over-taken of fat and sweet food, or spicy or alcohol, causes heat depression in the stomach, leading to pains due to stomach heat. Fourth, long-term abnormal hunger and fullness, irregular diet, causes dysfunction of stomach harmonizing and descending, dysfunction of spleen healthy transporting, which damages the spleen and stomach and resulting disease.

3.情志因素　肝主疏泄，性喜条达。忧思恼怒，情志不畅，肝郁气滞，疏泄失职，横逆犯胃，郁滞不行，不通则痛；忧思伤脾，脾气郁结，运化失常，水谷不化，也可见胃脘胀满、疼痛之症。

2.1.3 Emotional factors　Liver is mainly responsible for mood dispersing, it is used to the state of regulation and peace. Worry, contemplation, anxiety and rage and other unhealthy mood causes liver depression and qi stagnation, leading to dysfunction of liver dispersing, invading the stomach adversely, depression and stagnation results obstruction and then various pains; worry and contemplation hurt the spleen, stagnation of spleen qi causes dysfunction of spleen transporting, and indigestion of water and grains, resulting epigastric distension, pains.

4.劳倦过度　繁重的劳动，紧张的工作，皆可损伤脾胃而发病。

2.1.4 Over-fatigue　Heavy labor, intense work, can damage the spleen and stomach and cause disease.

5.外邪犯胃　浊毒可由外而入，或从皮毛，或从口鼻，侵入机体，对人体脏腑、经络、气血、阴阳均能造成严重损害。"浊"者，不清也，浊与湿紧密相关，外感湿浊，由表入里。

2.1.5 External evil attacks stomach　Turbid toxin can enter from the outside, or from the fur, or from the mouth and nose, invade the body, making severe damages to viscera, meridians, breath and blood, Yin and Yang. "turbidity", means "not clear", turbidity and wet are closely related, external wet turbidity, enter from the surface into the internal body.

（二）病机

2.2 Pathogenesis

1.胃气壅滞　腑气以通为用，胃气主降，脾胃功能受损，胃气不降，阻滞于中焦，则胃脘胀满疼痛；气或聚或散，故胀痛走窜不定；胃气失降而上逆，则嗳气、欲吐；胃肠之气不降则大便秘结；舌红苔黄，脉弦，为浊气内停，气机阻滞之象。

2.2.1 The stomach qi stagnation　Stomach qi is used to unblock, mainly controls descending. When spleen and stomach function is impaired, stomach qi does not descend, being blocked in middle energizer, epigastric distention fullness and pain occurs; the stomach qi sometimes gather sometimes scatter, so swelling pain wanders around without stopping; when stomach qi does not descend but go reversely, belching occurs with desire to vomit; when gastro-intestinal qi does not descend, constipation occurs; red tongue with yellow moss, string pulse, is the image indicating turbidity retaining inside and energy mechanism obstructed.

2.湿浊中阻　脾喜燥恶湿，湿浊中阻，湿困脾阳，运化失职，水湿内停，脾气郁滞，则脘腹痞胀或痛，食少；脾失健运，湿滞气机，则口中黏腻无味；水湿下渗则见大便稀溏，湿性重浊，也可见到大便黏腻不爽；湿性重浊，泛溢肌肤，则见头身困重，肢体肿胀等。舌红苔腻，脉濡或滑同为湿浊中阻之象。

2.2.2 Wet and turbidity obstructed in middle energizer　Spleen likes dryness but dislikes dampness. When dampness and turbidity is resisted in middle energizer, the dampness distresses spleen Yang, spleen transporting function does not work, water wet retains inside, spleen qi is stagnated and depressed, epigastric and abdominal swelling or pain occurs, the appetite becomes poor. When spleen looses healthy operation, wet stagnates the energy mechanism, patients feel sticky, greasy and tasteless in mouth. When water wet infiltrates downward, loose stool occurs. If the dampness is heavy with turbidity, the stool will be sticky and difficult to be discharged. Wet heavy turbidity overflows the skin, patients have head and body trapped, limb swelling, etc. Red tongue with greasy moss, weak or slippery pulse is the image indicating wet turbidity obstructed in middle energizer.

3.浊犯肝胃　情志不遂，肝失疏泄，肝气横逆犯胃，胃气郁滞，则胃脘、胸胁胀满疼痛，走窜不定；胃气上逆而见呃逆、嗳气；肝失条达，情志失调，则见精神抑郁，善太息；木郁作酸，肝气犯胃，则吞酸嘈杂；胃受纳失职，则不思饮食；肝气郁滞，则可见大便不爽；舌红苔薄黄，脉弦滑为肝气郁滞，肝气犯胃之象。

2.2.3 The turbidity invades liver and stomach　Unhealthy mood causes liver dysfunction in dispersing, liver qi invades stomach adversely, stomach qi turns to be depressed and stagnated, thus stomach chest distention full and pain occurs, and wanders around. Adverse flow of stomach qi causes hiccup and belching; liver dysfunction in dispersing, emotion turns to be irregular, patients see depressed mood, frequent sighing. Depressed wood generates acid, liver qi attacks stomach, patients have acid regurgitation and upset; stomach failure in receiving and acceptance, patient's appetite becomes poor. Liver depression causes difficult stool. Red tongue with thin and yellow moss, string and slippery pulse is the image indicating liver qi depression and stagnation, liver qi invading the stomach.

4.浊毒内蕴　胃病日久，湿浊之气留滞于中焦，郁久化热，则见胃脘胀满，胀痛灼热。湿热浊毒之气耗伤气阴，则见口干口苦；浊气犯胃，胃失和降，胃气上逆，则见恶心呕吐；胃气受浊毒影响，不主受纳，则见纳呆；中焦气机阻滞，浊毒内蕴，阳气不能输布于体表四肢，则见怕冷；浊毒之气内蕴于中焦脏腑，气机不通，可见到大便不爽或便溏；舌红或紫红，苔黄腻，脉滑或滑数为浊毒内蕴，湿热中阻之象。

2.2.4 The internal accumulation of turbid toxin　Stomach disease for a long time causes wet turbid substance remain and stagnate in middle energizer, sustainable depression turns to be heat, patients see stomach distension full, pain and burning hot. Wet heat and turbid toxic substance consumes qi Yin, patients feel dry and bitter in mouth; when turbidity substance invades stomach, stomach looses the function of harmonizing and descending, stomach qi flow adversely, patients feel nausea and vomiting; when stomach qi is affected by turbid toxin, fails to receive and accept, anorexia occurs; when energy mechanism in middle energizer is obstructed by accumulated turbid toxin, yang qi cannot be scattered over the body and limbs, patients will be afraid of coldness; when turbid toxin is accumulated in viscera of middle energizer, the energy mechanism cannot work normally, patients see bad or loose stool; red or purple red tongue with yellow and greasy moss, slippery or slippery and rapid pulse is the image indicating internal accumulation of turbid toxin and obstruction of dampness and heat in middle energizer.

5.浊毒壅盛　浊毒壅盛，中焦气机郁滞，可见脘腹胀满疼痛；浊毒上扰清窍，故见心烦躁扰，头晕胀痛，寐差；浊毒下注，大肠传导功能失司，故见大便秘结不通，小便短赤或黄；舌紫红，苔黄厚腻，脉滑数或弦滑数均为湿热中阻，浊毒壅盛之象。

2.2.5 Turbid toxin obstruction　Turbid toxin obstruction causes energy mechanism stagnation in middle energizer, patients feel abdominal distension and pain. Turbid toxin disturbs upper orifices, patients feel heart irritability, dizziness, distension pain, poor sleep. When turbid toxin attacks downwards, patients see difficult stool and constipation, short red or yellow urine. Purple red tongue with yellow thick greasy moss, slippery rapid or string slippery rapid pulse is the image indicating that damp and heat is resisted in middle energizer, turbid toxin is abundantly obstructed.

6.瘀血内结　瘀血阻滞，则可见胃脘部为刺痛，痛有定处，以夜间为甚。血瘀日久伤阴，阴伤则燥，胸满口燥，面色暗滞也较为常见。而舌质紫或紫暗，或有瘀点、瘀斑，脉弦涩均为瘀血内结之象。

2.2.6 Internal stagnation of blood stasis When blood stasis is blocked, it can be seen that the epigastric part feels tingling pain, the pain is fixed, more severe at night. Blood stasis for a long time hurt Yin, when Yin fluid is injured, patient feels dry, full in chest, dry in mouth, and usually dull in complexion. Purple or purple dark tongue, with petechia or ecchymosis, string astringent pulse is the image of internal stagnation of blood stasis.

7.**毒热伤阴** 胃病日久，毒热盛，耗伤阴液，常出现阴伤之象。胃阴不足，虚热内生，热郁于胃，气失和降，则见胃脘胀满，灼痛，嘈杂不舒，痞满不适；胃失阴滋，纳化迟滞，则饥不欲食或食少；胃阴亏耗，阴津不能上滋则口燥咽干，不能下润则大便秘结、小便短少；舌红少津，苔少或花剥，脉弦细或细数是毒热内结、耗伤胃阴之象。

2.2.7 Toxic heat hurt Yin Stomach disease for a long time, toxic heat generates abundantly, consumes and damages Yin liquid, the phenomenon of Yin injury appears. When stomach Yin is short, deficient heat generates endogenously, heat is accumulated in the stomach, stomach looses the function of harmonizing and descending, patients feel epigastric distension, burning pain, uncomfortable upset, ruffian discomfort. When stomach looses the nourishing of Yin, acceptance and digestion is late and stagnated, patient do not want to eat or eat little when they are hungry. When stomach Yin is severely consumed, Yin fluid fails to nourish upward, patients feel dry in mouth and throat; when Yin fluid fails to lubricate downward, constipation and short urine occurs. Red tongue with less fluid, less or lingua geographia moss, string thready or thready rapid pulse is the image indicating toxic heat stagnates internally and severely consumes the stomach Yin.

8.**脾胃虚弱** 脾胃功能虚弱，脾失健运，胃失和降，脾胃气机壅滞于中焦，则见胃脘部胀满或隐痛，胃部喜按喜暖；脾胃虚弱，其受纳腐熟水谷及运化功能失司，则见食少；而气血生化乏源，机体失于濡养，则见气短、懒言、口淡、乏力、大便稀溏等；而舌质淡，边有齿痕，脉细弱均为浊毒伤脾、脾胃虚弱之象。

2.2.8 Weak spleen and stomach When the function of spleen and stomach is weak, spleen fails to transport, stomach fails to harmonize and descend, the qi movement of spleen and stomach is stagnated in middle energizer, patients feel epigastric distension or hidden pain, the stomach likes to be pressed and warmed. Weak spleen and stomach fails to accept, digest food and transport grain essence, patients eat little; Human body is lack of resource to generate and transmit the breath and blood, physical body can not be sufficiently nourished, patients become short in breath, lazy to speak, tired of salty food, fatigue, loose stool, etc. Weak tongue with teeth mark in edge, weak thready pulse is the image indicating that the spleen is hurt by turbid toxin, spleen and stomach turns to be weak.

第二节 辨证要点
Section 2 Key Factors For Differentiation

一、辨缓急
1. To differentiate urgent or slow disease

凡胃痛暴作，起病急者，多因外受寒邪，或恣食生冷，或暴饮暴食，以致中阳受损；或积滞不化，胃失和降，不通则痛。胃胀突发者，多因暴怒伤肝，肝气失于疏泄，胃络失和；或饮食失宜，食滞胃脘，胃失和降所致。凡胃痛胃胀渐发，起病缓者，多因脾胃虚弱，胃络失其气血温煦或土壅木郁，而致肝胃不和，气滞血阻。

Abrupt occurrences of stomach pain are mostly due to external cold evil, or eating rough and cold food, or eating and drinking too much at one meal, making damages to middle Yang; or food stagnated without digesting, stomach looses the function of harmonizing and descending, obstruction leading to pain. Abrupt occurrence of stomach distension are due to violent anger hurting the liver, liver qi cannot be normally dispersed, stomach collateral is not in harmony; or irregular diet causes food stagnation in stomach, stomach looses the function of harmonizing and descending. All the gradual, slow occurrence of stomach pain and distension are mostly due to spleen and stomach weakness, stomach looses the warming of blood and breath, or accumulation of spleen qi causes liver depression, leading to disharmony of liver and stomach, qi stagnation and blood resistance.

二、辨虚实
2. Distinguish between deficiency and excess

胃痛而胀，大便秘结不通者多实，痛而不胀，大便不秘结者多虚；喜凉者多实，喜温者多虚；拒按者多实，喜按者多虚；食后痛胀甚者多实，饥则腹痛胀满者多虚；脉实气逆者多实，脉细弱者多虚；痛胀起病徐缓，按之濡软而不坚者多虚；新病体壮者多实，久病体衰者多虚。

Stomach pain and distension, stool closed or constipation, the disease is mostly excess; pain without distension, without constipation, the disease is mostly deficient; if patients are in favor of cool food or drink, their diseases are mostly excess, if patients are in favor of warm food and drink, the diseases are mostly deficient; patients refuse to be pressed, the diseases are mostly excess, patients like to be pressed, the diseases are mostly deficient. If the pain and distension becomes more severe after meal, the disease is mostly excess, if the pain and distension becomes more severe when hungry, the disease is mostly deficient. Patient with adverse flow of qi and excess pulse, the disease is mostly excess; patient with weak and thready pulse, the disease is mostly deficient. Pain and distension which occurs gradually, feels soft but not hard, is mostly deficient, pain and distension which occurs recently in strong body, the disease is mostly excess, pain and distension which has last for a long time in weak body, the disease is mostly deficient.

三、望颜面五官
3. Look at the facial features and five sense organs

浊毒蕴结，郁蒸体内，上蒸于头面，而见面色粗黄，晦浊。若浊毒为热蒸而外溢于皮肤则见皮肤油腻，患者每有面部洗不净的感觉，给人一种秽浊之象。浊毒上犯清窍则头晕，蕴于颜面则面红目赤。

When turbid toxin is accumulated and steaming depressed in head and body, patient will see coarse yellow, cloudy and turbid complexion. If the turbid toxin is hot steamed and spilled over the skin, the skin becomes greasy, the patient feels difficult to wash the face cleanly, presenting a impression of filthy. When turbid toxin invades upper lucid orifices, patients feel dizzy; when turbid toxin retains in faces, red faces and eyes appear.

四、望舌苔
4. Look at the tongue moss

患者以黄腻苔多见，但因感浊毒的轻重不同而有所差别。浊毒轻者舌红，苔腻、薄腻，或黄或白或黄白相间；浊毒重者舌质紫红、红绛，苔黄腻，或黄厚腻。因感邪脏腑不同苔位亦异，如浊毒中阻者，苔中部黄腻；浊毒阻于肝胆者，苔两侧黄腻。苔色、苔质根据病情的新久而变，初感浊毒、津液未伤时见黄滑腻苔，浊毒日久伤津时则为黄燥腻苔。

Patients with yellow greasy moss is more common, but the tongue moss is different due to the severity of turbid toxin. Patient with lighter turbid toxin has red tongue, greasy moss, or thin and greasy moss, or yellow, white, yellow and white moss; patient with heavier turbid toxin has heavy purple, or red purple tongue, yellow, greasy moss, or yellow thick and greasy moss. Moss is located in different area of the tongue due to the different viscera which is invaded by turbid toxin. For example, when turbid toxin is resisted in middle energizer, the yellow and greasy moss is located in middle part of the tongue; when turbid toxin is blocked in the liver and gallbladder, the yellow and greasy moss will be located in two sides of the tongue. The color and nature of tongue moss will change according to the course of the disease. At the beginning of turbid toxin invasion, body fluid is not yet hurt, yellow slippery and greasy tongue moss is seen; when turbid toxin lasts for a long time and injures the body fluid, yellow dry and greasy tongue moss is seen.

五、脉象
5. Pulse conditions

浊毒证患者滑数脉常见，尤以右关脉滑数突出。临床以滑数、弦滑、弦细滑、细滑多见。病程短，浊毒盛者，可见弦滑、或弦滑数脉。病程长、阴虚有浊毒者，可见细滑脉、沉细滑脉。但患者出现沉细脉时多为浊毒内蕴、络脉瘀阻，而不应仅仅认为是虚或虚寒脉。

Slippery rapid pulse, especially slippery rapid in the right guan pulse is common for the patients of turbid toxin disease. In clinical practices, slippery rapid pulse, string slippery pulse, string thin slippery pulse, thready slippery pulse is usually seen. Patients with short course of severe turbid toxin disease see string slippery, or string slippery rapid pulse. Patients with long course of turbid toxin disease accompanied by Yin deficiency see thready slippery, sunken thin slippery pulse. However, when patients show sunken thready pulse, they are mostly involved by internal turbid toxin accumulation and collateral stasis resistance, and should not be simply considered as deficient or deficient cold pulse.

第三节　治疗原则
Section 3 Principles of Treatment

一、正治反治
1. Routine treatment and contrary treatment

正治法，或称逆治法，寒者热之，热者寒之，虚者补之，实者泻之，均为正治法。如浊毒内蕴用化浊解毒法、肝胃郁热用疏肝泄热法等均为正治法。如寒因寒用（以寒治寒）、热因热用（以热治热）、塞因塞用（以补开塞）、通因通用（以泻下剂治泻利）均为反治法。

The routine treatment method or the reverse treatment method, to treat cold with heat, to treat heat with cold, to treat deficiency with tonic, to treat excess with purging. For example, using turbidity resolving and toxin removing method to treat internal accumulation of turbid toxin, using liver dispersing and pathogenic heat purging method to treat depressed heat in liver and stomach, the above method belong to routine treatment method. For example, to treat cold with cold (cold), to treat heat with heat, to treat block with block, to treat dredging with dredging are all contray-treatment methods.

二、标本缓急
2. The tip and root, slow and urgent

按照"急则治其标，缓则治其本"和"间者并行，甚者独行"的原则进行治疗。如胃溃疡并发大量吐血，治当先止其血，再治其胃之虚实。急则治其标，多为权宜急救之法，待急象缓解，则应转为治本，以除病根。

To treat diseases according to the principle of "to treat the tip first in acute disease, to treat the root first in chronic disease" and "simultaneous treatment for slow and lighter disease, focal treatment for urgent and serious disease". If the gastric ulcer is accompanied with a large amount of blood vomiting, the treatment should first stop its blood, and then cure the deficiency and excess of the stomach. "To treat the tip first in acute disease" is usually an expedient and emergency treatment method, when the emergency condition is relieved, treatment should be turned to the root, in order to remove the root of the disease.

三、扶正祛邪
3. To reinforce the healthy factor and dispel the pathogenic factor

扶正用于正虚邪不盛的病证；祛邪用于邪实正虚不显的病证。正虚邪实者，则宜扶正祛邪并举，总之以扶正不留邪，祛邪不伤正为原则。

The method to reinforce the healthy factor is used to treat the disease with the characteristic of deficient in healthy factor while the pathogenic factor is not excessive. The method to dispel the pathogenic factor is used to treat the disease with the characteristic of excess in pathogenic factor, while the healthy factor is not deficient. For the disease of deficient in healthy factor while the pathogenic factor is excess, it should be treated by using the method of reinforcing the healthy factor simultaneously with the method of dispelling the pathogenic factor. The general principle is, to reinforce the healthy factor without remaining the evil, and expel the pathogenic factor without hurt to healthy factor.

四、三因制宜
4. To treat disease according to three basic conditions

三因制宜即因时、因地、因人制宜，是指治疗疾病应根据季节、地区以及人体的体质、性别等不同而制定适宜的治疗方法。

The three basic conditions means the time, the place, and the nature of person in relation with the disease. It indicates to choose proper treating method according to different season, region, constitution and sex of the patient.

五、整体治疗与局部治疗相结合
5. Combination of wholistic treatment and local treatment

消化性溃疡不仅有全身性的表现，更有其独特的局部表现。由于脾胃纳化升降失常，气血运行受阻，造成胃络瘀阻，胃失所养，胃膜破溃，在局部形成溃疡，甚至造成络破血溢，溃破穿孔。所以，其局部表现更为突出和严重。因此，消化性溃疡的治疗，不仅要进行整体辨证治疗，更要注重局部治疗。如用一些祛腐收敛生肌、活血化瘀止痛的药物，促进局部溃疡愈合。

Digestive ulcer has not only systemic manifestations, but also unique local manifestations. Abnormal function of accepting, digesting, ascending and descending of the spleen and stomach resists breath and blood operation, causes stasis in gastric collateral. Without regular nourishment, gastric membrane is ulcerated, causing local ulcers and even collateral damage with blood overflowing, diabrotic and perforation. Thus the local performance of peptic ulcer is even more prominent and serious. Therefore, the treatment of peptic ulcer should not only carry out the overall syndrome differentiation treatment, but also pay more attention to the local treatment. For example, use some medicine to dispel putridity, astringent and promote tissue regeneration, activate blood, resolve stasis and relieve pain, in result to promote local ulcer healing.

六、以通为顺
6. Dredging is smoothing

胃脘痛的发病机制就是脾胃受纳运化升降失常，气血瘀阻不畅，即所谓"不通则痛"。故治疗上多用通法，使气血调畅，纳运复常，则其痛自止。但当辨虚实寒热，分别施治。如肝郁气滞者，当疏肝理气；肝郁化火者，当清肝泄热；血瘀者，当活血化瘀；阳气虚者，当温阳益气；阴津少者，当养阴益胃。

The pathogenesis of epigastric pain is that dysfunction of accepting, transporting, ascending and descending of the spleen and stomach obstructs the smooth circulation of breath and blood. So-called "pain is generated from blocking". Therefore, dredging method is usually used to treat the disease in order to regulate the operation of breath and blood, recover the function of digesting and transporting, thus the pain will stop itself. However, clinical treatment should be made differently according to deficiency, excess, cold and heat of the disease. For example, to treat liver depression and qi stagnation, method of liver soothing and qi regulating should be used. When liver depression is transformed into fire, the method of purging the fire to clear the liver should be used. To treat blood stasis, method of blood activating and stasis resolving should be used. To treat Yang deficiency, method of warming Yang to reinforce qi should be used; To treat the syndrome lack of Yin fluid, the method of benefiting stomach by Yin nourishing should be used.

第四节 常用治法
Section 4 Common Method of Treatment

一、化浊解毒法
1. Method to resolve turbidity and remove toxin

化浊解毒为治疗消化性溃疡的基本大法。浊毒致病具有难治性、顽固性的特点，若徒解其毒则浊难祛，徒化其浊则毒愈甚。因此分离浊毒，孤立邪势，是治疗的关键。化浊解毒可使浊化毒除，从而气行血畅，积除郁解，痰消火散，或给邪以出路，使浊毒从大便而出，从小便而去，从汗液而消，积除郁解，恢复脾升胃降之特性，而化浊解毒之法可随证灵活加减，或从根本截断浊毒生成，阻断湿、浊、痰、热、毒胶结成浊毒内蕴之势。

To resolve turbidity and remove toxin is the basic method to treat peptic ulcer. Disease caused by turbid toxin has the characteristics of refractory, stubborn, only removing toxin, turbidity is difficult to be resolved; only resolving the turbidity, toxin will be more severe. Therefore, the separation of turbidity and toxin, and the isolation of evil tendency is the key factor for treatment. The method to resolve turbidity and remove toxin can make turbidity dissipated and toxin disappeared, thus the circulation of breath and blood become normal, stagnation and depression is resolved, phlegm is cleaned and fire is dispersed, or leave a way out for pathogenic evil, discharge the turbid toxin along with stool, with urine, with sweat, without stagnation and depression, restore the function of spleen ascending and stomach descending is recovered. The prescription of turbidity resolving and toxin removing can be flexibly adjusted by adding or reducing medicine, or fundamentally cut off turbid toxin generation, block the combination and transmitting tendency from wet, turbidity, phlegm, heat, toxin into turbid toxin according to the development of syndrom.

（一）芳香化浊解毒法
1.1 To resolve turbidity and remove toxin with aroma

气味芳香之品，多具有醒脾运脾、化浊辟秽的作用，故临床症见脘腹胀痛、痞满、呕吐泛酸、大便溏薄、食少体倦、口干多涎、舌苔白腻等可选用此法。常用药物为藿香、佩兰、半夏、苍术、白术、砂仁、紫豆蔻、陈皮等品。

Most of the aromatic medicine has the function of activating and transporting spleen, resolving turbidity and stopping filthy, so the method of resolving turbidity and removing toxin with aroma is clinically used when the following symptom occur: such as abdominal distension, ruffian, vomiting with pantothenic acid, thin and loose stool, less eating and physically tired, dry mouth with more saliva, white and greasy tongue moss etc. Common medicines are: huo xiang (Herba Agastaches seu Pogostemonis), pei lan (Herba Eupatorii), ban xia (Rhizoma Pinelliae), cang zhu (Rhizoma Atractylodis), bai zhu (Rhizoma Atractylodis Macrocephalae), sha ren (Fructus Amomi), zi dou kou (Purple Cardamom Kernel), chen pi (Pericarpium Citri Reticulatae) and other products.

（二）通腑泄浊解毒法
1.2 To unblock the fu-organ, purge turbidity, and remove toxin

浊毒内停日久，可致腑气不通，邪滞壅盛。本法运用通泻药物荡涤腑气，保持腑气通畅，使浊毒之邪从下而走，属中医学下法范畴。临床用于胃脘胀满，疼痛，恶心呕吐，口气秽浊，大便秘结不通等症。药用大黄、川朴、枳实、芦荟等，常用方剂为小承气汤等。

When turbid toxin retains in patient's body for a long time, it can cause qi block of fu-organ, evil abundantly stagnate. This method uses purging medicine to cleanse the qi of fu-organ, ensuring the unobstruction of fu-organ, discharge the evil of turbid toxin along with stool. It belongs to the purgation method of TCM. It is clinically used to treat epigastric distension, pain, nausea and vomiting, foul breath, constipation and other diseases. Medicines generally used are da huang (Radix et Rhizoma Rhei), chuan po (Magnolia Officinalis), zhi shi (Frutus Aurantii Immaturus), lu hui (Aloe) the common prescription is Xiaochengqi Decoction.

（三）淡渗利湿解毒法

1.3 To dispel pathogenic dampness and remove toxin with bland medicines

湿浊同源，湿久凝浊，久则浊毒内蕴。使用甘淡利湿之品，可使浊毒之邪从下焦排出。临床用于肢体水肿，小便不利，身体困重，泄泻清稀，舌苔白，脉濡等症。常用茯苓、猪苓、泽泻、冬瓜子、薏苡仁等药。常用方剂为五皮饮、五苓散等。

As wet and turbidity are generated from the same resource, long - time dampness turns to be turbidity, then transmitted in to internal turbid toxin. To use sweet, light and damp-dispelling medicine, can discharge the turbid toxin evil from the lower energizer. This method is clinically used to treat limb edema, adverse urination, fatigued and heavy body, thin and loose diarrhea, white tongue moss, weal pulse and other symptoms. Medicines usually used in the above method include fu ling (Poria), zhu ling (Polygorus Umbellatus), ze xie (Rhizoma Alismatis), dong gua zi (Semen Benincasae), yi yi ren (Semen Coisis), etc. Prescriptions commonly used are Wupi Yin Decoction, Wuling Powder, etc.

（四）清热燥湿解毒法

1.4 To clear heat, eliminate dampness and remove toxin

湿久凝浊，热久生毒，凡湿热之证，缠绵不解，皆可化生浊毒。故清热燥湿法可从发病的来源上遏制浊毒的产生和传变。临床用于胃脘疼痛或胀满、口干口苦、恶心欲吐，或心烦焦躁，头身困重，纳呆，寐差等症。常用药物为黄连、黄柏、黄芩、栀子、龙胆草等，常用方剂为黄连解毒汤、葛根芩连汤等。

As long - time dampness will be coagulated into turbidity, long - time heat will generate toxin, so all linggering disease of damp and heat, can be converted to turbid toxin. Therefore, the method of heat - clearing, dampness eliminating can curb the generation and transmission of turbid toxin from the source of the disease. It is clinically used to treat epigastric pain or distension, dry and bitter mouth, nausea and vomitting, dysphoria and anxiety, fatigued and lazy in head and body, poor appetite and sleep and other diseases. Following drugs such as huang lian (Rhizoma Coptidis), huang bo (Cortex Phellodendri), huang qin (Radix Scutellariae), zhi zi (Fructus Gardeniae), long dan cao (Gentianae Radix et Rhizoma), etc. are commonly used. Prescriptions such as Huanglian Jiedu Decoction, Gegen Qinlian Decoction, etc. are generally used.

（五）以毒攻毒化浊法

1.5 Combat poison with poison and resolve turbidity

毒陷邪深，非攻不克，故常用有毒之品，借其性峻力猛以攻邪，即常用的"以毒攻毒法"。以毒攻毒之应用，应适可而止，衰其大半而止，要根据患者的体质状况和耐攻承受能力，把握用量、用法及用药时间，方能收到预期的效果。常用的药物有斑蝥、全蝎、水蛭、蜈蚣、蟾蜍、土鳖虫、守宫等。

When toxin evil sinks deep, it cannot be removed unless combating, so toxic medicines are commonly used to attack the evil by its powerful nature and acute strength, that is, the commonly used "combat poison with poison". The method of treating the virulent pathogen with poisonous agents should be stopped when most of the evil is eliminated. At the same time, to realize the expected medical effect, the dosage, usage and medication time should be decided according to the patient's physical condition and the ability to bear the attacking. Drugs commonly used are ban mao (Mylabris), quan xie (Scorpio), shui zhi (Herudo), wu gong (Scolopendra), chan chu (Bufo), tu bie chong (Eupolyphaga Steleophaga), shou gong (Gekko) and so on.

二、理气和胃法
2. Method to manage qi and harmonize the stomach

（一）行气法
2.1 The method of qi regulating

该法即通过理气、行气，使气机条达的治法。其主要用于气机不畅、气滞不行，致胃脘痞满、饭后尤甚、腹胀纳呆、大便不畅者。代表方为四磨饮、天台乌药散。

This method is a way of treatment to recover smooth operation of qi movement by regulating and moving qi. It is mainly used to treat epigastric ruffian full, especially after meals, abdominal distension, stool is not smooth due to unsmooth operation or stagnation of qi mechanism. Representative prescriptions include Simo Yin Decoction, Tiantai Wuyao Powder.

（二）疏肝法
2.2 Liver dispersing method

该法即通过解郁、理气使肝气条达，气机通畅的治法。其主要用于肝气不舒，横逆犯胃，致胃脘两胁攻撑者。代表方为柴胡疏肝散、逍遥散等。

The metnod is a treatment solution to harmonize the liver qi and smooth the operation of energy mechanism by resolving depression and regulating qi. It's mainly used for abnormal liver qi transverse stomach, causing epigastric distension in two lateral sides. The representative prescriptions are Chaihu Shugan Powder, Xiaoyao Powder, etc.

（三）降胃法
2.3 To downbear the counterflow and harmonize the stomach

该法即用顺气降逆的方药，以纠正胃气上逆的治法。代表方为橘皮竹茹汤、黄连苏叶汤。

This method is usually used to correct the counterflow of stomach qi by using prescription of unblocking the qi and correct the flow of gastric qi. The representative prescriptions are Jupi Zhuru Decoction and Huanglian Suye Decoction.

三、活血通络法
3. Promoting blood circulation and dredging collateral method

活血通络法即通过行血、活血、祛瘀使气血通畅的治法。主要用于血行不畅，脉络瘀阻所致诸瘀。代表方为膈下逐瘀汤、失笑散、丹参饮等。

The method of activating blood circulation and dredging collateral is to smooth and activate blood circulation and remove blood stasis to ensure the normal operation of breath and blood. It is mainly used to various stasis caused by poor blood flow and pulse obstruction. The representative prescriptions are Gexia Zhuyu Decoction (Decoction for Diaphragm Stasis Removing), Shixiao Powder (Powder for dissipating Blood Stasis), dan shen yin (Salivia Miltiorrhiza Juice), etc.

四、养阴益胃法
4. Nourishing the Yin and benefiting the stomach method

（一）养胃阴
4.1 Nourishing the stomach Yin

该法即通过养脾胃之阴，以恢复脾胃受纳、运化功能的治法。代表方为以益胃汤、甘露饮等。

It is a treatment method to restore the transporting and accepting function of spleen and stomach by nourishing the spleen and stomach Yin. The representative prescriptions are Yiwei Decoction (Decoction For Benefiting Stomach), Ganlu Yin Decoction , etc.

（二）柔肝法
4.2 Liver softening method

该法即通过滋养肝血、肝阴使升动无制的肝气、肝阳得到牵制的治法。其主要用于肝胃阴虚、肝血亏虚所致的眩晕，目赤，目涩而干，两胁胃脘隐痛，脉弦而细等症。代表方为一贯煎等。

It is the treatment method to restrain the ascending liver qi and function by nourishing liver blood, and liver Yin. It is mainly used for dizziness, astringent and dry eyes and hidden pain of epigastric and two lateral sides, string and thready pulse and other symptoms due to deficiency of liver, stomach Yin, and deficiency liver blood. The representative prescription is Yiguan Decoction.

五、健脾和胃法
5. Method to reinforce spleen and stomach

（一）健脾法
5.1 The spleen reinforcing method

该法即通过补益脾气，以恢复其运化的治法，包括补气健脾法、补气升陷法。代表方为四君子汤、香砂六君子汤、参苓白术散、补中益气汤等。

It is the way to restore the transporting function of spleen by tonifying spleen qi, including the method of tonifying qi to reinforce spleen, and the method to tonify qi and upraise the sunk. The representative prescriptions are Sijunzi Decoction, Xiangsha Liujunzi Decoction, Shenling Baizhu Decoction, Buzhong Yiqi Decoction (Decoction for Tonifying the Spleen and Stomach and Replenishing Qi), etc.

（二）和胃法
5.2 Stomach harmonizing method

该法即用消导食积的方药，消除气滞食积，以调和胃气的治法。其用于饮食积停聚中焦而生湿蕴热，症见脘腹痞满、嗳腐噫气、大便不畅。代表方为保和丸、枳实导滞丸等。

It is the way to eliminate qi stagnation and food accumulation to regulate the stomach qi by using prescriptions and medicines of promoting digestion and remove food stagnation. It is usually used to treat symptoms like abdominal ruffian full, fetic eructation and belching, difficult stool due to diet stagnation in middle energizer which generates dampness and heat. The representative prescriptions are Baohe Pill, Zhishi Daozhi Pill, etc.

六、敛酸制胃法
6. To constrain acid to harmonize the stomach

该法即通过用一些金石、动物类药以收敛胃酸的治法。其主要适用于反酸、呃逆等症，以乌贝散为代表方。

That is, to use some mineral stone, and animal drugs to constrain gastric acid. It is mainly used for acid reflux, hiccups and other diseases, with Wubei Powder as the representative prescription.

第五节　辨证治疗
Section 5　Treatment with Syndrome Differentiation

一、胃气壅滞证
1. Gastric qi obstruction syndrome

（一）证候
1.1 Symptoms

脘腹痞胀疼痛，痛而欲吐，或腹胀痛剧，肠鸣走窜不定，矢气频作，矢气后胀痛减轻，或胀痛剧而无肠鸣矢气，大便秘结，舌红，苔黄，脉弦。

Abdominal distentional pain, pain and vomiting, abdominal distention and abrupt pain, wandering gurgling, breaking wind frequently, swelling pain less severe after breaking wind, or abrupt distentional pain without wind-breaking, constipation, red tongue with yellow moss, string pulse.

（二）病机

1.2 Pathogenesis

浊蕴胃肠，气机阻滞。

Turbidity is accumulated in stomach and intestine, qi mechanism is blocked.

（三）治法

1.3 Method of treatment

理气和胃，降逆消痞。

Regulate qi and harmonize stomach, downbear counterflow and eliminate ruffian.

（四）常用药物

1.4 Medicines generally used

木香、枳实、厚朴、槟榔、炒莱菔子。

Mu xiang (Radix Aucklandiae), zhi shi (Fructus Aurantii Immaturus), hou po (Cortex Magnoliae Officinalis), bing lang (Arecae Semen), chao lai fu zi (fried Semen Raphani).

（五）加减运用

1.5 Addition and reduction principle

胃气上逆、食入则吐，加大黄、甘草；若伴胃脘疼痛，加延胡索、白芷；嗳气，加石菖蒲、郁金、紫苏叶、黄连；食积滞气、嗳腐吞酸，加鸡内金、焦三仙、茵陈；呃逆，加丁香、柿蒂。

Upward counterflow of gastric qi, vomiting samultaneously with eating, add da huang (Radix et Rhizoma Rhei), gan cao (Radix Glycyrrhizae); if accompanied by epigastric pain, add yan hu suo (Rhizoma Corydalis), bai zhi (Radix Angelicae Dahuricae); for belching, add shi chang pu (Rhizoma Acori Graminei), yu jin (Radix Curcumae), zi su ye (Folium Perillae), huang lian (Rhizoma Coptidis); for food accumulation and qi stagnation, fetic eructation and acid regurgitation, add ji nei jin (Endothlium Corneum Gigeriae Galli), jiao san xian (fried Hordei Fructus Germinatus, fried Massa Medicata Fermentata, fried Crataegi Fructus), yin chen (Cacuman Artemisiae Sccopariae); for hiccup, add ding xiang (lilac) and shi di (Calyx Kaki).

二、湿浊中阻证
2. Wet and turbidity resisted in middle energizer

（一）证候

2.1 Symptoms

胃脘隐痛或撑胀，胸闷，口中黏腻无味，恶心，纳呆食少，大便溏或大便不爽，肢体困重，舌暗红苔腻，脉濡或滑。

Epigastric vague pain or distension, chest distress, sticky and tasteless in mouth, nausea, anorexia, loose stool or difficult stool, tired and heavy limbs, dark red tongue with greasy moss, weak or slippery pulse.

（二）病机
2.2 Pathogenesis

湿浊内生，阻滞气机。

Wet and turbidity internally generated blocks the qi movement.

（三）治法
2.3 Method of treatment

除湿化浊，和胃消痞。

Remove dampness and resolve turbidity, and harmonize stomach and eliminate ruffian.

（四）常用药物
2.4 Medicines generally used

石菖蒲、郁金、茯苓、白术、茵陈、白豆蔻、砂仁、紫豆蔻、苍术。

Shi chang pu (Rhizoma Acori Graminei), yu jin (Radix Curcumae), fu ling (Poria), bai zhu (Rhizoma Atractylodis Macrocephalae), yin chen (Herba Artemisiae Scopariae), bai dou kou (Fructus Amomi Rotundus), sha ren (Fructus Amomi), zi dou kou (Purple Cardamom Kernel), cang zhu (Rhizoma Atractylodis).

（五）加减运用
2.5 Addition and reduction principle

胸骨后隐痛，痰多，恶心者加半夏、旋覆花、代赭石；烧心反酸者，加乌贼骨、瓦楞粉、煅龙骨、煅牡蛎；呕吐者加半夏、降香。

Patients with vague pain on the back of sternum, more phlegm, nausea, add ban xia (Rhizoma Pinelliae), xuan fu hua (Flos Inulae), dai zhe shi (Hematitum Seu Ochra); patients with symptom of heartburn and acid reflux, add wu zei gu (Os Sepiellae seu Sepiae), wa leng zi fen (Concha Arcae), duan long gu (Os Draconis) and duan mu li (Concha Ostreae); in case of vomiting, add ban xia (Rhizoma Pinelliae), jiang xiang (Ligum Dalbergiae Oderiferiae).

三、浊犯肝胃证
3. Turbidity attacking liver and stomach

（一）证候
3.1 Symptoms

胃脘胀满或胀痛，胁肋胀满，嗳气，泛酸，善太息，遇烦恼郁怒则症状加重，精神抑郁，寐差，大便不爽，舌红苔薄黄，脉弦滑。

Epigastric distensional fullness or pain, flank distension, belching, pantothenic acid, frequent sighing, more severe when involved in worry and stagnant anger, spiritual depression, poor sleep, difficult stool, red tongue with thin yellow moss, string and slippery pulse.

（二）病机
3.2 Pathogenesis

肝气不疏，肝胃不和。

Liver qi is not dispersed, liver and stomach discordant.

（三）治法
3.3 Method of treatment

疏肝理气，和胃消痞。

Disperse liver and regulate qi, harmonize stomach and eliminate ruffian.

（四）常用药物
3.4 Drugs generally used

柴胡、香附、青皮、荔枝核、佛手、白梅花、预知子、香橼。

Chai hu (Radix Bulpleuri), xiang fu (Rhizoma Cyperi) , qing pi (Pericarpium Citri Reticcutatae Viride), li zhi he (lychee core), fo shou (Fructus Citri Sarcodactylis), bai mei hua (Flos Mume), yu zhi zi (Fructus Akebiae), xiang yuan (Fructus Citron).

（五）加减运用
3.5 Addition and reduction principle

腹胀满加焦槟片、炒莱菔子、大腹皮；浊阻气机、脘痞苔腻，加茯苓、泽泻、石菖蒲；气郁化火、胃中灼热，加黄芩、黄连、生石膏；寐差加合欢皮、夜交藤。

For abdominal distension symptom, add jiao bing lang pian (burnt piece of Arecae), chao lai fu zi (fried Semen Raphani), da fu pi (Pericarpium Arecae); when turbidity blocks qi movement, epigastric ruffian occurs with greasy moss, add fu ling (Poria), ze xie (Rhizoma Alismatis), shi chang pu (Rhizoma Acori Graminei); When qi stagnation generates fire, stomach turns to be burning hot, add huang qin (Radix Scutellariae), huang lian (Rhizoma Coptidis) and sheng shi gao (Crude Gypsum Fibrosum); for patients with poor sleep, add he huan pi (Cortex Albiziae) and ye jiao teng (Caulis Polygoni Multiflori)..

四、浊毒内蕴证
4. Internal accumulation of turbid toxin

（一）证候
4.1 Symptoms

胃脘胀痛或灼痛，口干口苦，恶心呕吐，或牙龈肿痛，口舌生疮，或心烦不寐，纳呆，大便干燥或不爽或便溏，小便黄，舌红，苔黄厚或腻，脉弦滑或数。

Epigastric distensional pain or burning pain, dry and bitter in mouth, nausea and vomiting, or gingival swelling pain, oral sore, or upset and insomnia, anorexia, dry or difficult or loose stool, yellow urine, red tongue with yellow thick or greasy moss, string slippery or rapid pulse.

（二）病机

4.2 Pathogenesis

湿热中阻，浊毒内蕴。

Dampness and heat resisted in meddle energizer, turbid toxin internally accumulated.

（三）治法

4.3 Method of treatment

化浊解毒，和胃消痞。

To resolve turbidity and remove toxin, and harmonize stomach and eliminate ruffian.

（四）常用药物

4.4 Medicines generally used

黄芩、黄连、黄柏、蒲公英、生石膏、茵陈、藿香、佩兰。

Huang qin (Radix Scutellariae), huang lian (Rhizoma Coptidis), huang bo (Cortex Phellodendri), pu gong ying (Herba Taraxaci cum Radice), sheng shi gao (Crude Gypsum Fibrosum), yin chen (Herba Artemisiae Scopariae), huo xiang (Herba Agastaches seu Pogostemonis) and pei lan (Herba Eupatorii).

（五）加减运用

4.5 Addition and reduction principle

伴恶心加紫苏叶、黄连；伴肠化者，加半枝莲、半边莲、绞股蓝、薏苡仁、白英；伴不典型增生者，加三棱、莪术；伴幽门螺杆菌感染者，加蒲公英、虎杖、连翘、黄连等；心下痞者，加瓜蒌、黄连、半夏；胃黏膜充血水肿、有瘀血常加川芎、延胡索、三七以活血通络。

With nausea, add zi su ye (Folium Perillae), huang lian (Rhizoma Coptidis); Accompanied with intestinal metaplasia, add ban zhi lian (herba Portulacae Grabdiflorae), ban bian lian (Herba Lobaliae Radicantis), jiao gu lan (Gynostemma pentaphylia), yi yi ren (Semen Coisis), bai ying (Herba Solani Lyranti); accompanied with Atypical Hyperplasia, add san leng (Rhizoma Sparganii), e zhu (Rhizoma Curcumae); accompanied with Helicobacter pylori, add pu gong ying (Herba Taraxaci cum Radice), hu zhang (Rhizoma Polygoni Cuspidati), lian qiao (Fructus Forsythiae), huang lian (Rhizoma Coptidis); for patients with epigastric ruffian, add gua lou (Fructus Trichosanthis), huang lian (Rhizoma Coptidis), ban xia (Rhizoma Pinelliae); for patients with gastric mucosa congestion edema and blood stasis, add chuan xiong (Rhizoma Chuanxiong), yan hu suo (Rhizoma Corydalis), san qi (Radix Notoginseng) to promote blood circulation.

五、瘀血内结证
5. Internal stagnation of blood stasis

（一）证候
5.1 Symptoms

胃脘痛如针刺或如刀割，痛处不移，拒按，可痛彻胸背，肢冷汗出，可有呕血或黑便史，舌质暗红或紫暗，或见瘀斑，脉涩或沉弦。

Epigastric pain as severe as being needled or knife-cut, the pain is fixed, patient refuses to be pressed, the pain affects chest and back, makes limbs cold with sweating, might have a history of vomiting or black stool, dark red or purple dark tongue, perhaps with ecchymosis, astringent or sunk string pulse.

（二）病机
5.2 Pathogenesis

浊毒中阻，瘀血内结。

Obstruction of turbid toxin in middle energizer, internal stagnation of blood stasis.

（三）治法
5.3 Method of treatment

理气活血，化瘀消痞。

Regulate qi and promote blood circulation, resolve blood stasis and eliminate ruffians.

（四）常用药物
5.4 Medicines generally used

当归、川芎、延胡索、三七、蒲黄、五灵脂、姜黄、白芷、丹参、鸡血藤。

Dang gui (Radix Angelicae Sinensis), chuan xiong (Rhizoma Chuanxiong), yan hu suo (Rhizoma Corydalis), san qi (Radix Notoginseng), pu huang (Pollen Typhae), wu ling zhi (Faeces Trogopterorum), jiang huang (Rhizoma Curcumae Longae), bai zhi (Radix Angelicae Dahuricae), dan shen (Salviae Miltiorrhizae), ji xue teng (Caulis Spatholobi).

（五）加减运用
5.5 Addition and reduction principle

伴胃脘胀满气滞者，加柴胡、香附、木香；心血暗耗、虚火内浮所致眠差者，加酸枣仁；伴异型增生者，加三棱、莪术。

Accompanied with epigastric distention, fullness and qi stagnation, add chai hu (Radix Bulpleuri), xiang fu (Rhizoma Cyperi) , mu xiang (Radix Aucklandiae); poor sleep caused by blood consumption, deficient fire floating, add suan zao ren (Semen Zizyphi Jujubae); accompanied with Atypical Hyperplasia, add san leng (Rhizoma Sparganii), e zhu (Rhizoma Curcumae).

六、毒热伤阴证
6. Toxic heat injures Yin

（一）证候
6.1 Symptoms

胃脘隐痛不适，似饥而不欲食，口燥咽干，五心烦热，消瘦乏力，大便干结，舌红少津，苔少或花剥，脉弦细或细数。

Epigastric vague pain and discomfort, hungry but without desire to eat, dry mouth and throat, restless heat, emaciated and fatigue, dry stool, red tongue with less fluid, less or exploited tongue moss, string thready or thready rapid pulse.

（二）病机
6.2 Pathogenesis

毒热内结，耗伤胃阴。

Internal stagnation of toxic heat wastes and damages stomach Yin.

（三）治法
6.3 Method of treatment

滋养胃阴，和胃消痞。

To nourish the stomach Yin, and harmonize stomach to eliminate ruffian.

（四）常用药物
6.4 Medicines generally used

百合、乌药、沙参、麦冬、五味子、山萸肉、乌梅、玄参、玉竹、黄精。

Bai he (lily), wu yao (Radix Linderae), sha shen (Radix Adenophorrae Strictae), mai dong (Radix Ophiopogonis), wu wei zi (Fructus Schisandalis), shan yu rou (Corni Fructus), wu mei (Fructus Mume), xuan shen (Radix Scrophulariae), yu zhu (Rhizoma Poligonati Odorati), huang jing (Rhizoma Rolygonati).

（五）加减运用
6.5 Addition and reduction principle

伴胃中烧灼者，加生石膏、黄连；胃痛兼背痛，加沙参、威灵仙；伴胃酸缺乏者，加石斛；伴口干者，加天花粉；伴咽堵者，加射干、桔梗、板蓝根。

Accompanied with burning in stomach, add sheng shi gao (Crude Gypsum Fibrosum), and huang lian (Rhizoma Coptidis); stomach and back pain, add sha shen (Radix Adenophorae Strictae), wei ling xian (Radix Clematidis); lack of gastric acid, add shi hu (Dendrobium); with dry mouth, add tian hua fen (Radix Trichaosanthis); accompanied with congestion in throat, add she gan (Rhizoma Belamcandae), jie geng (Radix Platycodi), ban lan gen (Radix Isatidis).

七、脾胃虚弱证
7. The spleen and stomach weakness

（一）证候
7.1 Symptoms

胃脘隐痛，绵绵不断，空腹及劳累后尤甚，得食痛减，口泛清水，纳差，神疲乏力，大便溏，舌淡，苔白，脉细弱。

Epigastric vague lingering pain, even more severe when hungry and fatigue, the pain becomes less serious after eating, vomiting with lucid water, poor appetite, fatigue, loose stool, light tongue with white moss, weak thready pulse.

（二）病机
7.2 Pathogenesis

浊毒伤脾，脾胃虚弱。

Turbid toxin hurts the spleen, the spleen and stomach are weak.

（三）治法
7.3 Method of treatment

补气健脾，和胃消痞。

To tonify qi and reinforce spleen, harmonize stomach and eliminate ruffian.

（四）常用药物
7.4 Medicines generally used

党参、茯苓、白术、陈皮、白扁豆、山药。

Dang shen (Radix Codonopsitis Pilosulae),fu ling (Poria), bai zhu (Rhizoma Atractylodis Macrocephalae), chen pi (Pericarpium Citri Reticulatae), bai bian dou (Semen Dolichoris Album), shan yao (Tuber Dioscoreae).

（五）加减运用
7.5 Addition and reduction principle

脾阳不振、手足不温者，加附子、炮姜；气虚失运、满闷较重者，加木香、枳实、厚朴；气血两亏、心悸气短、神疲乏力、面色无华者，加太子参、五味子；脾胃虚寒者，加高良姜、荜茇。

When spleen Yang is not active, hands and feet are not warm, add fu zi (Radix Aconiti), pao jiang (prepared Ginger); for patients with heavier ruffian and distress, abnormal breath due to qi deficiency, add mu xiang (Radix Aucklandiae), zhi shi (Fructus Aurantii Immaturus), hou po (Cortex Magnoliae Officinalis); dual deficiency of qi and blood, palpitations with short breath, fatigue in mind and force, dull complexion, add tai zi shen (Radix Pseudostellariae), wu wei zi (Fructus Schisandalis); spleen and stomach deficiency and cold, add gao liang jiang (Rhizoma Aipiniae Officinari) and bi bo (Fructus Piperis Longi).

第四章 肝纤维化浊毒论
Chapter 4 On Turbid Toxin of Liver Fibrosis

第一节 病因病机
Section 1 Etiology and Pathogenesis

一、古代中医名家对肝纤维化的认识
1. The understanding of liver fibrosis by the ancient TCM masters

纵览古代医书，并无关于肝纤维化之名的论述，但是根据其临床表现特点，可将其归属于中医学的"胁痛""肝癖""臌胀""黄疸""肝积""肝著""腹痛""肝水""癥瘕""积聚"等范畴。其中对病因病机的认识，可谓百花齐放，各有芬芳。

In ancient medical books, there is no discussion on the name of liver fibrosis, but according to clinical manifestation, it can be attributed to the categories of "pain of lateral side of thorax", "liver addiction", "tympanities", "jaundice", "abnormal liver mass", "liver stagnation", "abdominal pain", "hepatic ascities", "abnormal abdominal mass" in traditional Chinese medicine. From the above, we can see the understanding of the etiology and pathogenesis are various like blossom of different kind of flowers with their own fragrance.

（一）先秦时期
1.1 Period of pre-Qin dynasty

先秦时期对肝纤维化的认识处于萌芽时期，虽然理论体系不完整，但其中蕴含的整体观以及运用阴阳、五行、六气、经脉学说指导药物、食物、艾灸等的治疗方法，对今天的临床诊治仍具有重要意义。如现存最早的医学专著马王堆汉墓帛书《足臂十一脉灸经》记载"足少阴脉……肝痛，心痛，烦心""臂少阴脉……其病胁痛""腹痛，腹胀……诸病此物者，皆灸足太阴脉"。《五十二病方》也有"瘠者，身热而数惊，颈脊强而腹大""蛊者，燔蝙蝠以荆薪，即以食邪者"的论述。这说明当时已经对其治疗方法进行了实践探讨。

The understanding of liver fibrosis in the pre-Qin period is in its embryonic period. Although the theoretical system is incomplete, the holistic view contained in it and the treatment methods of using Yin and Yang, five elements, six qi, meridian theory to guide the treatment by using drugs, food and moxibustion are still of great significance to present clinical diagnosis and treatment. For example, the extant earliest silk medical monograph found in Mawangdui Grave of Han dynasty *Eleven Meridian Moxibustion Treatments On Arms And Feet* says: "To moxibust Zushaoyin Meridian... can treat liver pain, heartache, upset", "Shoushaoyin Meridian... can treat lateral side pain", "diseases like abdominal pain, abdominal distension... can be treated by moxibusting Zushaoyin Meridian".The book *Prescriptions for Fifty-two Diseases* says: "Epileptic patient has the symptom of fever and repeated frightening, hard neck and abdominal distension", "Roundworm diseases can be treated by roasting bat with Herba Schizonepetae, that is, let the bat to eat the evil in patient's body". It shows that the treatment method had been discussed practically at that time.

（二）秦汉时期
1.2 In the Qin and Han dynasties

伴随着《黄帝内经》《难经》《神农本草经》《伤寒杂病论》四部中医经典的问世，这一时期中医学整体理论体系基本形成，对肝纤维化的认识也日趋深入。在疾病的治疗方面，调和阴阳为其必须遵循的治疗法则。因肝为阴脏，为阴中之阳，体阴而用阳；肝属厥阴，系于胆少阳，为阴阳之枢，故肝纤维化以调治阴阳枢机为特点。在具体治疗方面，张仲景首创辨证论治的诊疗体系，创立了诸如治疗血瘀肝络而致肝著的旋覆花汤、肝络瘀阻日久而致癥瘕（疟母）的鳖甲煎丸、虚寒侵入肝络而致疼痛的小建中汤、寒湿内蕴肝络的附子粳米汤、湿热蕴结肝胆而致黄疸的茵陈蒿汤等行之有效的良方。

With the publication of four classical Chinese Medical Works, including *The Medical Classic of the Yellow Emperor, Nan Jing (Classic of Questioning), Shennong's Classic of Materia Medica* and *Treaties on Febrile and Miscellaneous Diseases,* the overall theoretical system of traditional Chinese medicine was basically formed in this period, and the understanding of liver fibrosis became deeper. To reconcile Yin and Yang is the fundamental treatment principle which must be implemented in clinical practice. Because the liver is Yin (zang-organ), Yang in Yin, i.e. the Yang function of Yin organ; liver belongs to Jueyin Jing, and is closely related with gallbladder, Shaoyang Jing, which is the large articulation of Yin and Yang. So the characterisic of liver fibrosis treatment is to regulate the articulation of Yin and Yang, For the specific treatment, Zhang Zhongjing first created the syndrome differentiation treatment system, invented effective prescriptions as Xuanfuhua Decoction to treat blood stasis in liver which causes liver stagnation, Biejia Jian Pills to treat abnormal abdominal mass due to long-time liver stasis stagnation, Xiaojianzhong Decoction (Little Decoction for Reinforcing the Middle Energizer) to treat liver pain dueto deficiency and cold invasion, Fuzi Jingmi Decoction to treat internal accumulation of cold and dampness in liver collateral, and Yinchenhao Decoction to treat jaundice caused by damp and heat stagnation.

（三）魏晋时期至清代
1.3 From Wei and Jin dynasties to Qing dynasty

这一时期是对肝纤维化认识的成熟时期，这一时期的认识流派纷呈，百家争鸣。西晋王叔和认为肝病以胃气为要，与五脏相关，如在《脉经》中指出"胃者，土也，万物禀土而生，胃亦养五脏，故肝王以胃气为本也"。说明肝脏安和，有赖于后天之本脾胃的濡养。此外，《脉经·肝足厥阴经病证》言："病先发于肝者，头目眩，胁痛支满；一日之脾，闭塞不通，身痛体重；二日之胃，而腹胀；三日之肾，少腹腰脊痛。"指出肝纤维化病证循经脉演化，传变至脾胃肾。魏晋皇甫谧亦认为不同肝病合并肝纤维化发展演化及转归，病变常累及胃腑，如《针灸甲乙经·五脏大小六腑应候》言："肝小则安，无胁下之病；肝大则逼胃迫咽，迫咽则善膈中，且胁下痛；肝高则上支贲加胁下急，为息贲；肝下则逼胃，胁下空，空则易受邪。"

The understanding of liver fibrosis became gradually matured. In this period, various schools of understanding was established and each school tried to express its independent thought. Wang Shuhe of the Western Jin dynasty believed that liver disease is mainly affected by stomach qi and related to the five zang- organs. For example, he pointed out in the book of *Mai Jing (The Pulse Classic)* that "the stomach is the earth of human body, all things are born from the earth, and the stomach also nourishes the five zang- organs, so the liver king is based on stomach qi".It shows that the liver peace depends on the nourishment of the spleen and stomach. Besides, *Mai Jing (The Pulse Classic)- The Syndrome of Liver, Zu Jue Yin Jing* says: "Patients with the liver disease which is firstly generated in the liver meridian, usually feel vertiginous in head and eyes, with hypochondriac pain and limbs distension; on the first day, evil attacks spleen, patients feel obstructed in spleen, painful and heavy in body; on the second day, evil attacks stomach, patients feel abdominal distension; on the third day, evil attacks kidney, patients feel painful in lower abdomen and lumbar." It is pointed out that the liver fibrosis will evolute and be transmitted to spleen, stomach and kidney along with the meridian. Huang Fumi of Wei and Jin dynasty also believed that different liver diseases with liver fibrosis will develop and evolute, the lesions will often involve the stomach fu-organ, just as *Classic of Acupuncture and Moxibustion A and B-Treatment on Different Diseases in Five Zang-organs and Six Fu-organs says*: "If the liver is small, it is safe, no hypochondriac disease occurs; if liver is macromized, it will force throat to swallow, forced swallowing will cause dysphagia and hypochondriac pain; if the liver is at higher position,it will prop up the diaphragm and cause hypochondriac distress and distension, hypochondrium lumps occurs; if the liver is at lower position, it will press the stomach, causing hypochondriac empty,which is easy to be attacked by evil."

二、现代中医名家对肝纤维化的论述
2. The discussion of modern traditional Chinese medicine masters on liver fibrosis

现代医家继承了古代医家的理论思想，但又有创新之处，在对病因病机、辨证分型和治疗方面各有不同。在对肝纤维化的病因病机认识上，姚希贤认为气滞血瘀贯穿于肝纤维化的各个阶段，血瘀是肝纤维化病理过程的最终结局。刘绍能认为湿热疫毒是本病的始发因子和持续活动因素，正是由于湿热与疫毒胶着难祛，导致疾病的持续存在和慢性过程。吕志平认为湿热疫毒入侵与正气不足是慢性肝炎肝纤维化的主要病因，肝郁脾虚血瘀兼湿热是病机关键。可见，虽然对病因病机有不同的观点，但是可以肯定的是，在肝纤维化的初期，湿热疫毒和气机郁滞为主，而在肝纤维化的后期，血瘀与正气不足当为主要的病理过程。

Modern doctors inherit the theoretical thought of ancient doctors, but there are innovations including differences in the etiology, syndrome differentiation and treatment. In the understanding of the etiology of liver fibrosis, Yao Xixian believes that qi stagnation and blood stasis runs through all stages of liver fibrosis, and blood stasis is the final outcome of the pathological process of liver fibrosis. Liu Shaoneng believes that hot and humid epidemic virus is the initiating factor and the continuous active factor of the disease. Just because it is difficult to resolve the stalemate of hot and dampness and the epidemic virus, the liver fibrosis becomes lingering and chronic. Lv Zhiping believes that the invasion of dampness and heat epidemic virus and the deficiency of healthy qi are the main causes of chronic hepatitis liver fibrosis, liver depression, spleen deficiency, blood stasis and dampness and heat are the key pathogenic factors of the diseases. Although there are different views on the etiology and pathogenesis, it is certain that in the early stage of liver fibrosis, dampness and heat plague and qi stagnation are the main factors, while in the late stage of liver fibrosis, blood stasis and insufficient healthy qi mainly cover the pathological process.

可见，现代医家对肝纤维化的认识虽然有所不同，但其理论精髓基本一致。李佃贵教授结合自己的临床经验，创造性地提出了"浊毒"致肝纤维化的理论。其理论有专篇论述，此处不再赘述。

It can be seen that although modern doctors have different understandings of liver fibrosis, their theoretical essence is basically the same. Professor Li Diangui creatively put forward the theory that liver fibrosis is caused by "turbid toxin". As the theory has special discussion in this book, it will not be repeatedly discussed here.

三、基于浊毒理论对肝纤维化病因病机的认识
3. The understanding on the etiology of liver fibrosis according to the theory of turbid toxin

浊毒既可为外邪，亦可为内邪。作为外邪，由表侵入；作为内邪，由内而生。浊毒病邪作用于人体，循人体络脉体系由表入里，由局部至全身。浊毒之邪胶结，可导致人体细胞、组织和器官的浊化，即致病过程；浊化的结果导致细胞、组织和器官的浊变，即形态结构的改变，包括现代病理学中的肥大、增生、萎缩、化生和癌变，以及炎症、变性、凋亡和坏死等变化。浊变的结果是毒害细胞、组织和器官，使之代谢和功能失常，乃至功能衰竭。浊毒病邪入侵机体，克正气而致病；浊毒之邪猖獗，发病急重，或病情加重；浊毒之邪滞留不去，疾病迁延不愈；浊毒之邪被战胜克制，则疾病好转，机体得以康复。因此，浊毒病邪有轻、中、重相对量化的划分。

Turbid toxin can be both external evil and internal evil. As external evil, it invades human body from outside; as internal evil, it is generated from internal body. Turbid toxin evil invades human body following human system from the surface into the inside, from local area to the whole body. The stalemate of turbid toxin evil can corrupt human cells, tissues and organs, forming the pathogenic process. The result of corruption make the cells, tissues and organs transmit towards turbidity, i.e. change from form structure, including hypertrophy, hyperplasia, atrophy, metaplasia and carcinogenesis in modern pathology, as well as inflammation, degeneration, apoptosis and necrosis. The result of turbid transmission is to poison cells, tissues and organs, make their metabolism and function disorder, and even functional failure. The evil invades human body, restrict the healthy qi and causes disease; the evil of turbid toxin is rampant, causes urgent and serious disease, or worsen the disease. If the evil lingers, the disease will be delayed and difficult to recover. If the turbid toxin evil is defeated and resolved, the disease will take a favorable turn, the patient will recover. Therefore, there is a quantitative division of turbid toxin evil as light, medium and heavy.

浊毒证形成的内在因素，包括中气的虚实、阳气的盛衰、体质的强弱和内生湿浊的有无等。人体是否易患，内生浊毒起决定作用，而内生浊毒多责之于脾胃功能，如叶天士所言之湿热病，"又有酒客，里湿素盛，外邪入里，里湿为合"，即指出嗜食酒肉，影响脾胃运化而湿热内生，是湿热类温病发生的重要因素。后薛生白取叶氏之意，提出了"太阴内伤，湿饮停聚，客邪再至，内外相引，故病湿热"的观点。《医宗金鉴》云："人感受邪气虽一，因其形脏不同，或从寒化，或从热化，或从虚化，或从实化，故多端不齐也。"浊毒证的发展，有热化和寒化的不同，从而形成伤阴伤阳之病理机转，不同的病机转化与病邪、体质及治疗恰当与否密切相关。

The internal factors to generate turbid toxin include the sthenia and asthenia of the middle qi, the abundant and declining of Yang qi, the strength and weakness of the constitution and the presence of endogenous dampness and turbidity. Whether the human body is easy to be invaded by disease, endogenous turbid toxin plays a decisive role, and the generation of endogenous turbid toxin depend on the spleen and stomach function, just as Ye Tianshi's view when he described the disease of dampness and heat: "some wine drinkers who are endogenously wet usually, when external evil invades, it stagnates with the endogenous wet", taking-in of wine and meat affect the transporting of spleen and stomach, generates endogenous dampness and heat, is an important factor in the occurrence of warm disease in category of dampness and heat. Later, Xue Shengbai took the meaning of Ye Tianshi, and put forward the view of "When Taiyin (the spleen) has been internally injured, more wet drinking retained bring in guest evil again, interaction of the inside and outside evil, causes the disease of dampness and heat". *Goden Mirror of Medicine* says: "Although people feel almost the same evil, actually its shape and source is different, either transformed from cold, from heat, or from asthenia, or from sthenia, so it is not uniform." The development of turbid toxin syndrome has difference in heat transmission and cold transmission, thus forming the pathological tendency of injuring Yin or injuring Yang, which is closely related to the disease evil, constitution of patient and proper or improper treatment.

（一）外感淫疠毒邪

3.1 Exterior pathogenous pestilence and toxic evil

浊毒可由外而入，或从皮毛，或从口鼻，侵入机体，对人体脏腑、经络、气血、阴阳均能造成严重损害。"浊"者，不清也，浊与湿紧密相关，外感湿浊，由表入里。外界湿浊之邪侵入人体的途径大致有三条：一是通过呼吸由口鼻进入人体，先影响人体的上焦，进而影响到中、下焦。正如《医原·湿气论》所说："湿之化气，多从上受，邪自口鼻吸入，故先传天气，次及地气。"二是通过肌肉皮肤渗透进入人体，先客于肌表关节，次阻经络，最终深入脏腑。清代张璐说，"湿气积久，留滞关节"。《素问·调经论》曰："风雨之伤人也，先客于皮肤，传入于孙脉，孙脉满则传入于络脉，络脉满则输入于大经脉。"又曰："寒湿之中人也，皮肤不收，肌肉坚紧，荣血泣，卫气去，故曰虚。"三是湿邪中伤脾胃。

Turbid toxin can enter from the outside, either from the fur, or from the mouth and nose, invade the body, make severe damages to the human body viscera, meridians, qi and blood, Yin and Yang. "Turbid", not clear, turbidity and wet are closely related, external wet turbidity, from the surface into the inside. There are three ways for the evil of external damp turbidity to invade the human body: first, to enter the human body along with breath from the mouth and nose, which first affects the upper energizer of human body, and then affects the middle and lower energizer. As *Yi Yuan (Root of Medical Science)-Discussion on Moisture* says: "Dampness enters human body, mostly from the top, evil is absorbed with breath from the mouth and nose, so the weather enters first, the moisture of earth enters the second." Second, penetrates the muscle skin into the human body, first stays in the joint of muscle surface, then obstructs meridians, and finally invades deep into the viscera. Zhang Lu of Qing dynasty said: "Moisture accumulates for a long time, retains in the joint." *Simple Conversation-Discussion on Meridian Regulation* says: "Wind and rain hurt people, first in the skin, enters the fine collaterals, then transmits into the collaterals, when the collaterals are full, it will get into the large channels." It also says: "When cold and wet attacks people, the skin can not contract, muscles will be hard and tight. blood will be astringent, the defensive qi leaves away, so- called deficiency syndrome occurs"; third, dampness evil hurt the spleen and stomach.

（二）饮食失节

3.2 Uncontrolled Diet

《素问·脏气法时论》指出："五谷为养，五果为助，五畜为益，五菜为充，气味合而服之，以补精益气。"这就要求我们以植物性食物为主，动物性食物为辅，并配合果、蔬，使饮食性味柔和，不偏不倚，以保证机体阴阳平衡，气血充沛。然而，随着人们生活水平的不断提高，传统的饮食习惯已被打破，过去偶尔食之的鸡鸭鱼肉等副食品已经成为普通百姓的日常饮食，高热量、高蛋白、高脂肪的"西式快餐"被国人奉为美味佳肴，强食过饮现象非常普遍。而过食肥甘厚味，超出脾胃运化功能，则湿聚食积，化为痰饮，蕴郁日久，化为浊毒之邪。正所谓"肥者令人内热，甘者令人中满"（《素问·奇病论》），"多食浓厚，则痰湿俱生"（《医方论·消导之剂》）。

Simple Conversation-Zangqi Fashi Lun (Discussion on the Association of the Zang-Qi with the Four Seasons) points out: "Five kinds of grain are used to nourish the human body, five kinds of fruit are used to assist the nourishment, five kinds of livestock are used to improve the nourishment, five kinds of vegetable are used to enrich the nourishment, harmonic mixture of smells and tastes can to tonify the essence and benefit qi." It requires us to take plant food as main diet, animal food as assistant diet, fruit and vegetables as supplement, make the diet softly delicious, impartial, in order to ensure the balance of Yin and Yang, the abundance of qi and blood. However, with the continuous improvement of people's living standards, the traditional eating habits have been broken. Chicken, duck, fish and other non-staple foods which are seldom eaten in the past have become the daily diet of ordinary people. The "Western fast food" with high calories, high protein and high fat is regarded as delicious food by Chinese people, and the phenomenon of strong eating and over-drunk is very popular. Over-taken of fat and thick taste without considering the function and ability of spleen and stomach causes accumulation of dampness and food, with time going, the accumulation turns to be phlegmatic retention, then into the evil of turbid toxin. As the saying goes, "Fat food generates internal hot, sweet food generates abdominal fullness" (*Discussion on Special Diseases, Simple Conversation*), "More thick and fat food generates phlegm and dampness" (*The Agent of Elimination, Discussion on Prescriptions*).

（三）情志不畅

3.3 Unhealthy mood

《素问·八正神明论》说："血气者，人之神，不可不谨养。"神态是内在气血的总体体现，因此所谓"清静"，是指的人体精神状态的安详，是一个人内在脏腑气血功能正常的外在表现。人体在精神上能够长期保持清静，营卫之气运行有序，肌肉腠理的功能状态正常，表现为致密而柔顺，邪气难以进犯肌体，人体就不会得病。正所谓"正气存内，邪不可干"。

Simple Conversation-Bazheng Shenming Lun (Discussion on the Mysterious Influence of the Eight Directions on Acupuncture) says: "Vigor and vitality, as the spirit of man, must be nourished." Appearance is the overall embodiment of the internal qi and blood, so the so-called "quietness" refers to the serenity of the human mind, and is the external expression of the normal operation of a person's internal qi and blood and viscera. If a man can keep quiet in spirit for a long time, the nourishing and defensive qi runs in order, muscle and striae perform densely and softy, evil is difficult to invade the body, he will not get sick. As the saying goes, "When healthy qi is sufficiently stored inside, evil can not attack".

（四）环境改变

3.4 Environmental changes

《素问·宝命全形论》指出："人以天地之气生，四时之法成。"人只有顺应自然气候的变化规律才能保持健康。随着各种现代化的生活设施不断地介入人类的生活，人们不必再"动作以避寒，阴居以避暑"，悠然地生活在人工营造的舒适环境之中。即使夏季室外酷暑炎热，室内也可以冷气习习；冬季户外冰雪凛冽，屋内也可以暖气融融。人们出入于这样乍热乍凉，或乍寒乍暖，温度悬殊的环境，使肌体腠理汗孔骤开骤闭，卫外功能难以适应，久而久之，闭阻体内的浊气即可化为浊毒而致病。

Simple Conversation-Discussion on Preserving Health and Life points out: "Man exists depending on the energy of heaven and earth, grows up in accordance with the rules of four seasons." People can only keep healthy by conforming to the changing rules of natural climate. With variety of modern living facilities constantly intervene in human life, people leisurely live in the artificial comfortable environment, no longer need to "do exercises to get away coldness, live in shade place to escape form the hotness of summer". Even in specially hot summer, we can keep cool indoors; in terribly cold winter, the house can be filled with warm air. People are involved in such an environment with temperature changing abruptly from cool to hot, and from warm to cold, making the striae and sweat holes of human body suddenly open and suddenly close, the defensive function can hardly be adapted, with time going, the turbidity within the body will be turned into turbid toxin and diseases.

（五）运动缺乏

3.5 Lack of Exercises

《素问·宣明五气》云："久视伤血，久卧伤气，久坐伤肉。"若长年伏案，以车代步，室外活动减少，不仅可以导致气血亏虚，而且还可以使气机阻滞，津液运化、布散失常，从而浊毒之邪难免滋生。多食少动，对于浊毒体质的产生具有重要作用。颜元在《颜习斋言行录》中写道："习行、礼、乐、射、御之学，健人筋骨，和人气血，调人情绪，长人仁义……为其动生阴阳，下积痰郁气，安内抒外也。"这充分表明：体育运动既可强身健体，娱乐身心，磨炼意志，促进德智发展；又可防病治病，帮助身体早日康复。

Simple Conversation-Discussion on the Elucidation of Function of Five Storing Organs says: "Seeing for a long time impairs blood, lying for a long time impairs breath, sitting for a long time impairs flesh." If we sit at the desk year by year, tour by car instead of walking, with outdoor activities reduced, it will not only lead to deficiency of breath and blood, but also induce the obstruction of energy mechanism, disorder of fluid transmission and spreading, thus the evil of turbid toxin will inevitably breed. Eating more and moving less plays an important role in the production of turbid toxin constitution. Yan Yuan wrote in Words and Behavior Record of Yan Xi Zhai: "Learning and Practicing skills and arts like ritual, music, archery, horse-riding will strengthen people's muscles and bones, harmonize human breath and blood, regulate people's mind, increase people's benevolence and righteousness... because exercises produce Yin and Yang, unload accumulated phlegm and depressed mood, make peace inside and defend evil-attacking from outside." This fully shows that sports can strengthen human body, entertain the body and mind, temper the will, promote moral and intellectual development, and can prevent and cure diseases, and help recovering the patient as early as possible.

（六）虚损劳倦
3.6 Deficiency and fatigue

人体是否发病，主要取决于人体的正气强弱。"正气存内，邪不可干""邪之所凑，其气必虚"，是中医药贡献给人民大众的养生智慧。《灵枢·百病始生》说："风雨寒热不得虚，邪不能独伤人。卒然逢疾风暴雨而不病者，盖无虚，故邪不能独伤人。此必因虚邪之风，与其身形，两虚相得，乃客其形。两实相逢，众人肉坚。其中于虚邪，也因于天时，与其身形，参以虚实，大病乃成。气有定舍，因处为名。"

Whether the person will be attacked by diseases mainly depends on the strength of healthy qi in his body. "when (abundant) healthy qi exists inside, evil can not attack", "if evil can gather together in one's body, its healthy qi must be deficient", of this is the health nourishing wisdom contributed by traditional Chinese medical science to the people. Spiritual Pivot-The Occurrences of all Diseases says: "If the human body is not deficient, the evil of wind, rain, cold and heat itself can not hurt people. People who do not fall ill when they were suddenly involved in abrupt wind and hard rain, are not deficient, so evil can not hurt people itself. This is because when the wind of deficient evil come across deficient human body, the wind evil wins the attack, and stays as the guest of the body. But the evil of wind will fail the attack, if the human body is strong enough. The occurrence of serious disease of deficient evil is because the abnormal weather further weaken the deficient human body. The pathogenic evils retain in different region of the body, and are named according to the region they stays."

（七）他邪转化
3.7 The evil transformed from other evils

浊毒之邪为与内生五邪、外感六淫密切相关，又有不同。浊毒兼具浊与毒的特性，可以由他邪转化，且为诸邪致病之甚者也。如食积，本为伤食，食积日久则生湿聚痰，湿与痰即具浊之性，湿痰蕴积日久则生毒，至此浊毒生焉。浊毒生则导致胃病渐重，甚至癌变。饮食若超过自身耐受量，则可转化成浊毒。如过饮久饮为酒浊毒；过食为病之食积化浊毒；

大便干燥影响毒素排出，吸收毒素过多成粪毒；血糖、血脂过高形成糖浊毒、脂浊毒等。

The evil of turbid toxin is different from but closely related with endogenous five evil and external six evil. Turbid toxin with characteristics of both turbidity and toxin which can be transformed by other evils is more powerful to cause diseases than other evils. For example, food accumulation, originally is simply impairment of overeating, but accumulation of food for a long time produces wet and phlegm with characteristic of turbidity, stagnation of wet and phlegm over a long time produces toxin, so far turbidity and toxin arises. The arising of turbid toxin makes stomach disease gradually become more and more severe, or even develop to cancer. If the diet exceeds the tolerance of stomach, it will be converted into turbid toxin. Other examples such as turbid toxin of over drunk or long-time drinking of wine, turbid toxin of accumulated food, turbid toxin of excrement (some dry excrement absorb in instead of discharging excessive toxin finally turn to be excrement toxin); sugar toxin transformed from high blood glucose, grease toxin transformed from high blood fat.

第二节　治疗原则
Section 2　Principles of Treatment

在肝纤维化的治疗方面，总的治疗原则应以"调和阴阳"为主，恢复机体的"阴平阳秘"状态。在具体治疗上，根据患者表现的临床证型，选以不同的治法。李佃贵教授认为，肝纤维化的发生，其基本病机为浊毒内蕴，故其治则不离"调和阴阳"和"化浊解毒"。

In the treatment of liver fibrosis, the general treatment principle should be to "reconcile Yin and Yang", and restore the "dynamic balance of Yin and Yang" in the body. In the specific clinical practice, different treatment will choose according to the type of syndrome manifested by the patient. Professor Li Diangui believes that the basic pathogenesis of liver fibro is internal accumulation of turbid toxin, so the treatment is not far from the principle "to reconcile Yin and Yang" and "to resolve turbidity and remove toxin".

一、辨证与辨病相结合
1. Combination of syndrome differentiation and disease differentiation

只有将辨证与辨病很好地结合起来，才能从宏观上和微观上整体把握疾病的程度及发展变化趋势。由于个体差异和病机不同，将辨证与辨病结合起来，可以纵观全局，既了解疾病的情况，又了解辨证的依据，更好地指导治疗。

Only by combining syndrome differentiation and disease differentiation well can we grasp the degree and development trend of the disease from the macro and micro levels. Due to the individual differences in constitution and pathogenesis, the combination of syndrome differentiation and disease differentiation can review the whole situation, not only understand the disease, but also understand the basis of syndrome differentiation, and better guide the treatment.

二、基本原则
2. Basic principles

治疗肝纤维化的基本原则应是化浊解毒，祛邪扶正。参考先贤对于积的治法，如《医宗必读·积聚》曰："初者，病邪初起，正气尚强，邪气尚浅，则任受攻；中者，受病渐久，邪气较深，正气较弱，任受且攻且补；末者，病魔经久，受病渐久，邪气侵凌，正气消残，则任受补。"

The basic principles to treat liver fibrosis should be to resolve turbidity and remove toxin, dispel pathogenic qi and reinforce the healthy qi. Referring to the treatment principles of accumulation carried out by former generations, such as *Discussion on Accumulation, Necessary Reference For Doctors* says: "At first, the attack of evil starts only, healthy qi is still sufficient, pathogenic evil is weak, human body can bear attacking; in the middle period, human body suffers from the the disease for a long time, pathogenic evil is deep, healthy qi turns to be weak, patients need to be tonified as well as being attacked; at the end, the patient suffers from the disease for too long a time, disease, the pathogenic evil abuses, healthy qi is worn down, patients should be tonified."

第三节 常用治法
Section 3 The Common Treatment Method

根据肝纤维化的治则，结合患者的不同病情，确定不同的治疗方法。根据肝纤维化的临床分型，其具体治法包括化浊解毒法、以毒攻毒法、疏理气机法、活血化瘀法、化痰除湿法、清热利湿法、软坚散结法等。

According to the treatment of liver fibrosis, combined with the different conditions of the patients, the different treatment methods are determined. According to the clinical classification of liver fibrosis, the specific treatment methods include turbidity resolving and toxin removing method, fighting poison with poison method, regulating qi method, blood circulation promoting and blood stasis removing method, phlegm resolving and dampness eliminating method, heat clearing and dampness eliminating method, hardness softening and bind dissipating method, etc.

一、化浊解毒法
1. Method of turbidity resolving and toxin removing

化浊解毒法针对浊毒内蕴及其所致的肝纤维化。情志内伤或其他因素所导致的郁火、邪热郁结日久而成为浊毒，浊毒内蕴肝胆，导致气血瘀滞津停，凝结成块。浊毒内蕴与肝纤维化的发生、发展与转移有密切关系。化浊解毒法适应于肝纤维化兼有浊毒内蕴征象者。临床上常用化浊解毒药有漏芦、露蜂房、白花蛇舌草、山豆根、菝葜、泽漆、蜀羊泉、藤梨根、猫爪草、龙葵、白毛夏枯草、夏枯草、石打穿、红豆杉、半枝莲、半边莲、穿心莲、重楼、板蓝根、大青叶、虎杖、紫草、蒲公英、紫花地丁、黄连、黄芩、黄柏、苦参、龙胆草、土茯苓等。

The turbidity resolving and toxin removing method targets the internal accumulation of turbid toxin and the related result — liver fibrosis. The depression fire and evil heat caused by internal injury or other factors will become turbid toxin after a long - time stagnation. Turbid toxin retains in liver and gallbladder causes qi stagnation and blood stasis, which will condense into masses. The internal accumulation of turbid toxin is closely related with the occurrence, development and metastasis of liver fibrosis. The turbidity resolving and toxin removing method is adapted to liver fibrosis with signs of internal accumulation of turbid toxin. Drugs generally used to resolve turbidity and remove toxin in clinical practice are: lou lu (Radix Rhapontici seu Echinopsis), lu feng fang (Nidus Polistis), bai hua she she cao (Herba Oldenlandiae Diffusae), shan dou gen(Subprostrate Sophora), ba qia (Smilacis Chinae Rhizoma), ze qi (Herba Euphobiae Heliscopiae), shu yang quan (Solanum Lyratum Thunb), teng li gen (Radix Actinidae Chinensis), mao zhua cao (Radix Ranunculi Ternati), long kui (Herba Solani Nigri), bai mao xia ku cao (Herba Ajugae Decumbentis), xia ku cao (Spica Prunellae), shi da chuan (Herba Salviae Chinensis), hong dou shan (Taxus), ban zhi lian (Scutellariae Barbatae Herba), ban bian lian (Herba Lobeliae Chinensis), chuan xin lian (Herba seu Folium Andrographidis), chong lou (Rhizoma Paridis), ban lan gen (Radix Isatidis), da qing ye (Folium Isatidis), hu zhang (Rhizoma Polygoni Cuspidati), zi cao (Radix Arnebiae), pu gong ying (Herba Taraxaci cum Radice), zi hua di ding (Herba Violae), huang lian (Rhizoma Coptidis), huang qin (Radix Scutellariae), huang bo (Cortex Phellodendri), ku shen (Sophorae Flavescentis), long dan cao (Gentianae Radix et Rhizoma), tu fu ling (Rhizoma Smilacis Glabrae), etc.

二、以毒攻毒法
2. Method of fighting poison with poison

以毒攻毒法是指使用有毒之品、性峻力猛之药解除癌毒而抗癌的一种方法。如《素问·五常政大论》曰："大毒治病，十去其六，常毒治病，十去其七，小毒治病，十去其八，无毒治病，十去其九。"本法是针对肝纤维化深伏于内、凶险恶劣、非攻难克的特点而设立的。临床常用的以毒攻毒药有全蝎、蜈蚣、蟾皮、土鳖虫、炮山甲、独角蜣螂、露蜂房、半夏、马钱子等。

It indicates to use toxic products and powerful drugs to remove cancer toxin and fight against cancer. For example, *Simple Conversation-Major Discussion on the administration of Five-Motions* says: "To treat diseases with drugs of great toxin, 60% of the disease could be cured, to treat the disease with drugs of moderate toxin, 70% of the disease could be cured, to treat the disease with drugs of mild toxin, 80% of the disease could be cured, to treat the disease with non-toxic drugs, 90% of the disease could be cured." This method is set up regarding the deep-located, dangerous and nasty liver fibrosis which cannot be defeated unless attacking. Drugs generally used to attack toxic disease in clinical practice are: quan xie (Scorpio), wu gong (Scolopendra), chan pi (Cutis Bufonis), tu bie chong (Eupolyphaga Steleophaga), pao shan jia (prepared Squanma Manitis), du jiao qiang lang (Unicorn Catharsius), lu feng fang (Nidus Polistis), ban xia (Rhizoma Pinelliae), ma qian zi (Semen Strychni) and so on.

三、疏理气机法
3. Method of regulating qi

疏理气机法针对肝纤维化以气滞为主而设，对肝郁气滞、脾虚气滞较为合适。肝癌病位于肝胆，肝失疏泄，气机不畅则津液血液代谢运行障碍。气滞是肝纤维化发生发展过程中最基本的病理变化。其他病理因素如血瘀、湿阻、痰凝、湿热、热毒的生成与变化无不与气滞相关，故与气滞密切相连。因此，理气药在肝纤维化的治疗中贯穿全程，必不可少，至关重要。对肝癌，临床常用的理气药有柴胡、青皮、预知子、陈皮、枳壳、制香附、郁金、炒延胡索、川楝子、大腹皮、佛手、乌药、沉香、玫瑰花、九香虫、绿萼梅、厚朴、旋覆花等。

The method of regulating qi is mainly designed for liver fibrosis, which is more suitable for liver stagnation, qi stagnation and spleen deficiency and qi stagnation. Liver cancer is located in the liver and gallbladder, liver loss and drainage, qi is not smooth, body fluid blood metabolism dysfunction. Qi stagnation is the most basic pathological change in the development of liver fibrosis. Other pathological factors such as blood stasis, wet resistance, phlegm coagulation, dampness and heat, and heat poison are all related to qi stagnation, so they are closely related to qi stagnation.Therefore, it is essential and crucial for the treatment of liver fibrosis throughout the whole process of regulating qi medicine. For liver cancer, the commonly used clinical drugs are: chai hu (Radix Bulpleuri), qing pi (Pericarpium Citri Reticcutatae Viride), yu zhi zi (Fructus Akebiae), chen pi (Pericarpium Citri Reticulatae), zhi qiao (Fructus Aurantii), zhi xiang fu (prepared Rhizoma Cyperi) , yu jin (Radix Curcumae), chao yan hu suo (fried Rhizoma Corydalis), chuan lian zi (Fructus Toosendan), da fu pi (Pericarpium Arecae), fo shou (Fructus Citri Sarcodactylis), wu yao (Radix Linderae), chen xiang (Lignum Aquilariae Resinatum), mei gui hua (Rosae Rugosae Flos), jiu xiang chong (Aspongopus), lv e mei (Green Calyx Plum), hou po (Cortex Magnoliae Officinalis), xuan fu hua (Flos Inulae), etc.

四、活血化瘀法
4. Method of activating blood circulation and removing blood stasis

活血化瘀法是针对肝纤维化以瘀血为著而设。历代医家皆重视瘀血与有形结块的关系。如王清任在《医林改错》中说："肚腹结块，必有形之血。"肝癌与古称"癥"互参，其形成的病理机制与瘀血凝滞有密切关系，因为瘀血停滞、气行不畅、气滞血瘀经久不散。对于肝癌的治疗，临床上常用的活血化瘀药有当归尾、赤芍、川芎、丹参、莪术、郁金、虻虫、水蛭、水红花子、红花、石见穿、乳香、没药、炮山甲、全蝎、蜈蚣、血竭、老鹳草、土鳖虫、九香虫、王不留行、大黄等。

The method is mainly used to treat liver fibrosis with the characteristic of blood stasis. Doctors in former generations attached great importance to the relationship between blood stasis and tangible lumps.For example, Wang Qingren said in *Errors Correction In Medical Classics*: "Belly lump must be caused by tangible blood." Liver cancer is similar to so-called "lump" in ancient TCM. The pathological mechanism has close relationship with blood stasis stagnation, because blood stasis is stagnated, qi flow is blocked, qi stagnation and blood stasis linger year in and year out. Drugs generally used for activating blood circulation and removing blood stasis in liver cancer treatment are: dang gui wei (Radix

Angelicae Sinensis), chi shao (Radix Paeoniae Rubra), chuan xiong (Rhizoma Chuanxiong), dan shen (Salviae Miltiorrhizae), e zhu (Rhizoma Curcumae), yu jin (Radix Curcumae), meng chong (Tabanus Bivittatus), shui zhi (Herudo), shui hong hua zi (Fructus Polygoni Orientalis), hong hua (Flos Carthami), shi jian chuan (Herba Salviae Chinensis), ru xiang (Resina Boswelliae Carterii seu Masticis), mo yao (Resina Commiphorae Myrrhae), pao shan jia (prepared Squanma Manitis), quan xie (Scorpio), wu gong (Scolopendra), xue jie (Resina Draconis), lao guan cao (Erodii Herba), tu bie chong (Eupolyphaga Steleophaga), jiu xiang chong (Aspongopus), wang bu liu xing (Semen Vaccariae), da huang (Radix et Rhizoma Rhei), etc.

五、化痰除湿法
5. Method of phlegm resolving and dampness eliminating

朱丹溪曾曰："凡人身上中下有块者，多是痰。"痰凝湿聚是致使肝纤维化形成的基本病理之一，化痰除湿法正是针对痰湿这个病理因素而设立的。化痰除湿不仅对因，而且可以减轻临床症状，使肝癌发展转移得以控制。在肝纤维化的治疗中，常用的化痰除湿药物有泽漆、山慈菇、茯苓、猪苓、泽泻、车前子、薏苡仁、木防己、大贝母、皂角刺、半夏、葶苈子、苍术、厚朴、藿香、佩兰、蚕砂、煨草果等。

Zhu Danxi once said: "Masses or lumps in any of the triple energizers of human body, most probably are phlegm disease." Phlegm condensation and dampness aggregation is one of the basic pathologies resulting in the formation of liver fibrosis, phlegm resolving and dampness eliminating method is established precisely for the pathological factor of phlegm and dampness. This method can not only eliminate the disease cause, but also reduce clinical symptoms, so that the development of liver cancer metastasis can be controlled. In the treatment of liver fibrosis, drugs generally used to resolve phlegm and eliminate dampness are: ze qi (Herba Euphorbiae Heliscopiae), shan ci gu (Pseudobulbus Cremastrae Variabilis), fu ling (Poria), zhu ling (Polygorus Umbellatus), ze xie (Rhizoma Alismatis), che qian zi (Semen Plantaginis), yi yi ren (Semen Coisis), mu fang ji (Radix Cocculi Trilobi), da bei mu (Fritillaria Thunnbergii), zao jiao ci (Spina Gleditsiae), ban xia (Rhizoma Pinelliae), ting li zi (Semen Lepdii seu Descurainiae), cang zhu (Rhizoma Atractylodis), hou po (Cortex Magnoliae Officinalis), huo xiang (Herba Agastaches seu Pogostemonis), pei lan (Herba Eupatorii), can sha (Faeces Bombycis), wei cao guo (simmered Fructus Tsaoko), and so on.

六、清热利湿法
6. Method of heat clearing and dampness eliminating

湿热亦是致使肝纤维化形成的基本病理之一。清热利湿法是针对湿热毒邪，或湿浊蕴而化热成毒设立的。因肝胆、脾胃位于中焦，湿热蕴结极为常见。本法可缓解临床症状，改善实验室指标，保护肝功能，部分药物具有直接抑制、杀伤肝癌细胞的作用。故肝癌治疗使用清热利湿法具有重要意义。在肝癌治疗中，常用的清热化湿药有黄连、黄芩、黄柏、夏枯草、田基黄、茵陈、垂盆草、苦参、虎杖、凤尾草、鸡骨草、酢浆草、白鲜皮、地肤子、金钱草、海金沙等。

Dampness and heat is also one of the basic pathologies of liver fibrosis. The method of clearing heat and eliminating dampness is established to treat dampness and heat toxic evil, or accumulated dampness and turbidity transmitted into heat and toxin. Because the liver and gallbladder, spleen and stomach are located in the middle energizer, accumulation and stagnation of dampness and heat is very common. This method can alleviate clinical symptoms, improve laboratory indicators, and protect liver function. Some drugs can directly inhibit and kill liver cancer cells. Therefore, it is of great significance to treat liver cancer with heat clearing and dampness eliminating method. In the treatment of liver cancer, drugs generally used to clear heat and disinhibit dampness are: huang lian (Rhizoma Coptidis), huang qin (Radix Scutellariae), huang bo (Cortex Phellodendri), xia ku cao (Spica Prunellae), tian ji huang (Grangea Maderaspatana), yin chen (Cacumen Artemistae Scopariae), chui pen cao (herba Sedi Sarmentosi), ku shen (Sophorae Flavescentis Radix), hu zhang (Rhizoma Polygoni Cuspidati), feng wei cao (Herba Pterdis Multifidae), ji gu cao (Herba Abri), cu jiang cao (Oxalis Corniculata), bai xian pi (Cortex Dictamni Radicis), di fu zi (Kochiae Fructus), jin qian cao (Herba Lysmachiae), hai jin sha (Herba Lygodii) and so on.

七、软坚散结法
7. Method of hardness softening and mass dissipating

软坚散结法是针对肝纤维化结块坚硬所设，是使用软坚散结药物使肿块软化、缩小、消散的治疗方法。味咸中药能够软化坚块，如鳖甲的咸平、龟甲的甘咸、海螵蛸的咸涩、海浮石的咸寒等都有软坚作用。散结则常通过治疗产生聚结的病因而达到散结的目的，如清热散结药治热结，理气散结药治气结，化瘀散结药治瘀结等。在治疗肝纤维化时常用的软坚散结类药物有龟甲、鳖甲、牡蛎、海浮石、海藻、瓦楞子、昆布、海蛤壳、夏枯草、穿山甲、地龙、白芥子、半夏、胆南星、瓜蒌、天葵子、山慈菇等。

The method is set up to treat the hard lump of the liver fibrosis, to soften, shrink and dissipate the mass by using hardness softening and bind dissipating drugs. According to TCM, salty drugs can soften the hard lumps, such as the mild salty of the turtle nail, the sweet salty of the turtle plate, the astringent salty of the octopus, the salty coldness of the pumstone have the function of soften hard lumps. Mass dissipating indicates to achieves the purpose of mass dissipating through resolving the cause of polyknot, for example, to treat heat bind with heat clearing and bind dispersing medicine, to treat qi bind with qi regulating and bind dispersing medicine, to treat stasis bind with blood stasis resolving and bind dispersing medicine, etc. In the treatment of liver fibrosis, drugs generally used to soften hardness and dissipating mass are: gui jia (Plastrum Testudinis), bie jia (Carapax Trionycis seu Amydae), mu li (Ostreae), hai fu shi (Os Costaziae), hai zao (Herba Sargassi), wa leng zi (Choncha Arcae), kun bu (Thallus Laminariae seu Eckloniae), hai ge qiao (Concha Cyclinae), xia ku cao (Spica Prunellae), chuan shan jia (Squanma Manitis), di long (Lumbricus), bai jie zi (Semen Sinapis Albae), ban xia (Rhizoma Pinelliae), dan nan xing (Arisaema Cum Bile), gua lou (Trichosanthis Fructus), tian kui zi (Semiaquilegiae Radix), shan ci gu (Pseudobulbus Cremastrae Variabilis) and so on.

第四节　辨证治疗
Section 4　Treatment with Syndrome Differentiation

肝纤维化并不是一种独立的病症，而是由肝脏原发病引起肝内结缔组织异常增生，导致肝内弥散性细胞外基质过度沉淀的病理过程，可以说是肝硬化的前奏，是可以治愈的肝病。但像一些患有肝炎、酒精肝、药物与毒物肝病、血吸虫病、代谢和遗传病、胆汁淤积、自身免疫性肝病等的患者，如果对此放松警惕，就会转化为肝硬化而难以治愈。肝纤维化的基本证候病机为正虚血瘀。但在肝纤维化病变的不同阶段、不同患者，可表现为不同的证候类型，在辨证治疗时，应病证结合，基本治法与辨证论治结合灵活运用。

Liver fibrosis is not an independent disease, but a pathogenic process in which connective tissue dysplasia caused by the primary disease of the liver leads to excessive precipitation of disseminated extracellular matrix in the liver, it can be said to be the prelude to liver cirrhosis, is a curable liver disease. But some patients with hepatitis, alcoholic liver, drug and toxic liver disease, schistosomiasis, metabolic and genetic diseases, cholestasis, autoimmune liver disease, if they relax their vigilance, will turn into cirrhosis and difficult to be cured. The basic syndrome of liver fibrosis is deficiency of healthy qi and blood stasis. However, different patients, in different stages of liver fibrosis lesions manifest different types of syndrome, disease and syndrome should be considered simultaneously, basic treatment method and syndrome differentiation should be combined flexibly in clinical practice.

一、基本病机与基本治法
1. Basic pathogenesis and basic treatment method

基本病机为正虚血瘀，正虚主要表现为气阴两虚，血瘀则主要表现为瘀血阻络。其基本证型为气阴虚损，瘀血阻络。典型表现有疲倦乏力、食欲缺乏、大便异常、肝区不适或胀或痛、面色晦暗、舌质暗红、舌下静脉曲张、脉弦细等。基本治法为益气养阴、活血化瘀。益气药可选用黄芪、白术、炙甘草等；养阴药可选用生地黄、沙参、麦冬、白芍等；活血化瘀药可选用丹参、桃仁、当归、赤芍、川芎等。

The basic pathogenesis is deficiency of healthy qi and blood stasis. Healthy qi deficiency is mainly manifested by qi and Yin deficiency. Blood stasis is mainly manifested by blood stasis resist the collaterals. Its basic syndrome classification is qi and Yin deficient loss, blood stasis resists. Typical manifestations are fatigue, poor appetite, abnormal stool, liver discomfort either distension or pain, dark complexion, dark red tongue, sublingual varicosis, string thready pulse and so on. The basic treatment method is to replenish qi and nourish Yin, to promote blood circulation and resolve blood stasis. Medicines for replenishing qi are: huang qi (Radix Astragali seu Hedysari), bai zhu (Rhizoma Atractylodis Macrocephalae), zhi gan cao (fried Radix Glycyrrhizae). Medicines for yin nourishing are: sheng di huang (Radix Rehmanniae), sha shen (Radix Adenophorae Strictae), mai dong (Radix Ophiopogonis), and bai shao (Radix Paeoniae Alba). Medicines for promoting blood circulation and resolving blood stasis are: dan shen (Salviae Miltiorrhizae), tao ren (Semen Persicae), dang gui (Radix Angelicae Sinensis), chi shao (Radix Paeoniae Rubra), chuan xiong (Rhizoma Chuanxiong).

二、主要证型与治法方药
2. The main syndrome classification, treatment method, prescription and drugs

在治疗方面，在中医的整体观和辨证施治原则指导下立足化浊解毒，科学运用中医理论，辨病与辨证结合，宏观与微观结合，综合全身整体调理，采用化浊解毒为大法，兼疏肝理气、活血化瘀、软坚散结、养肝和胃等治疗方法。

Under the guidance of the holistic view and therapy syndrome differentiation of TCM, based on turbidity resolving and toxin removing, scientifically using TCM theory, combining disease differentiation, syndrome differentiation, macro and micro, treatment is made comprehensively according to the constitution of the patient, using turbidity resolving and toxin removing method, and the method of liver dispersing and qi regulating, method of blood circulation promoting and blood stasis resolving, method of hardness softening and mass dissipating, method of liver nourishing and stomach harmonizing.

（一）浊毒内蕴
2.1 Internal accumulation of turbid toxin

1.主要症状 胁肋胀痛或灼热疼痛，腹胀如鼓，胸闷纳呆，口渴而苦，小便黄赤，大便不爽，舌质红，苔黄燥，脉弦数。

2.1.1 Main symptoms Hypochondrium distending pain or burning pain, abdominal distension, chest distress with anorexia, thirsty and bitter in mouth, yellow urine, difficult stool, red tongue with yellow and dry moss, string rapid pulse.

2.病机 由于脾胃虚弱，肝气不疏肝，木克脾土，脾失健运，湿浊内生，浊邪内蕴，日久化热成毒，浊毒使气、血、水搏结，水湿内停，肝络瘀阻，肝体失养，硬结变性。

2.1.2 Pathogenesis As the spleen and stomach are weak, liver qi cannot be dispersed, wood (liver) restricts spleen soil, spleen looses the normal function of transporting, wet and turbidity is generated endogenously, internal accumulation of turbidity evil is transmitted into heat and then toxin over time, turbid toxin makes qi, blood, water condensed, water dampness retain, liver collateral blocked by stasis, liver is short of nourishment, degeneration of induration occurs.

3.治则 化浊解毒，软肝化坚。

2.1.3 Treatment principles Turbidity resolving and toxin removing, liver softening and hardness resolving.

4.方药 化浊解毒软肝方。药用白花蛇舌草，半枝莲，半边莲，茵陈，板蓝根，苦参，黄芩，黄连，栀子，黄柏，猪苓，茯苓，白术，泽泻，陈皮，木香，车前子，泽兰，甘鳖甲，山甲珠。

2.1.4 Prescriptions and drugs Prescriptions of turbidity resolving and toxin removing and preccription of liver softening. Medicines: bai hua she she cao (Herba Oldenlandiae Diffusae), ban zhi lian (Scutellariae Barbatae Herba), ban bian lian (Herba Lobeliae Radicantis), yin chen (Herba Artemisiae Scophriae), ban lan gen (Radix Isatidis), ku shen (Sophorae Flavescentis Radix), huang qin (Radix Scutellariae), huang lian (Rhizoma Coptidis), zhi zi (Fructus Gardeniae), huang bo (Cortex

Phellodendri), zhu ling (Polygorus Umbellatus), fu ling (Poria), bai zhu (Rhizoma Atractylodis Macrocephalae), ze xie (Rhizoma Alismatis), chen pi (Pericarpium Citri Reticulatae), mu xiang (Radix Aucklandiae), che qian zi (Semen Plantaginis), ze lan (Herba Lycopi), gan bie jia (Carapax Tronysis), shan jia zhu (Carapace Bead).

5.加减　肝功能异常者，常选用龙胆草、五味子、垂盆草保肝降酶。

2.1.5 Addition and reduction principles　Patients with abnormal liver function, long dan cao (Gentianae Radix et Rhizoma), wu wei zi (Fructus Schisandalis) and chui pen cao (Herba Sedi Sarmentosi) are often used to protect liver and descend transaminase.

（二）痰瘀互结

2.2 Binding of phlegm and blood stasis

1.主要症状　身困体倦，头晕眼花，两胁隐痛，肌肤甲错，食少便溏，胁肋下或见癥块，舌质淡紫有瘀斑，脉滑数。

2.2.1 Main symptoms　Fatigue, dizziness, hypochondrium vague pain, scaly skin, poor appetite and loose stool, abnormal hypochondrium mass, pale purple tongue with ecchymosis, slippery rapid pulse.

2.病机　由于体内邪毒内侵，阻滞肝络，化热灼津，脾不运化，水湿成痰，气滞血瘀而致。

2.2.2 Pathogenesis　As the toxin evil invades in the body, blocks the liver collateral, transmits into heat and hurt the fluid, spleen does not transport, water and dampness turns to be phlegm, qi stagnation and blood stasis causes the binding of phlegm and stasis.

3.治则　健脾化痰，活血祛瘀。

2.2.3 Treatment principles　To invigorate the spleen and reduce phlegm, promote blood circulation and remove blood stasis.

4.方药　二陈汤合四物汤加减。药用陈皮，半夏，茯苓，当归，川芎，赤芍，生地黄，红景天，桃仁，红花，甘草。

2.2.4 Prescriptions and drugs　Addition and reduction on the basis of Er chen Decoction and Siwu Decoction combination. Medicines: chen pi (Pericarpium Citri Reticulatae), ban xia (Rhizoma Pinelliae), fu ling (Poria), dang gui (Radix Angelicae Sinensis), chuan xiong (Rhizoma Chuanxiong), chi shao (Radix Paeoniae Rubra), sheng di huang (Radix Rehmanniae), hong jing tian (Rhodiolae Crenulatae Radix et Rhizoma), tao ren (Semen Persicae), hong hua (Flos Carthami), gan cao (Radix Glycyrrhizae).

（三）肝肾阴虚

2.3 Liver and kidney Yin deficiency

1.主要症状　面色黧黑，胁肋隐痛，口干咽燥，潮热盗汗，心烦易怒，失眠多梦，悠悠不休，头晕目眩，舌红少苔，脉细弦而数。

2.3.1 Main symptoms　Dark complexion, hypochondrium vague pain, dry mouth and throat, hectic fever with night sweating, irritability, insomnia, more dreams in a trance, dizziness, red tongue with less moss, thready string rapid pulse.

2.病机　由于肝肾同源，肝病日久，势必伤及肾脏，耗伤阴液，是肾阴亏虚而致。

2.3.2 Pathogenesis　As liver and kidney are homology, long-time liver disease will surely hurt the kidney and consume Yin fluid, leading to kidney Yin deficiency.

3.治则　养肝肾，育阴清热。

2.3.3 Treatment principles　Nourishing the liver and kidney, nourishing Yin and clearing heat.

4.方药　一贯煎加减。药用沙参，麦冬，生地黄，枸杞子，川楝子，白蒺藜，牡丹皮，栀子，知母，黄柏，赤芍，甘草。

2.3.4 Prescriptions and drugs　Addition and reduction on the basis of Yiguan Decoction. Medicines: sha shen (Radix Adenophorae Strictae), mai dong (Radix Ophiopogonis), sheng di huang (Radix Rehmanniae), gou qi zi (Lycii Fructus), chuan lian zi (Fructus Toosendan), bai ji li (Fructus Tribuli), mu dan pi (Cortex Moutan), zhi zi (Fructus Gardeniae), zhi mu (Rhizoma Anemarrhennae), huang bo (Cortex Phellodendri), chi shao (Radix Paeoniae Rubra), gan cao (Radix Glycyrrhizae).

（四）肝脾阳虚
2.4 Liver, spleen and Yang deficiency

1.主要症状　两胁胀痛，胸腹满闷，嗳气纳差，畏寒肢冷，倦怠乏力，面色萎黄，大便溏薄，脉弦细，舌质淡，苔黄。

2.4.1 Main symptoms　Hypochondrium distension pain, chest and abdominal fullness and distress, belching, poor appetite, fear of cold with cold limbs, fatigue, fading yellow complexion, thin and loose stool, string thready pulse, light tongue with yellow moss.

2.病机　由于肝主疏泄，脾主运化，功能失职，木横克土，致水湿停滞，气机不畅而致。

2.4.2 Pathogenesis　Liver controls dispersing, spleen controls transporting, when liver and spleen dysfunctions, wood restricts soil, causes water dampness stagnation and the abnormal operation of qi movement.

3.治则　疏肝健脾，温阳利湿。

2.4.3 Treatment principles　To disperse liver and reinforce spleen, warm Yang and diminish wet.

4.方药　柴胡疏肝散。药用柴胡，白芍，枳壳，白术，香附，川芎，厚朴，茯苓，桂枝，干姜，甘草。

2.4.4 Prescriptions and drugs　Chaihu Shugan Powder. Medicines: chai hu (Radix Bulpleuri), bai shao (Radix Paeoniae Alba), zhi qiao (Fructus Aurantii), bai zhu (Rhizoma Atractylodis Macrocephalae), xiang fu (Rhizoma Cyperi) , chuan xiong (Rhizoma Chuanxiong), hou po (Cortex Magnoliae Officinalis), fu ling (Poria), gui zhi (Cmnamomi Mmulus), gan jiang (Zingiberis Rhizomar), gan cao (Radix Glycyrrhizae).

第五章　胃癌浊毒论
Chapter 5　On Turbid Toxin of Gastric Cancer

第一节　病因病机
Section 1　Etiology and Pathogenesis

一、古代医家对本病的认识
1. The ancient medical understanding of this disease

中医学虽无胃癌的名称，但根据胃癌的临床表现，可归属于"胃脘痛""反胃""噎膈""伏梁""癥瘕积聚"等范畴。其最早记载，可追溯到《黄帝内经》。如《素问》指出："胃脘当心而痛，上支两胁，甚则呕吐，膈咽不通。"《难经》云："心之积名曰伏梁，起脐上，大如臂，上至心下，久不愈，令人病烦心。"《金匮要略》曰："朝食暮吐，暮食朝吐，宿谷不化，名曰反胃。"这些都类似于胃癌症状的描述。

Although there is no "gastric cancer" in TCM vocabulary, according to the clinical manifestations of gastric cancer, it can be attributed to "epigastric pain", "stomach nausea", "choking", "diaphragm" and "accumulation of lump". The earliest record can be traced back to *The Medical Classic Of the Yellow Emperor*. For example, *Simple Conversation* points out: "Epigastric pain affects hypochondrium, even causes vomiting, diaphragmatic pharynx." *Nan Jing (Classic of Questioning)* says: "Abdominal mass is called fu liang, over the umbilical cord, as big as the diameter of arms, up to the heart. It can not be cured for a long time which makes people vexed." *Synopsis of Golden Chamber* says: "When patients eat in the morning, vomit in the evening, or eat in the evening, vomit in the morning, dyspepsia fails to be digested, we call it dysphagia." These are all similar symptoms to describe gastric cancer.

历代医家有较多发挥。清代吴谦等著《医宗金鉴》中记载："三阳热结，谓胃、小肠、大肠三腑热结不散，灼伤津液也。胃之上口为贲门，小肠之上口为幽门，大肠之下口为魄门。三腑津液既伤，三门自然干枯，而水谷出入之道不得流通矣。贲门干枯，则纳入水谷之道路狭隘，故食不能下，为噎塞也。幽门干枯，则放出腐化之道路狭隘，故食入反出为翻胃也。二证留连日久，则大肠传导之路狭隘，故魄门自应燥涩难行也。胸痛如刺，胃脘伤也。便如羊粪，津液枯也。吐沫呕血，血液不行，皆死证也。"很像胃癌贲门梗阻、幽门梗阻产生的症状和晚期的证候及不良预后。在病因病机上，隋代《诸病源候论》云："荣卫俱虚，其血气不足，停水积饮，在胃脘则脏冷，脏冷则脾不磨，脾不磨则宿谷不化，其气逆而成胃反也。"明代《景岳全书》指出："（反胃）或以酷饮无度，伤于酒湿，或以纵食生冷败其真阳，或因七情郁竭中气，总之无非内伤之甚，致损胃气而然。"在治疗方面，《景岳全书》曰："治反胃之法……必宜以扶助正气，健脾养胃为主。"历代医家对胃癌的预后也有所认识。《石室秘录》曰："反胃之证，虽一时不能遽死，然治之不得其宜，亦必死而后已。"

Doctors in different dynasties have provided further more descriptions. In the Qing dynasty, Wu Qian and others wrote in *Golden Mirror of Medicine*: "Heat binding of Three Yang, indicates the heat is stagnated in stomach, small intestine, large intestine three Fu-organs and cannot be eliminated, it burns the body fluid. The upper orifice of the stomach is the cardia, the upper orifice of the small intestine is the pyloric, and the orifice under the large intestine is the anus. As the fluid of three fu-organs are damaged, three orifices are naturally dry, and the channel for water and grain entering and exiting are blocked. As the cardia is dry, the entrance channel of the water and grain becomes narrow, so food can not be swallowed down, 'dysphagia' occurs. As the pyloric is dry, the road to release the corrupt becomes narrow, so the swallowed food counterflow, so-called 'regurgitation' occurs. If the syndrome of 'dysphagia' and 'regurgitation' linger for days, the conduction way of large intestine turns to be narrow, so the anus should be dry, astringent and difficult to run through. When chest is painful as being needled, the stomach has been damaged. The stool is as dry as sheep excrement, the body fluid is dried up. The patient spits foam and vomits blood, blood does not flow, all the above phenomenon are signs of death." It is similar to gastric cancer cardia obstruction, pyloric obstruction symptoms, late gastric cancer with unfavourable prognosis. About the etiology and pathogenesis of the disease, the Sui dynasty *General Treatise on Causes and Menifestation of all Diseases* said: "deficiency of Rong qi (nourishing qi) and Wei qi (defending qi), its blood and breath is insufficient, retained water and accumulated drinking in the stomach makes viscera cold, cold viscera causes dysfunction of spleen grinding, the spleen does not grind, the grain cannot be digested, its qi counterflows, leading to regurgitation." The Ming dynasty *Jing Yue Complete Works* points out: "Regurgitation is caused by overdrinking, hurt by the dampness of wine, or by over - taking of raw and cold food, which damages its kidney Yang, or because seven feelings depresses and exhausts stomach-qi, in short, nothing more than internal injury, damages the stomach qi." In terms of treatment, *Jing Yue Complete Works* says: "The method of treating stomach regurgitation... must be to reinforce healthy qi, tonify spleen and nourish stomach." Doctors of former generations have also had some understanding on the prognosis of gastric cancer. *The Secret Record of the Stone Room* says: "Although the patient with syndrome of regurgitation might not die suddenly, but if it can not be treated appropriately, the patient will die later."

总之，历代医家多认为胃癌的病因较为复杂。中医学认为，邪之所凑，其气必虚，胃癌的发病系先天不足、后天失养、饮食不节、嗜烟饮酒、六淫侵袭、忧思过度、脾胃损伤、脏腑失调等内外因素综合作用的结果。胃癌肿瘤的形成，可能与气结、邪热、食积、痰湿、瘀血等瘀滞及脾胃虚寒有关。其病例特点为本虚标实。本虚多为脾胃阳虚、脾肾阳虚、气血亏虚等，而标实多为气结、血瘀、湿热、痰浊等夹杂互见。

In short, most doctors in all former generations believe that the cause of gastric cancer is complicated. TCM believes that wherever evil concentrates, qi will surely be deficient. The cause of gastric cancer is the result of comprehensive actions of internal and external pathogenic factors such as congenital deficiency, acquired loss of nourishment, diet, smoking, drinking, excessive worry and thinking, spleen and stomach damage, and disorders of zang-organs and fu-organs. The formation of gastric cancer tumor may be related to the qi stagnation, evil heat, dyspepsia, phlegm and dampness, blood stasis, and the cold deficiency of spleen and stomach. The characteristics of the syndrome are asthenia in root and sthenia in tip. Asthenia in root is mostly Yang deficiency of spleen and stomach, Yang deficiency of spleen and kidney, qi and blood deficiency, and sthenia in top indicates mostly qi stagnation, blood stasis, dampness and heat, phlegm turbidity and other factors which might be found as mixed or mutual transformed.

二、基于浊毒理论对本病的认识
2. The understanding of gastric cancer according to the theory of turbid toxin

在胃癌的发病中，浊毒既是一种病理产物，又是其重要的致病因素。胃癌病因不外有三：饮食不节或不洁；情志不畅，肝气犯胃；或受外邪。肠胃为市，无所不受，三者皆可使胃腑损伤，胃气不行，胃失和降，脾亦不运，脾胃气机壅滞，功能失调，水反为湿，谷反为滞，日久则出现气滞、血瘀、湿阻、浊聚、食积、痰结及郁火诸症。而最重要的莫过于浊、毒之邪。因积湿成浊，积滞化热，郁热内生，蕴热入血而为毒。毒热伤阴耗血，浊邪中阻，气机不利，肝失疏泄，脾胃升降失司，水津不布，水湿、痰饮、食积不化而形成积聚。可见，胃癌以气血津液亏虚为本，浊毒内壅为标，而浊毒相关为害乃病机关键之所在。从临床表现看，胃癌患者舌质多红或紫暗，舌苔黄燥或黄腻，脉多弦滑或滑数，均为浊毒中阻之明征。从胃镜表现看，胃癌患者癌肿呈菜花状突入胃腔，表面有污秽的苔覆盖，或溃疡型，黏膜糜烂，底部有细小颗粒或覆盖白薄苔，与"浊"性质相似，而肿块隆起，黏膜充血、糜烂、溃疡，透见红色血管纹，与热"毒"伤阴性质相似。我们发现，以解毒化浊为主，辅以健脾和胃法指导胃癌的临床用药后，患者舌质转淡红，苔转薄白，脉象趋于和缓，临床症状减轻或消失，能明显延长患者生存期，提高生活质量。

In the pathogenic process of gastric cancer, turbid toxin is a pathological product as well as an important pathogenic factor. There are no more than three causes of stomach cancer: uncontrolled or untidy diet; unhealthy mood, liver qi attacks stomach; or external evil. Intestines and stomach are like sea, they can accept almost everything. The above three causes can make damages to stomach, when the stomach qi does not flow, the stomach looses the function of harmonizing and descending, spleen looses the function of transporting, qi mechanism of spleen and stomach is stagnated, disorder in function, adverse flow of water turns to be dampness, adverse flow of grain turns to be stagnation, with time going, qi stagnation, blood stasis, dampness resistance, turbidity accumulation, dyspepsia, phlegm binding and depressed fire occur. But nothing is more important than the evil of turbid toxin. Because moisture accumulates into turbidity, stagnation accumulates into heat, depressed heat is generated endogenously, accumulated heat will be transformed into toxin when it enters the blood. Toxic heat injures Yin and wears out blood, turbidity evil is obstructed in middle energizer, causes abnormal operation of energy mechanism, liver looses the function of dispersing, spleen and stomach loose the function of ascending and descending, fluid cannot be irrigated, water dampness and phlegm retention, dyspepsia forms accumulation. It can be seen that the deficiency of qi, blood, fluid and liquid is the root, the internal accumulation of turbid toxin is the tip. And the related harm made by turbid toxin is the key factor of the pathogenesis of gastric cancer. From the clinical manifestations, gastric cancer patients are with red or purple dark tongue, yellow dry or yellow greasy moss, string slippery, or slippery rapid pulse, clearly signifying the retention of turbid toxin. Referring gastroscope performance, the cancer edema of gastric cancer patients is with cauliflower shape, abruptly projects into the stomach cavity, the surface is covered by dirty coating, or ulcer, mucous membrane erosion, small particles at the bottom or thin white moss, similar to "turbidity" properties, and mass bulge, mucous membrane congestion, erosion, ulcer, see red blood veins, and heat "poison" injury Yin properties. We found that after using the method of removing toxin and resolving turbidity, supplemented by the method of spleen reinforcing and stomach harmonizing, the tongue of the patient turned light red, the moss turned thin white, the pulse tended to be reconciled, and the clinical symptoms decreased or disappeared, which significantly prolong the survival of patients and improve the quality of life.

第二节　治疗原则
Section 2　Principles of Treatment

本病多由气、痰、湿、瘀、浊毒互结所致，故理气、化痰、燥湿、活血化瘀、化浊解毒是本病主要治标之法，尤其是化浊解毒是中晚期胃癌的重要治疗原则之一；后期出现胃热伤阴、脾胃虚寒、气血两虚者，则应标本兼顾，扶正与祛邪并进。本病病位在胃，多有脾胃气机阻滞，气化不利，运化无权，在治疗中应始终重视顾护脾胃，勿损正气，也是应遵从的治疗原则。这一点对中晚期患者和放化疗患者更为重要。只有胃气得充，脾气得健，才能使气血生化有源，也才能助药以祛邪。但补虚时，用药也不可过于滋腻，以免呆滞脾胃，应在辨证论治的基础上，结合选用具有一定抗胃癌作用的中草药。

This disease is mostly caused by co-stagnation of qi, phlegm, wet, blood stasis, turbid toxin, so qi regulating, phlegm resolving, dampness drying, blood circulation promoting and blood stasis resolving, turbidity resolving and toxin removing are the main methods to treat the top of the disease, especially the method of turbidity resolving and toxin removing is one of the important treatment principles of mid and late period of gastric cancer; for late gastric cancer patients, when stomach heat injures Yin, spleen and stomach become deficient cold, qi and blood are both deficient, treatment should be made considering both the tip and the root, reinforcing the healthy qi as well as dispelling the evil. This disease is located in the stomach, qi mechanism of spleen and stomach is blocked, obstruction of qi activity, transporting and digesting function does not work, in the treatment we should always care and protect the spleen and stomach, do not damage the healthy qi, complying with the treatment principle. This is more important for patients in advanced stage and patients with chemoradiotherapy treatment. Only when the stomach qi is sufficient. Spleen qi is reinforced, can we ensure abundant source to generate qi and blood and help medicine to dispel evil. But when we tonify deficiency, medication should not be too greasy, so as not to dull the spleen and stomach, selecting some Chinese herbal medicine with a certain anti-gastric cancer effect on the basis of syndrome differentiation therapy.

第三节　常用治法
Section 3　The Common Treatment Methods

一、化浊解毒（化浊毒）法为治疗胃癌之总则
1. Turbidity resolving and toxin removing method is the general rule of the treatment of gastric cancer

　　浊毒理论认为，疾病发生发展的根本病机在于机体组织的"浊毒化"，浊毒病邪胶结作用于人体，导致人体细胞、组织和器官的浊化，即致病过程；浊化的结果导致细胞、组织和器官的浊变，即形态结构的改变，包括现代病理学中的肥大、增生、萎缩、化生和癌变，以及炎症、变性、凋亡和坏死等变化。浊变的结果是毒害细胞、组织和器官，使之代谢和功能失常，乃至功能衰竭。癌症也概莫能外。其产生归根结底还是由于不同的内因和外因导致脏腑气血阴阳失衡，浊毒内蕴，日久不能排出体外，结于某处而成，其实就是机体组织的"浊毒化"，因而"化浊解毒"实为治疗肿瘤之总则。在此总则的指导下，"坚者消之，结者散之，留者攻之，损者益之"，以期取得满意效果。我们在总结古人宝贵经验的基础之上，总结了健脾化浊法、补肾化浊法、养阴化浊法、养血化浊法、清热解毒法、解毒散结法、祛湿化浊法、活血化浊法、泄浊解毒法和以毒攻毒法这十大法则，这十种治法不是孤立存在的，而是相辅相成，临床上当根据患者具体病情灵活运用。

According to the turbid toxin theory, the fundamental pathogenesis is the "turbid toxin change" of the body, and the disease evil of turbid toxin binding affects human body, causes turbid transmission of body cells, tissues and organs, that is, the pathogenic process. The result of turbid toxin transmission leads to the turbid change of cells, tissues and organs, i.e. the change of forming structures, including the changes of inflammation, degeneration, apoptosis and necrosis. The result of turbid change is to poison cells, tissues and organs, and make the metabolism and function disorder, functional failure, and even unavoidable cancer. In final analysis, the disease is resulted from the imbalance of qi, blood, Yin and Yang in the viscera due to different internal and external causes, from internal accumulation of turbid toxin, which cannot be discharged from the body over time, and stagnated in certain area of the body. It is actually the "turbid toxin change" of the body tissue, so "to resolve turbidity and remove toxin" is actually the general principle for the treatment of tumors. In order to achieve satisfied results, we should "soften the hardness, dispel the binding, eliminate the retention, and tonify the deficiency" under the guidance of the general principle. On the basis of absorbing the valuable experiences of the ancients, we summarizes ten methods as the following: the method to resolve the turbidity by reinforcing the spleen, to resolve the turbidity by reinforcing kidney, to resolve turbidity by nourishing Yin, to resolve turbidity by nourishing blood, to remove toxin by clearing heat, to dispel binding by detoxification, to resolve turbidity by dispelling humidity, to resolve turbidity by promoting blood circulation, to remove toxin by turbidity purging and to attack poison by using poison agents, the ten methods of treatment is not isolated, but complement each other, they should be used flexibly in clinical practice according to specific condition of the patients.

二、健脾化浊法
2. The method to resolve turbidity by reinforcing the spleen

脾在中医生理病理中占有相当重要的位置，中医学认为"脾胃为后天之本"，主运化、升清而统血液，机体的消化运动主要依赖于脾胃的生理功能，机体生命活动的持续和气血津液的生化都有赖于脾胃运化，故称其为气血生化之源。一旦脾的正常生理功能的每个环节遭到阻断或运行不畅则产生脾的病理变化，就恶性肿瘤的发生发展过程中的各方面变化与脾之功能密切有关。因此，健脾化浊法在恶性肿瘤治疗中有重要地位，凡恶性肿瘤见有神疲乏力、纳食减少、脘腹作胀、形体消瘦、大便溏薄和脾虚之舌象、脉象的均可运用健脾化浊法治疗，而消化道恶性肿瘤应用健脾化浊方法在治疗中尤为重要，健脾以去湿浊之源为治本之法，其治法贯穿治疗胃癌的各个阶段。

Spleen occupies an important position in the physiology and pathology of TCM, which believes that "spleen and stomach is the root of body acquired after birth", mainly controlling transporting, lucidity ascending and blood circulation, the digestive movement mainly depends on the physiological function of the spleen and stomach, the sustainability of life activity and the generation and change of qi and blood, fluid and liquid depend on the transporting function of spleen and stomach, so spleen and stomach are called the source of generation and change of qi and blood. Once every link of the normal physiological function of the spleen is blocked or abnormal, pathological changes of the spleen will surely occur. As the development of malignant tumors is closely related to the function of the spleen, the method to resolve turbidity by reinforcing spleen has an important position in the treatment of malignant tumors. Whenever malignant tumors see fatigue complexion and force, poor appetite, epigastric and abdominal distension, thin and loose stool and spleen deficiency in tongue and pulse image, the method to resolve turbidity by reinforcing spleen can be used. In treatment of digestive tract malignancy, the above method is particularly important, to reinforce the spleen and remove the source of wet turbidity is the method of root curing, the method is carried out through all stages of gastric cancer treatment.

三、补肾化浊法
3. Method to resolve turbidity by reinforcing the kidney

补肾化浊法在恶性肿瘤的治疗方面有广泛的应用基础，中医学认为"肾为先天之本"，而"先天之本"的肾与恶性肿瘤有密切关系，在临床上使用补肾化浊法治疗恶性肿瘤其例不胜枚举。肾主二便，为水之下源，肾气不足，蒸腾气化不足，湿浊内盛，日久蕴化浊毒。

Kidney reinforcing and turbidity resolving method is widely used in the treatment of malignant tumors. TCM believes that "kidney is the foundation of congenital", while as "congenital foundation", kidney is closely related to malignant tumors. There are numerous cases of using kidney reinforcing and turbidity resolving method in clinical practice to treat malignant tumors. Kidney controls double stools, is the lower source of water, when kidney qi is insufficient, the ability of transpiration and gasification is insufficient, wet turbidity is generated inside, will be accumulated into turbid toxin over time.

四、养阴化浊法
4. Method to resolve turbidity by nourishing yin

阴是相对于阳而言的中医概念，阴液也是人体内的基本生命物质，所谓"阴平阳秘，精神乃治"。疾病的状态必然是体内阴阳平衡关系的失衡，而阴液的亏损更较为多见。朱丹溪倡言"阳常有余，阴常不足"，恶性肿瘤患者，较多见到神疲乏力、午后低热、夜烦不眠、舌红苔剥、脉细之征象，故养阴化浊法在中医药诊治恶性肿瘤的过程中具有不可忽视的作用。气、阴的盛衰与五脏都有关，尤与肺、脾、肝、肾关系密切。

Yin is a TCM concept opposite to Yang, Yin liquid is also the basic life material in human body, the so-called "Only when Yin is at peace, Yang is impact, can Jingshen (Essence-Spirit) be normal." The state of the disease is inevitably the imbalance of Yin and Yang in the body, and the loss of Yin fluid is more common. Zhu Danxi advocated that "Yang is often surplus, but Yin is often insufficient". More patients with malignant tumors see fatigue in complexion and force, low fever in the afternoon, restless and sleepless at night, with red tongue, peeling moss and thready pulse, so the method of resolving turbidity by nourishing Yin plays a significant role in the diagnosis and treatment of malignant tumors with traditional Chinese medicine. The rise and fall of qi and Yin are related to the five zang organs, especially to the lung, spleen, liver and kidney.

五、养血化浊法
5. Method to resolve turbidity by nourishing blood

从现代分子生物学观点来看，癌症的形成是由于抑癌基因的失活和癌基因的被激活所致。从传统中医学理论上来分析，肿瘤形成的原因不外乎外邪与内伤。外邪包括环境中的"六淫"和毒物，内伤则主要是脏腑的功能虚衰和气血津液的亏损。根据病因，中医对肿瘤的治则可主要分为扶正与祛邪，扶正的主要内容如健脾、补肾、益肺，或理气、养血、养阴等。中医治疗尤为注意扶正，所谓"养正积自除""正气存内，邪不可干"。养血化浊的治疗方法在肿瘤的治疗中得到广泛应用。另外通过中医扶正治疗增强患者免疫功能，改善机体内环境的平衡，已成为中医抗肿瘤的一大特色。

In the view point of modern molecular biology, the formation of cancer is due to the inactivation of tumor suppressor genes and the activation of oncogenes. According to the analysis of traditional Chinese medicine theory, the cause of tumor formation is nothing more than external evil and internal injury. External evil includes the "six evils" and toxic materials in the environment, while the internal injury is mainly the function deficiency and failure of viscera and the loss of qi, blood and fluid and liquid. According to the etiology, the treatment of tumors in traditional Chinese medicine can be mainly divided into healthy qi reinforcing and pathogenic factor eliminating, the main contents of healthy qi reinforcing, including reinforcing spleen, reinforcing kidney, nourishing lung, or regulating qi, nourishing blood, nourishing Yin, etc. TCM treatment pays special attention to reinforcing healthy qi, so-called "Masses will certainly be eliminated when healthy qi is reinforced.""when healthy qi sufficient, evil can not attack". The method of turbidity resolving by blood nourishing is widely used in the treatment of tumors. In addition, it has become a major characteristic of TCM anti-tumor practice to enhance the immune function of patients and improve the internal balance of the patient by the treatment of reinforcing healthy qi.

六、清热解毒法
6. Method to remove toxin by clearing heat

热毒是恶性肿瘤的主要病因病理要素之一，因而清热解毒法亦为当代中医治疗恶性肿瘤的一种被广泛运用并取得好的疗效的方法之一。在临床上所见之恶性肿瘤患者常有邪实之表现，其中不乏表现为邪毒热郁之症状，故临床上见到恶性肿瘤患者肿块增大、发热或午后潮热、局部灼热疼痛拒按、口渴欲饮或不欲饮、大便干燥或秘结、小便黄赤、舌质红或绛红、苔黄或薄黄、脉细数或弦数证候者，即认为有邪热蕴毒之征象，可以配合清热解毒方法给予治疗。实热者应用清热解毒法，伴有虚热者则须在清热解毒的同时配合补虚，清热解毒法还可作为恶性肿瘤治疗的不同时期或采用不同方法治疗时的配合与辅助。当代中医肿瘤治疗中清热解毒方法大量在临床应用并进行实验研究，取得了成绩。

Heat toxin is one of the main etiological and pathological factors of malignant tumors, so the method of removing toxin by heat-clearing is one of the effective methods to treat malignant tumors widely used in contemporary TCM clinical practice. Many patients with malignant tumor see sthenia evil symptom, such as symptom of heat depression of evil toxin, the size of malignant tumor mass is larger, fever or hectic fever in afternoon, feels local burning pain and refuses to be pressed, thirsty in mouth but with no want to drink, dry stool or constipation, yellow red urine, red or crimson tongue, yellow or thin yellow moss, thready rapid or string rapid pulse, that is signs of accumulated toxin caused by evil heat, can be treated cooperating the method of toxin removing by heat clearing. Sthenia heat patients should be treated with the method of toxin removing by heat clearing, sthenia heat patients accompanied by asthenia heat should use the method of toxin removing by heat clearing cooperating with deficiency reinforcing. The method of toxin removing by heat clearing heat can also be used as assisting or complementary manner to treat different periods of malignant tumor. The method of removing toxin by clearing heat has been widely used and experimented in contemporary TCM clinical practice of tumor treatment and made significant achievements.

七、解毒散结法
7. Method to dissipate binding by removing toxin

解毒散结，顾名思义即解其毒邪、消散其结，而肿块是为癥积。癥积其表现为固定不移、坚硬如石、痛有定处、疼痛拒按，故临床上见有癥积症状而正气尚强，能够承受祛邪之药物者可以采用解毒散结方法治疗。对恶性肿瘤术后复发或未能采取手术治疗者，或有恶性肿瘤周围及远处脏器转移、淋巴结转移者均可应用解毒散结法治疗。在当今中医治疗恶性肿瘤方面，解毒散结方法为公认的较有效的治疗法则之一，被大量应用于临床治疗中并取得相应疗效，而且进行了一些实验研究，证明解毒散结中药具有抗肿瘤的作用，为临床使用提供了有力的实验依据，因此解毒散结法也是肿瘤治疗的途径之一。

The method of dissipating bind by removing toxin, as the name implies, to remove toxin, and dissipate binding, and the abnormal abdominal mass is fixed as hard as stone, patient feels painful and refuses to be pressed, so clinically patient with abdominal mass are still strong in healthy qi, those who can bear the evil-dispelling drugs can use bind dissipating by toxin removing method. Patients of post-operative recurrence or failure to take surgical treatment of malignant tumors, or those with metastasis around malignancy and distant organs or lymph node metastasis can be treated with the method of dissipating bind by removing toxin. The method of dissipating bind by removing toxin is recognized as one of the more effective treatment method in today's TCM treatment of malignant tumors, and has been widely used in clinical treatment and obtained corresponding curative effect, and completed some experimental studies, it is proved that the Chinese medicine of dissipating bind by removing toxin has anti-tumor effect, provides a powerful experimental basis for clinical use, so The method of dissipating bind by removing toxin is one of the ways for tumor treatment.

八、祛湿化浊法
8. Method to resolve turbidity by dispelling dampness

痰饮湿浊是体内水液失于正常输布而产生的病理物质，其不但是水液输布代谢失常而产生的病理物质，本身又会反过来阻滞气机，妨碍水液正常运行。临床上常见肿瘤患者至疾病晚期表现出不思饮食，腹胀如鼓，下腹坠胀，身重如蒙，下肢水肿，按之皮肤凹陷，小溲短少，大便溏薄，舌淡胖，苔白厚腻，脉濡无力，此与脏腑功能虚衰，水液代谢输布失常有关，由湿浊作祟，水邪泛滥所致。因此，祛湿化浊法在中医药防治恶性肿瘤的临床工作中，具有十分重要的地位。

Phlegmatic retention and damp turbidity is the pathological substance produced by the abnormal transportation of water liquid in the body. It is not only the pathological substance produced by the abnormal transportation and metabolism of water and liquid, it will also block the energy mechanism and hinder the normal operation of water and liquid. Tumor patients with advanced disease usually show poor appetite, abdominal swelling distension as drum, somatic heaviness, lower limb edema, the skin is caved in when being pressed, little and short urine, loose and thin stool, light and fat tongue, white thick greasy moss, weak pulse, resulting from the viscera function deficiency and abnormal metabolism and transportation of water liquid, caused by water evil is in flood due to haunting and plaguing of wet turbidity. Therefore, using the method to resolve turbidity by dispelling dampness is very important in TCM clinical practice to prevent and treat malignant tumors.

九、活血化浊法
9. Method to resolve turbidity by promoting blood circulation

活血化浊法是现代中医肿瘤治疗学中广泛应用的一种抗恶性肿瘤的方法。临床上凡中医辨证属血瘀者，症见疼痛如针刺刀割，痛有定处拒按，夜间加剧；肿块在体表呈青紫，在腹内坚硬按之不移；出血反复不止，色泽紫暗，中夹血块或大便色黑如柏油；面色暗黑，肌肤甲错，口唇爪甲紫青，皮下紫斑，肤表丝状如缕，腹部青筋外露或下肢筋青胀痛；舌质紫暗或见有瘀斑瘀点，脉细涩者，均可运用活血化浊法治之。瘀血是中医学中特有的病理病因之一，是在中医理论与实践的发展过程中形成的一个极为宝贵的重要理论和经验，为后世所继承与发展，对恶性肿瘤的临床治疗起着指导作用，并取得了成效，在现代实验研究中获得了一定的成果。

The method is a widely used in modern TCM malignant tumor preventing therapy. Clinically, all TCM syndrome differentiated as blood stasis with symptoms as follows can be treated with the to resolve turbidity by promoting blood circulation: fixed pain as painful as being pricked and knife- cut, the patient refuses to be pressed, the pain becomes more severe at night; the lump is dark purple in body surface, hard and fixed in the abdomen, repeated bleeding with dark purple blood mingled with, blood lump, asphalt-black stool; dark black complexion, scaly skin, purple green mouth lips and finger nails, cyan macule under the skin, the skin surface is scattered with silk-thread like varicosity, bluish tendon exposed at abdomen, or bluish tendon and distension pain on lower limbs; purple dark tongue perhaps with ecchymosis and petechia, thready astringent pulse. Blood stasis as one of the characteristic pathological etiology in TCM, is a very valuable important theory and experience formed in the development of TCM theory and practice. It plays a guiding role in the clinical treatment of malignant tumors for inheritance and development by later generations, and has obtained significant results, made certain achievements in the modern experimental research.

十、泄浊解毒法
10. Method to remove toxin by purging turbidity

泄浊解毒法作为恶性肿瘤治疗方法的一种，在临床上常为使用，但泄浊解毒法的应用必须具有使用攻下的适应证。故凡中医辨证为邪实而正气不虚者，邪实而正气虚尚可承受攻下者，可以运用该方法治疗。因此在临床上见有里热积滞实证，热盛伤津，水饮停留胸胁者都可通过通便、下积、泻实、逐水的方法加以治疗。泄浊解毒法的使用以邪去为度，不宜过量，以防正气受伤。在恶性肿瘤的临床治疗中，泄浊解毒法的运用取得了一定疗效，并且在实验研究中也取得了成果，成为恶性肿瘤治疗的方法之一。

The method is often used clinically for malignant tumors treatment, but the application of the method must have the indication for purging. Therefore, all syndromes differentiated by TCM as sthenia evil but healthy qi is not deficient, sthenia evil and healthy qi deficient, but still can bear purging, can use this method. Therefore, in clinical practice, all patients with sthenia syndrom of internal heat accumulation and stagnation, excessive heat injures fluid, thoracic accumulation of fluid can be treated by stool dredging, accumulation lowering, excess purging, water expelling. The application of removing toxin by purging turbidity method should stop when evil is removed, in order not to injure the healthy qi. In the clinical treatment of malignant tumors, the application of toxin removing by turbidity purging method has achieved certain curative effect, and has also achieved results in experimental research.

十一、以毒攻毒法
11. Method to attack poison with poison

在中医药治疗各种恶性肿瘤的治则中，以毒攻毒法一直受到历代医家的重视。关于癌瘤的发生，中医学认为是人体脏腑阴阳失调、六淫、七情、饮食、劳倦、外伤等多因素综合作用的结果，即可分为内外两方面。而这两方面的致病因素在人体内导致了气滞、血瘀、痰凝、湿聚、热毒、浊毒等多种"毒"，在人体正气亏虚的情况下长期作用，最终导致肿瘤形成。现代医学对于癌症成因的研究正不断深入，已经肯定的致癌物质包括许多化学物质如苯、黄曲霉毒素、亚硝胺等，以及许多病原微生物如EB病毒、乙型肝炎病毒、乳头状瘤病毒、反转录病毒等，这些"毒"均有较强的致癌型。如乙型肝炎病毒的感染被认为是若感染者有足够的生存期则必将发展成原发性肝癌。中医理论中以毒攻毒法的运用，正是在中医学认为"邪去则正安"的基础上发展充实起来的。

In the treatment of various malignant tumors by TCM, the method of attacking poison with poison has been valued by doctors of all dynasties. As for the occurrence of cancer tumor, traditional Chinese medicine believes that it is the result of comprehensive action of multiple factors, which can be divided into internal and external aspects, including imbalance of Yin and Yang, six evils, seven emotions, (uncontrolled) diet, fatigue and trauma. The pathogenic factors of these two aspects in human body cause qi stagnation, blood stasis, phlegm coagulation, wet fusion, heat toxin, turbid toxin and other "toxins", and eventually lead to the formation of tumor after long-term effect in case of deficient healthy qi. The study of cancer pathogenesis in modern medical science is continuously deepening, carcinogens which has been affirmed including many chemicals such as benzene, aflatoxin, nitroamine, as well as many pathogenic microorganisms such as EB virus, hepatitis B virus, papillomoma virus, retrovirus, etc. these "toxins" have strong carcinogenic character. For example, hepatitis B virus infection is considered will unavoidably develop into primary liver cancer if the infected patient has enough time of surviving. The application of the method to attack poison with poison is developed on the basis of TCM theory that "healthy qi is safe when evil is kept away".

第四节　辨证治疗
Section 4　Treatment with Syndrome Differentiation

一、肝胃不和型
1. Disharmony of liver and stomach

（一）证候

1.1 Symptoms

胃脘胀痛或窜及两胁，嗳气频繁，嘈杂泛酸，呃逆呕吐，口苦口干，大便不畅，舌质淡红，苔薄白或薄黄，脉沉或弦细。

Epigastric distension pain or hypochondrium distension pain, frequent belching, upset, pantothenic acid, hiccup, vomiting, bitter and dry in mouth, difficult stool, light red tongue with thin and white moss or thin and yellow moss, sunk or string thready pulse.

（二）治法

1.2 Treatment method

疏肝和胃。

Disperse the liver and harmonize the stomach.

（三）方药

1.3 Prescriptions and drugs

柴胡疏肝散。若口干口苦，胃脘痞胀伴灼热感，属郁热不宣，去当归、柴胡、生姜，加吴茱萸、黄连、黄芩，以清热消痞满；若便秘燥结，腑气不通者，加瓜蒌仁、郁李仁、火麻仁，润燥通便；服药后大便仍不畅者，去半夏、茯苓、生姜，加大黄、芒硝，以峻下通腑泄实；若嗳腐吞酸，矢气臭，胃内停食者，加山楂、神曲、连翘、莱菔子，消食化积除滞。

Chaihu Shugan Powder. If the mouth is dry and bitter, stomach is ruffian and burning hot, it belongs to heat depression failing to be dispersed, reduce dang gui (Radix Angelicae Sinensis), chai hu (Radix Bulpleuri), sheng jiang (Rhizoma Zingiberis Recens), add wu zhu yu (Euodiae Fructus), huang lian (Rhizoma Coptidis), huang qin (Radix Scutellariae), to clear heat and dispel ruffian; for symptom of constipation and qi block in Fu-organs, add gua lou ren (Semen Trichosanthis), yu li ren (Pruni Semen), huo ma ren (Semen Cannabis), to lubricate the dryness and dredge the stool. If the stool is still difficult after taking the above medicines, reduce ban xia (Rhizoma Pinelliae), fu ling (Poria), sheng jiang (Rhizoma Zingiberis Recens), add da huang (Radix et Rhizoma Rhei), mang xiao (Mirabilite), to purg, unblock the fu-organ and discharge the accumulation in stomach and intestines. For patient with symptom of fetid eructation and acid regurgitation, foul wind-breaking, dyspepsia in stomach, add shan zha (Crataegi Fructus), shen qu (Massa Medicata Fermentata), lain qiao (Forsythia Fructus), lai fu zi (Semen Raphani), to promote digesting and resolve the dyspepsia.

二、浊毒内蕴型
2. Internal accumulation of turbid toxin

（一）证候

2.1 Symptoms

面色晦暗，胃脘部痞满或胀痛，口干口黏，或口舌生疮，渴不欲饮，畏寒与五心烦热同时出现，纳呆，寐欠佳，大便黏腻不爽，舌质暗红，苔黄厚腻，脉弦滑。

Dark complexion, epigastric ruffian full or pain, dry and sticky mouth, oral sore, thirsty but with no want to drink, fear of cold while upset hot in heart, hands and feet, anorexia, poor sleep, sticky and difficult stool, dark red tongue with yellow thick and greasy moss, string slippery pulse.

（二）治法

2.2 Treatment method

化浊解毒。

Turbidity resolving and toxin removing.

（三）方药

2.3 Prescription and drugs

自拟化浊解毒汤。药用黄芩、黄连、黄柏、蒲公英、生石膏、茵陈、藿香、佩兰、全蝎、蜈蚣等。神疲乏力者，加黄芪、党参，补气健脾；服后泛恶纳减者，加神曲、藿香，化湿浊助消化；可加白花蛇舌草、半枝莲、露蜂房、仙鹤草解毒祛瘀。若出血兼见舌质光红，口咽干燥，脉细数者，加沙参、地黄、麦冬滋阴养血；失血日久，心悸少气，多梦少寐，体倦纳差，唇白舌淡，脉虚弱者，加酸枣仁、黄芪、茯苓、远志补气养血、宁心安神。

Turbidity Resolving and Toxin Removing Decoction. Medicines: huang qin (Radix Scutellariae), huang lian (Rhizoma Coptidis), huang bo (Cortex Phellodendri), pu gong ying (Herba Taraxaci cum Radice), sheng shi gao (Crude Gypsum Fibrosum), yin chen (Herba Artemisiae Scophoriae), huo xiang (Herba Agastaches seu Pogostemonis), pei lan (Herba Eupatorii), quan xie (Scorpio), wu gong (Scolopendra), etc. For symptom of fatigue, add huang qi (Radix Astragali seu Hedysari) and dang shen (Radix Codonopsitis Pilosulae), to tonify qi and reinforce the spleen; for symptom of nausea and poor appetite after taking the said prescription, add shen qu (Massa Medicata Fermentata), huo xiang (Herba Agastaches seu Pogostmonis), to dispel dampness and promote digesting; add bai hua she she cao (Herba Oldenlandiae Diffusae), ban zhi lian (Herba Portulacae Grandiflorae), lu feng fang (Nidus Polistis), xian he cao (Herba Agrimoniae), to remove toxin and eliminate stasis. If the patient see bleeding, red and bright tongue, dry oropharynx, thready and rapid pulse, add sha shen (Radix Adenophorae Strictae), di huang (Radix Rehmanniae), mai dong (Radix Ophiopogonis) to tonify Yin and nourish blood; patients with blood loss over time, palpitation and short breath, poor sleep with more dreams, phisycally fatigue with poor appetite, white lip, light tongue, weak and deficient pulse, add suan zao ren (Semen Zizyphi Jujubae), huang qi (Radix Astragali seu Hedysari), fu ling (Poria), yuan zhi (Radix Polygalae), to tonify qi and nourish blood, and tranquilize the heart and nourish the mind.

三、瘀毒内阻型

3. Internal resistance of stasis toxin

（一）证候

3.1 Symptoms

症见胃脘刺痛不移，胃痛日久不愈，大便潜血或黑便，心下痞硬，吐血，皮肤甲错，舌质暗紫，可见瘀斑，脉沉细涩。

Epigastric fixed tingling pain for a long time, latent blood in stool or black stool, epigastric ruffian hard, blood vomiting, scaly skin, dark purple tongue with ecchymosis, sunk thready and astringent pulse.

（二）治法
3.2 Treatment method

活血解毒。

To promote blood circulation and remove toxin.

（三）方药
3.3 Prescription and drugs

失笑散合丹参饮。局部痛甚者，加延胡索、木香，以行气止痛；胃脘部积块明显者，加三棱、莪术、丹参，以消积破瘀散结；伴便血者加仙鹤草、地榆炭、三七以止血活血，使血止而不留瘀。

Combination of Shi xiao Powder and Danshen Yin Decoction. Local severe pain, add yan hu suo (Rhizoma Corydalis), mu xiang (Radix Aucklandiae), to promote qi flow and relieve pain; epigastric obvious mass, add san leng (Rhizoma Sparganii), e zhu (Rhizoma Curcumae), dan shen (Salviae Miltiorrhizae), to resolve retention, eliminate stasis and disperse binding; with blood stool, add xian he cao (Herba Agrimoniae), di yu tan (Radix et Rhizoma Sanguisorbae Carbon), san qi (Radix Notoginseng), to stop bleeding and promote blood circulation, in order to stop bleeding without stasis retention.

四、胃热伤阴型
4. The stomach heat injures Yin

（一）证候
4.1 Symptoms

胃脘灼热，食后疼痛，口干欲饮，大便干燥，胃脘嘈杂，五心烦热，食欲不振，舌红少苔或苔黄少津，脉弦细数。

Epigastric burning, pain after eating, dry mouth, dry to drink, dry stool, noisy stomach, five upset heat, loss of appetite, red tongue less moss or moss yellow less jin, detailed pulse string.

（二）治法
4.2 Treatment method

养阴清热。

To nourish Yin and clear heat.

（三）方药

4.3 Prescription and drugs

沙参麦冬汤。可加玄参、地黄、石斛以助养阴之力，加栀子、黄连、黄芩以清肺胃之热。若肠燥失润，大便干结，可加火麻仁、瓜蒌仁、何首乌润肠通便；若腹中胀满，大便不通，胃肠热盛，可用大黄甘草汤泻热存阴，但应中病即止，以免重伤津液；若食管干涩，口燥咽干，可饮五汁安中饮以生津养胃。

Shashen Maidong Decoction. The prescription can add xuan shen (Radix Scrophulariae), di huang (Rehmannia), shi hu (Dendrobii Caulis) to help nourish Yin, add zhi zi (Fructus Gardeniae), huang lian (Rhizoma Coptidis), huang qin (Radix Scutellariae) to clear the heat of lung and stomach. If the intestines are dry, with dry and retained stool, add huo ma ren (Semen Cannabis), gua lou ren (Semen Trichosanthis), he shou wu (Radix Polygoni Multiflori) to lubricate the intestine and unblock the constipation; if the abdomen is distension full, with difficult stool, and excess gastrointestinal heat, can use the prescription of Rhei and Glycyrrhizae Decoction to purge heat while preserving Yin, but using of the prescription should be stopped once symptom is controlled, so as not to seriously hurt the body fluid; if the esophagus is dry, with dry mouth and throat, can use the prescription of Wuzhi Anzhong Decoction to generate fluid and nourish the stomach.

五、痰湿凝滞型
5. Coagulation and stagnation of phlegmatic hygrosis

（一）证候

5.1 Symptoms

脘腹痞闷胀痛，恶心欲呕或呕吐痰涎，不欲进食，或进食不畅，甚至反食夹有多量黏液，口淡不欲饮，头晕身重，便溏，面黄虚肿，舌淡苔白腻或白滑，脉滑或缓或细缓。

Abdominal ruffian swelling pain, nausea with want to vomit or vomiting phlegm saliva, no want to eat, or difficult to eat, or even dysphagia with a large amount of mucus, light tasty with no want to drink, dizziness and stubborn in body, loose stool, yellow swelling face, light tongue with white or white smooth moss, slipper or slow or thready slow pulse.

（二）治法

5.2 Treatment method

化湿祛痰。

To resolve dampness and dispel phlegm.

（三）方药

5.3 Prescription and drugs

二陈汤。气短乏力，可加黄芪、党参，健脾扶正；呕恶频繁，为痰气上逆，加生姜、藿香，行气化浊止呕。

Erchen Decoction. Fatigue and short of breath, can add huang qi (Radix Astragali seu Hedysari), dang shen (Radix Codonopsitis Pilosulae), to reinforce spleen and strengthen healthy qi; frequent nausea, phlegmatic qi reverse, add sheng jiang (Rhizoma Zingiberis Recens), huo xiang (Herba Agastaches seu Pogostemonis), to promote qi flow, resolve turbidity and stop vomiting.

六、气血双亏型
6. Dual deficiency of qi and blood

（一）证候
6.1 Symptoms

胃脘隐痛，绵绵不断，腹胀纳差，乏力，气短，心悸倦怠，面色萎黄，舌质淡嫩，薄白苔，脉细弱。

Epigastric continuous vague pain, abdominal distension, poor appetite, fatigue, short of breath, palpitation and lassitude, pale yellow complexion, light and tender tongue with thin white moss, and thready weak pulse.

（二）治法
6.2 Treatment method

益气养血。

To reinforce qi and nourish blood.

（三）方药
6.3 Prescription and drugs

十全大补汤。该方以四君子汤补气健脾，以四物汤补血调肝，在此基础上更配伍黄芪益气补虚，肉桂补元阳、暖脾胃。诸药共奏气血双补、补虚暖中之效。此证型多属胃癌晚期，以虚为主，气血两亏，不任攻伐，当以救后天生化之源、顾护脾胃之气为要，待能稍进饮食与药物，再适当配合行气、化痰、活血等攻邪之品，且应与补益之品并进，或攻补两法交替使用。若气血亏虚损及阴阳，致阴阳俱虚，阳竭于上而水谷不入，阴竭于下而二便不通，则为阴阳离决之危候，当积极救治。

Shiquan Dabu Decoction (All Nourishing Decoction). The prescription uses Sijunzi Decoction to replenish qi and reinforce spleen, with Siwu Decoction to tonify blood and regulate the liver, on this basis, add huang qi (Radix Astragali seu Hedysari) to reinforce qi and tonify deficiency, add rou gui (Cortex Cinnamomi) to tonify kidney Yang, warm the spleen and stomach. These drugs can realize the effect of dual reinforcement of qi and blood, and warm the middle energizer by reinforcing deficiency. This type of syndrome mostly belongs to advanced gastric cancer, mainly deficiency, dual deficiency of qi and blood, can not bear attacking, so it is more important to save acquired vital genesis, and care and reinforce the qi of the spleen and stomach. When the patient can gradually take in food and drugs, and then appropriately use evil-attacking medicines to regulate qi, resolve phlegm, promote blood circulation, and these medicines should be used together with the tonic substances, or the two methods of attacking and reinforcing be alternatively used. If the deficiency of qi and blood affects Yin and Yang and caused dual deficiency of both Yin and Yang, when Yang is worn out on the top, water and grain can not enter, when Yin is worn out at the bottom, two feces are blocked, danger of Yin and Yang separation occurs, emergent and active treatment should be made.

七、肝郁脾虚型
7. Liver depression and spleen deficiency type

（一）证候
7.1 Symptoms

上腹胀痛，纳呆，便秘或有恶心，口黏口苦，倦怠乏力，舌苔白腻，脉弦。

Upper abdominal distention and pain, fatigue, constipation or nausea, bitter mouth sticky mouth, fatigue, white and greasy tongue coating, string pulse.

（二）治法
7.2 Treatment method

疏肝健脾。

To disperse liver and reinforce spleen.

（三）方药
7.3 Prescription and drugs

逍遥散。郁久化热，易伤肝阴，应慎用香燥之品，可选用香橼、佛手等理气而不伤阴的解郁止痛之品，也可用金铃子、郁金等偏凉性的理气药。若火热内盛，灼伤胃络，而见吐血，并出现脘腹灼热痞满、心烦便秘、面赤舌红、脉弦数有力等症者，可用泻心汤，苦寒泄热，直折其火。

Xiaoyao Powder. When long-time depression is transmitted into heat, it will easily hurt liver Yin, thus using of aromatic and dry medicines should be strictly controlled, we can choose xiang yuan (Fructus Citron), fo shou (Fructus Citri Sarcodactylis), and other depression resolving and pain stopping medicine to regulate qi without hurt to Yin, or using cool - natured medicines for regulating qi as jin ling zi (Fructus Rosae Laevigotae), yu jin (Radix Curcumae). If internal heat is excess, which burns stomach collateral, leading to blood vomiting, and abdominal burning ruffian, upset and constipation, red face, red tongue, powerful string and rapid pulse, we can use Heart-Purging Decoction, to purg heat with bitter cold medicine, straightly discharging the fire.

八、气阴两虚型
8. Dual Deficiency of Qi and Yin

（一）证候
8.1 Symptoms

可见恶病质，卧床不起，贫血，纳差，口干，自汗盗汗，或有浮肿，舌红少苔或光红，脉细沉。

Cachexia, bedridden, anemic, poor appetite, dry mouth, night sweat, or edema, red tongue with less or no moss, thin and sunk pulse.

（二）治法
8.2 Treatment method

益气养阴。

Reinforcing qi and Nourishing Yin.

（三）方药
8.3 Prescription and drugs

生脉饮合玉女煎加味。恶心呕吐，吐痰涎，兼见痰气上逆者，去知母，加法半夏、黄连降逆祛秽止呕；脘痛腹胀，气血不和者，加木香、大腹皮、延胡索，行气活血除胀；便结，加大黄，泻下通便。

Combination of Shengmai Decoction and Yunv Decoction. For symptom of nausea, vomiting, spitting of phlegm-saliva, together with the counter-flow of phlegmatic qi, to reduce zhi mu (Rhizoma Anemarrhennae), add fa ban xia (Rhizoma Pinelliae Preparata), huang lian (Rhizoma Coptidis) to downbear counterflow, dispel filthy and stop vomiting; epigastric pain and abdominal distention, with dishamony of qi and blood, add mu xiang (Radix Aucklandiae), da fu pi (Arecae Pericarpium), yan hu suo (Rhizoma Corydalis), to regulate qi, promote blood circulation and resolve distention; for constipation, add da huang (Radix et Rhizoma Rhei) to unblock the stool by purging.

九、痰凝气滞型
9. Phlegm coagulation and qi stagnation type

（一）证候
9.1 Symptoms

进食梗阻，脘膈痞满，甚则疼痛，情志舒畅则减轻，精神抑郁加重，嗳气呃逆，呕吐痰涎，口干咽燥，大便干涩，舌红，苔薄腻，脉弦滑。

Eating obstruction, epigastric and diaphragm ruffian full, even painful, lighter in case of healthy mood, more severe in case of spiritual depression, belching hiccup, vomiting phlegm and saliva, dry mouth and throat, dry astringent stool, red tongue, thin and greasy moss, string slippery pulse.

（二）治法
9.2 Treatment method

理气化痰。

To regulate qi and resolve phlegm.

（三）方药
9.3 Prescription and drugs

启膈散，可酌加瓜蒌、半夏、天南星以助化痰之力，加麦冬、玄参、天花粉以增润燥之效。若津伤便秘，可加增液汤和白蜜，以助生津润燥之力；若胃失和降，泛吐痰涎者，加半夏、陈皮、旋覆花以和胃降逆。

Qige Powder, can add gua lou (Trichosanthis), ban xia (Rhizoma Pinelliae), tian nan xing (Arisaematis Rhizoma) to help resolving phlegm, add mai dong (Radix Ophiopogonis), xuan shen (Radix Scrophulariae), tian hua fen (Radix Trichosanthis) to increase the effect of moistening the dryness. If the fluid is injured with constipation, can add Fluid Increasing Decoction with white honey, to help increasing fluid and lubricating dryness; if the stomach is in disharmony, spitting phlegm saliva, add ban xia (Rhizoma Pinelliae), chen pi (Pericarpium Citri Reticulatae), xuan fu hua (Flos Inulae), to harmonize the stomach and downbear the counterflow.

十、脾胃虚寒型
10. Deficiency and coldness of the spleen and stomach

（一）证候
10.1 Symptoms

胃脘隐痛，喜温喜按，腹部可触及积块，朝食暮吐，或暮食朝吐，宿食不化，泛吐清涎，面色㿠白，肢冷神疲，面部、四肢浮肿，便溏，大便可呈柏油样，舌淡而胖，苔白滑润，脉沉缓。

The patient feels epigastric vague pain, likes to be warmed and pressed, with abdominal mass which can be felt by touching, eat in morning vomit in evening, or eat in evening vomit in morning, dyspepsia, spitting lucid saliva, white pale complexion, cold limbs, fatigue in spirit, swelling in face and limbs, loose stool like asphalt, light and fat tongue, white and smooth lubricant moss, sunk slow pulse.

（二）治法
10.2 Treatment method

温中散寒，健脾和胃。

To warm the middle energizer and disperse the coldness, reinforce the spleen and harmonize the stomach.

（三）方药

10.3 Prescription and drugs

理中汤，可加丁香、吴茱萸温胃降逆止吐。若肢冷、呕吐、便溏等虚寒症状明显者，可加肉桂、附子即桂附理中汤，以增加温阳补虚散寒之力。全身浮肿者，可合真武汤以温阳化气利水。便血者，可合黄土汤温中健脾，益阴止血。

Lizhong Decoction adding ding xiang (Clove), wu zhu yu (Euodiae Fructus) to warm stomach, downbear counterflow and stop vomiting. For obvious deficient and cold symtoms like cold limbs, vomiting, loose stool, add rou gui (Cortex Cinnamomi), fu zi (Radix Aconiti) forming Guifu Decoction for Regulating Middle Energizer to increase the strength of warming Yang and tonifying deficiency and dispelling the coldness. For patient with edema in whole body, combine the Decoction for Regulating Middle Energizer with Zhenwu Decoction to warm Yang, regulate qi and improve urination. If there is blood in the stool, combine the prescription with huang tu tang (Terrae Flavae Decoction) to warm the middle energizer, reinforce the spleen, benefit Yin and stop bleeding inside.

经现代药理及临床研究，已筛选出一些较常用的抗胃癌及其他消化道肿瘤的中药，如清热解毒类的白花蛇舌草、半枝莲、菝葜、肿节风、藤梨根、拳参、苦参、野菊花、野葡萄藤等，活血化瘀类的鬼箭羽、丹参、虎杖、三棱、莪术、铁树叶等，化痰散结类的牡蛎、海蛤、半夏、瓜蒌、石菖蒲等，利水渗湿类的防己、泽泻等。上述这些具有一定抗癌作用的药物，可在辨证论治的基础上，结合胃癌的具体情况，酌情选用。

Modern pharmacological and clinical studies have screened some Chinese medicines for treating gastric cancer and other digestive tract tumors, such as medicines for heat clearing and toxin removing like bai hua she she cao (Herba Oldenlandiae Diffusae), ban zhi lian (Scutellariae Barbatae Herba), ba qia (Smilacis Chinae Rhizoma), zhong jie feng (Sarcandrae Herba), teng li gen (Radix Actinidae Chinensis), quan shen (Sophorae Flavescentis Radix), ku shen (Chysanthemi Indici Flos), ye ju hua (Flos Chrysanthemi), ye pu tao teng (Caulis et Folium Vitis). Medicines for promoting blood circulation and resolving blood stasis: gui jian yu (Ramulus Euonymi Atali), dan shen (Salviae Miltiorrhizae), hu zhang (Rhizoma Polygoni Cuspidati), san leng (Rhizoma Sparganii), e zhu (Rhizoma Curcumae), Tie shu ye (Folium Lordylines Fruticosae). Medicines for resolving phlegm and dissipating binds: mu li (Ostreae Concha), hai ge (Concha Merietricis seu Cyclinae), ban xia (Rhizoma Pinelliae), gua lou (Trichosanthis Fructus), shi chang pu (Rhizoma Acori Graminei). Medicines for Disinhibit water and drain dampness: fang ji (Radix Stephaniae Tetrandrae), ze xie (Rhizoma Alismatis). These drugs have certain anti-cancer effect, and can be used on the basis of syndrome differentiation treatment according to the specific situation of gastric cancer.

晚期出现合并症及转移，可参见有关章节，辨证论治。病情危重者还应中西医结合积极救治。

In the late stage of gastric cancer, when complication and metastasis occur, we should refer to the relevant chapter of this book, to make syndrome differentiation treatment. For patients with critical syndrome, we should make active treatment by integrating TCM with western medicine.

第六章　肝癌浊毒论
Chapter 6 On Turbid Toxin of Liver Cancer

第一节　病因病机
Section 1 Etiology and Pathogenesis

一、古代医家对本病的认识
1. The ancient medical understanding of this disease

在中医学文献中，没有"原发性肝癌"的病名，但根据临床症状，其相当于中医的"胁痛""黄疸""肥气""息贲""癥瘕""积聚""臌胀""肝积""痞气""脾积"等。《金匮要略》论"黄疸"病因为"黄家所得，从湿得之"。《张氏医通》谓："嗜酒之人，病腹胀如斗……此得之湿热伤脾阴……胃虽受谷，脾不输运，故成痞胀。"《诸病源候论》曰："寒温失节……食饮不消，聚结在内，染渐生块段……人即柴瘦，腹转大……""积聚者，由阴阳不和，脏腑虚弱，受于风邪，搏于腑脏之气所为也。"

In the Chinese medical literature, there is no disease name of "primary liver cancer", but according to the clinical symptoms, it is equivalent to "hypochondrium pain", "jaundice", "hypochondrium mass", "hypochondrium lumps", "abnormal abdominal mass", "abdominal mass", "tympanites", "hepatic retention", "mass", "splenic abdominal mass". *Synopsis of Golden Chamber* thinks that the etiology of "jaundice" is "characterized by yellow complexion, generated from dampness". *Zhangshi Yitong (Zhang's Medical View)* says: "Alcoholic people, with disease of abdominal distension... this is because dampness and heat hurt the spleen Yin... Although the stomach can accept grain, the spleen does not transport, thus ruffian distension occurs. *Zhubing Yuanhou Lun (General Treatise on Causes and Manifestations of All Diseases)* says: "Affected by abnormal cold and warm climatic... diet fails to be digested, accumulates and stagnates in the body and gradually generates masses... the patient is as thin as firewood, but the abdomen turns big..." "Abnormal abdominal masses are caused by disharmony of Yin and Yang, resulted from the fighting of wind evil against the qi of weak viscera."

沈金鳌在《杂病源流犀烛》中论述臌胀的病机，认为是"由怒气伤肝，渐蚀其脾，脾虚之极，故阴阳不交，清浊相混，隧道不通"而致，指出"从湿得之""湿热伤脾""寒温失节""饮食不消""七情所伤"是肝癌的主要病因，但是正气亏虚、脏腑失调是发病的内在条件。按气血辨证而言，多数学者认为气滞血瘀是肝癌产生的病理基础。司富春认为，肝癌产生的机制为各种原因导致气血失调，气滞血结，肿大成积，留而不去所致，而气滞血瘀，日久积聚成块是肝癌的基本病理。陈树森等指出原发性肝癌属本虚标实之证，"本虚即气血不足，正气亏损；标实即邪气内蕴，血瘀火毒"。周宜强等提出正虚不运，邪毒水湿停留，痰热蕴积可见标实之疾；标实之邪恋而不去，戕伤正气，损伤阴液乃见正虚之变。其或由虚致实，或由实致虚而呈或虚或实，而成虚实夹杂之证。苑淑芳等则提出热灼阴液，炼液成痰。阴虚聚毒成癌；或气滞血瘀，脉络阻塞，邪聚毒凝乃成。其中，湿热为启动子，血瘀和阴虚是主要病理基础。傅凤霞等认为：肝癌的发生，既有内在因素，又有外邪侵袭，使肝脾功能失调，邪毒蕴结于经络脏腑，引起气血瘀滞、痰湿凝聚等病理改变，日久不愈而成癥积。曾水成等认为：无论肝郁、血瘀、湿热、热毒，还是脾虚和肝肾阴虚，肝癌的发生机制则是在脾虚肝郁、痰瘀互结等病变基础上，机体受到一种或多种因素的影响，改变了机体的内在环境，使原有的痰、湿、瘀等病理产物发生质变，凝聚为癌毒，留滞于肝，形成恶肉，即癌肿。综观文献，中医学认为肝的生理特点是体阴而用阳，主疏泄，喜条达，恶抑郁，主藏血。因而肝癌的病位在肝，关于肝癌的病机，以肝郁、脾虚、血瘀、湿热、肝肾阴虚多见。

Shen Jinao discussed on the etiology of tympanites in his book *Cause Study on Miscellaneous Diseases*, believing that it begins "from the anger hurting the liver, gradually eroding the spleen, the spleen becomes extremely deficient, so Yin and Yang are separated, lucidity and turbidity are mixed, and the tunnel is blocked". It is pointed out that "generated from the dampness", "dampness hurt the spleen", "extreme cold and warm climatic phenomenon", "dyspepsia" and "hurt from seven kind of emotions" are the main causes of liver cancer, however, healthy qi deficiency, viscera disorder is the internal etiology of the disease. According to the syndrome differentiation theory, most scholars believe that qi stagnation and blood stasis is the pathological basis of liver cancer. Si Fuchun et al. believes that the pathogenesis of liver cancer is irregular operation of qi and blood, qi stagnation and blood bind, distended and enlarged to be mass, lingering without leaving, long-time accumulation of qi stagnation and blood stasis becoming masses is the basic principle of liver cancer. Chen Shusen et al. point out that primary liver cancer is the syndrome of sthenia tips with asthenia root "the asthenia root indicates the deficiency of healthy qi, and short of breath and blood; sthenia tips indicates that internal accumulation of evil qi, blood stasis and fire toxin." Zhou Yiqiang et al. put forward the deficient healthy qi does not transport, evil toxin and water dampness retains, phlegmatic heat accumulation can see the sthenia tip disease; the evil of sthenia tips lingers without leaving, further harms healthy qi, damages Yin liquid, causes the change of the deficiency of healthy qi. Either from asthenia to sthenia, or from sthenia to asthenia, or sometimes asthenia, sometimes sthenia, syndrome mingled with sthenia and ashenia. Yuan Shufang, et al. put forward that heat burns Yin liquid, refining liquid into sputum. Yin deficiency accumulates toxin into cancer; or qi stagnation and blood stasis, and vein obstruction, causes evil accumulation and toxin coagulation, lead to cancer. Among them, dampness and heat is the promoter, and blood stasis and Yin deficiency are the main pathological basis. Fu Fengxia et al. believe that the occurrence of liver cancer, has both internal factors, and the invasion of external evil, which make the liver and spleen dysfunction, evil toxin accumulated in the meridians and viscera, causing pathological changes as qi stagnation and blood stasis, condensation of phlegmatic hygrosis, lingering without recovery for long-time, turns to be hepatic retention. Zeng Shuicheng et al. think: among all the causes like the liver depression, blood stasis, dampness and heat, heat toxin, or spleen deficiency and liver Yin deficiency, the generating mechanism of liver cancer is that on the basis of fundamental pathological changes of spleen deficiency liver depression, co-binding of sputum and stasis, human body is affected by one or more factors, which change the internal environment, cause the original sputum, wet, stasis and other pathological products, make qualitative changes, and finally condensed into cancer toxin, retains in the liver, become evil meat, namely cancerous swelling. Based on the above literature, TCM believes that the physiological characteristics of the liver are that the organ is Yin and the function is Yang, it controls dispersing, likes peace and free, dislikes depression, is in charge of blood storing. Therefore, the location of liver cancer is in the liver, the symptom of liver cancer usually see liver depression, spleen deficiency, blood stasis, dampness and heat, liver and kidney Yin deficiency.

总之，历代医家多认为肝癌的病因较为复杂。中医学认为"邪之所凑，其气必虚"，肝癌发病系先天不足、后天失养、饮食不节、嗜烟饮酒、六淫侵袭、忧思过度、脾胃损伤、脏腑失调等内外因素综合作用的结果。肝癌肿瘤的形成，可能与肝郁、气结、湿热、痰湿、瘀血、热毒等瘀滞及肝肾阴虚有关。其病例特点为本虚标实。本虚多为脾胃阳虚、肝肾阴虚、气血亏虚等，而标实多为肝郁、血瘀、湿热、热毒等夹杂互见。

In short, most doctors in all dynasties believe that the cause of liver cancer is complicated. TCM believes that "Wherever evil accumulates, the qi must be deficient". The incidence of liver cancer is the result of comprehensive action of internal and external factors such as congenital deficiency, acquired loss of nourishment, irregular diet, favor of smoking and drinking, invading of six evils, excessive worry, spleen and stomach damage. The formation of liver cancer tumor may be related to the stasis and stagnation such as liver depression, qi binding, dampness and heat, phlegmatic hygrosis, blood stasis, heat toxin, and Yin deficiency of liver and kidney. The pathological characteristics are the asthenia root and sthenia tips. The asthenia root indicates the Yang deficiency of spleen and stomach, Yin deficiency of liver and kidney, dual deficiency of qi and blood, ect. while the sthenia tips indicates mingling of liver depression, blood stasis, dampness and heat, heat toxin.

二、基于浊毒理论对本病的认识
2. Understanding of liver cancer based on turbid toxin theory

在肝癌的发病中，浊毒既是一种病理产物，又是其重要的致病因素。浊毒是由感染病毒、饮酒过多、饮食不节及其他疾病转变所致，使肝脾受损，脏腑失和，肝失疏泄，气机郁滞，脾失健运，水湿不化，湿浊中阻，郁而不解，蕴积成热，热壅血瘀而成毒，形成"浊""毒"内壅之势。肝癌发生的病因，不外乎内、外两个方面的原因。外因是浊毒之邪外侵，蕴积中焦，脾失健运；内因为情志不舒、气机不畅或正气虚损，肝气疏泄失职，肝郁乘脾或脾虚肝乘，内外合邪，肝脾失调，成为肝癌发生发展变化的基础。肝癌的发生首先责之于浊毒内蕴。肝藏血而以疏泄为用，肝气调达，气机通畅，五脏乃和，六腑则安。若外感六淫或七情内伤，致肝气郁结，疏泄无权，则脏腑经络失调，气机不畅，造成气滞血瘀，脾虚湿困，日久湿、热、气、血、毒结聚成块，浊毒内蕴，形成肝积。

In the pathogenesis of liver cancer, turbid toxin is a pathological product as well as an important pathogenic factor. Turbid toxin is caused by infection of viruses, over-drinking, un-controlled diet and transmission from other diseases, which damage the liver and spleen, lead to viscera disharmony, liver looses the function of dispersing, qi mechanism is depressed and stagnated, spleen looses the function of transporting, water moisture can not be vaporized, wet turbidity is obstructed in middle energizer, depressed and confused, and then accumulated into heat, abundant heat and blood stasis are transmitted into toxin, forming the tendency of internal abundance of "turbidity" and "toxin". The cause of liver cancer is no more than internal and external causes.External cause is the invasion of turbid toxin evil from outside, accumulated in middle energizer, spleen looses the normal function of transportation; The internal causes include abnormal mood state, abnormal operation of qi mechanism, or deficiency of healthy qi, dysfunction of liver dispersing, liver depression over-restricts the spleen, or spleen deficiency is over-restricted by liver. The combination of internal and external evil, and the irregular liver and spleen, become the basis of the generation and development change of liver cancer. The generation of liver cancer is first because the internal accumulation of turbid toxin. Liver controls blood storing and disperse the liver qi, when liver qi is peaceful and free, the qi movement is in normal operation, five zang-organ are in harmony, six fu-organ are in peace. If human body is attacked by the external six evil or internal injured by seven emotions, liver qi will be stagnated, dispersing function does not work, the viscera and meridians will be disordered, energy mechanism operation will be abnormal, causing qi stagnation and blood stasis, spleen deficiency and dampness obstruction, with time passes, wet, heat, qi, blood, and toxin are aggregated into blood lumps, internal accumulation of turbidity poison generates hepatic retention.

　　从临床表现看，初期肝癌患者舌质多红，舌苔黄腻或黄厚腻，脉多弦细滑或弦滑，均为浊毒内蕴之征。中期患者舌质多暗红或紫暗，舌苔黄或黄腻，脉多弦细或涩，均为浊毒瘀阻之明征。后期患者舌质多红或红绛，舌苔少或无苔，脉多弦细或沉细，均为浊毒伤阴之征。因此，我们发现，以化浊解毒为主，辅以软肝散结、滋补肝肾法指导肝癌的临床用药后，患者舌质转淡红，苔转薄白，脉象趋于和缓，临床症状减轻或消失，能明显延长患者生存期，提高生活质量。

Observing the clinical manifestations, patients with the initial liver cancer usually have red tongue, yellow greasy or thick yellow greasy moss, string thready slippery pulse or string slippery pulse, this is the syndrome of internal accumulation of turbid toxin. Patients with mid-term liver cancer usually have dark red or purple dark tongue with yellow or yellow greasy moss, and string thready or astringent pulse, these are significant signs of congestion of turbid toxin. In the late stage of the disease, patients have red or red purple tongue, less or no moss, and string thready or sunk thready pulse, these are signs of turbid toxin injuring Yin.Therefore, we found that after the clinical use of prescriptions under the guidance of the method of turbidity resolving and toxin removing, assisted by the method of liver softening and bind dissipating, and nourishing of liver and reinforcing of kidney, conditions of patients have changes as follows, the tongue turns to be light red, tongue moss turns to be thin white, pulse tends to reconcile, clinical symptoms are reduced or disappeared, the above solution could significantly prolong the survival of patients and improve the quality of life.

第二节　治疗原则
Section 2　Principles of Treatment

　　肝癌的病理性质是邪实正虚、本虚标实、虚实夹杂，故治疗的基本原则应是祛邪扶正。同时，在肝癌的不同阶段，要掌握运用祛邪与扶正的时机。

The pathological nature of liver cancer is evil sthenia and healthy qi asthenia, root ashtenia and tip sthenia, mixed with ashenia and sthenia, so the basic principle of treatment should be to dispel evil and strengthen the healthy qi. At the same time, in the different stages of liver cancer, we should master to grasp the right time either to dispel evil or to reinforce the healthy qi.

肝癌早期，重在祛邪；肝癌中期，癌肿发展到一定程度，癌毒耗损机体正气，邪盛正虚，故宜攻补兼施；肝癌晚期，正气大伤，机体不能任受攻伐，治疗宜采用大补小攻的措施，补虚扶正为主，兼以祛邪抗癌，重施补益以增强患者体质，提高机体耐受能力，提高抗癌能力，配合施以抗癌祛邪使癌毒消散、肿瘤停止发展。

In the early stage of liver cancer, we should focus on removing evil. In the middle stage of liver cancer, the tumor has developed to certain degree, the cancerous evil consumes healthy qi of human body, evil is excess, healthy qi is deficient, so the treatment should combine purging with supplementing. In the late stage of liver cancer, healthy qi is mostly worn out, patient's body can not bear purging, the treatment should use the strategy of more reinforcing and less purging, mainly reinforcing the deficiency and strengthen the healthy qi, assisted with dispelling the evil and preventing the further development of cancer, make more effort on reinforcement to improve the constitution, raise up the ability of tolerance and cancer -preventing. Assisted with cancer preventing and evil dispelling in order to eliminate the cancerous toxin and stop the development of cancer.

第三节　常用治法
Section 3　The Common Method of Treatment

一、祛邪除因法
1. The method to eliminate the cause and dispel the evil

肝癌的癌毒炽盛，为多种病理因素合并，故祛邪之法当贯穿治疗的始终。因为邪能伤正，祛邪则正安。只有强化祛邪抗癌，才能消除多种病理因素，消解癌毒，减小瘤体体积，防止病情进一步发展，所以应特别强调祛邪抗癌在肝癌中的运用。在祛邪治疗中，有抗癌解毒法、疏理气机法、活血化瘀法、化痰除湿法、软坚散结法等具体治疗方法。肝癌癌毒为多因复合、交结错杂。因此，在相应病理因素存在的前提下，诸多治法可结合使用。

The cancerous toxin of liver cancer is abundant and flourishing due to combination of a variety of pathological factors, so the method of removing evil should be carried out throughout the whole process of the treatment. Because evil can hurt healthy, to dispel evil can ensure the safty of healthy qi. Only by strengthening the evil dispelling and cancer preventing, can we eliminate a variety of pathological factors, eliminate the cancer toxin, reduce the size of the tumor body, and prevent the further development of the disease. Therefore, special emphasis should be layed on the application of evil dispelling and cancer preventing in liver cancer treatment. In the treatment of evil dispelling, there are specific treatment methods such as anti-cancer and removing toxin method, regulating qi method, promoting blood circulation and resolving blood stasis method, resolving phlegm and dampness dissipating method, and softening the hardness and dissipating the binding method. The viruses of liver cancer is a mingled and mixed combination of multi cause compounds, therefore, under the premise of the existence of the corresponding pathological factors, many treatment methods can be used in combination.

（一）抗癌解毒法

1.1 The manner of removing toxin to prevent cancer

该法的目的在于攻克癌毒，抗击、解除凶、险、痼、顽邪毒。针对癌毒及其不同性质的病理因素，本法具体包括以毒攻毒、清热解毒、消瘀解毒、化痰解毒、化湿解毒、搜风解毒、散寒解毒等。如上所述，肝癌是由于气滞、血瘀、湿浊、痰凝、湿热、热毒等因素胶合，内生癌毒，癌毒袭人，凝滞气血津液，肝胆恶肉生成所致，故祛除相关病理因素，消除癌毒为治疗的关键。在临床运用中，以毒攻毒、清热解毒为常用抗癌解毒法，而消瘀解毒、化痰解毒、除湿解毒诸法又常被涵括于活血化瘀、化痰除湿、软坚散结等治法之中。

The purpose of the manner is to counteract cancer evil by removing toxin, fighting against and relieving fierce, dangerous, obstinate and chronic evil toxin. Aiming at the pathological factors of different nature, the manner includes the following methods: attacking toxin with toxic agent, removing toxin by clearing heat, removing toxin by dispelling stasis, removing toxin by dissipating phlegm, removing toxin by dissipating dampness, removing toxin by expelling wind, removing toxin by dissipating cold. As mentioned above, liver cancer is internally generated by combination of factors including qi stagnation, blood stasis, dampness retention, phlegm coagulation, dampness and heat, heat toxin and other factors. The cancer toxin attacks human body, coagulates and retains qi, blood, fluid and liquid, the evil meat of liver and gallbladder generates, so to remove related pathological factors, eliminate cancer toxin is the key for treatment.In clinical application, attacking toxin with toxic agent, removing toxin by clearing heat are the methods generally used. Methods of removing toxin by dispelling blood stasis, removing toxin by resolving phlegm, removing toxin by dampness elimination are often included in the treatment method of promoting blood circulation and removing blood stasis, resolving phlegm and eliminating dampness, softening the hardness and dispersing binds.

1.以毒攻毒法　是指使用有毒之品、性峻力猛之药解除癌毒而抗癌的一种方法。本法是针对癌毒胶结，深伏于内，凶险恶劣，非攻难克的特点而设立的。对于肝癌，临床常用的以毒攻毒药有全蝎、蜈蚣、蟾皮、土鳖虫、炮山甲等。此类药物多具有毒性，属于虫类药，多具有开结拔毒的功效。在临床使用时，应注意审视患者的体质情况、病程病期，注意药物的具体选择。另外，因为许多毒性药的中毒剂量与治疗剂量相近，且毒药伤正，故应慎重选择剂量、剂型，注意观察服药后的反应，中病即止，防止毒副反应的产生。必要时可配合扶正，防止毒副反应的药物共同使用。

1.1.1 Attacking toxin with toxin　The method refers to using toxic products, fierce and powerful

drugs to remove cancer toxin to fight against cancer. This method is established aiming at the characteristics of cancer toxin as agglutinated, deeply hidden, fierce and dangerous, and incurable unless being attacked. For liver cancer, medicines generally used in clinical practice for attacking toxin with toxic agent are quan xie (Scorpio), wu gong (Scolopendra), chan pi (Toad skin), tu bie chong (Eupolyphaga Steleophaga), pao shan jia (prepared Squanma Manitis). Most of these drugs are toxic insect herbs and have the effect of opening bind and removing toxin. In clinical use, attention should be paid to the patients' physical condition, course and stage of disease and the specific choice of herbs. In addition, because the poisoning dose of many toxic drugs is near to the treatment dose, further more, the toxic medicine injure healthy qi, so the dosage and form of medicine should be carefully selected, doctors should pay attention to observe the patient's reaction after taking the drug, the medicine should be stopped as soon as the disease is controlled, so as to prevent the occurrence of toxic and side effect. If necessary, drugs to reinforce the healthy qi can be used in cooperation to prevent toxic and side effect.

2.化浊解毒法　该法针对浊毒内蕴及其所致的肝癌癌毒。情志内伤或其他因素所导致的郁火、邪热郁结日久而成为浊毒，浊毒内蕴肝胆，导致气血瘀滞津停，凝结成块。浊毒内蕴与肝癌的发生、发展与转移有密切关系。化浊解毒法适应于肝癌兼有浊毒内蕴征象者。临床上常用清热解毒药有漏芦、露蜂房、白花蛇舌草、山豆根、藤梨根、猫爪草、龙葵、白毛夏枯草、夏枯草、石见穿、半枝莲、半边莲、穿心莲、重楼、板蓝根、大青叶、虎杖、紫草、蒲公英、紫花地丁、黄连、黄芩、黄柏、苦参、龙胆草、土茯苓等。清热解毒类药物性多偏凉、味苦，故选择使用时应注意药味数量和剂量，防止苦寒伤正、苦寒败胃。

1.1.2 Method of resolving turbidity and removing toxin　The method is set up for the internal accumulation of turbid toxin and the cancerous toxin of liver cancer which is generated from the form. When the depression fire and evil heat caused by internal injury of emotions or other factors stagnate for a long time, they will become turbid toxin. The turbid toxin accumulates internally in liver and gallbladder, causes qi stagnation and blood stasis and fluid block, which coagulates into masses. The internal accumulation of turbid toxin is closely related to the generation, development and metastasis of liver cancer. The method of removing toxin by resolving turbidity is adaptable to liver cancer with syndrome of internal accumulation of turbid toxin. Medicines generally used to remove toxin by clearing heat in clinical practice are: lou lu (Rhapontici Radix), lu feng fang (Nidus Polistis), bai hua she she cao (Herba Oldenlandiae Diffusae), shan dou gen (Radix Sophorae Tonkinensis), teng li gen (Radix Actinidae Chinensis), mao zhua cao (Radix Euophobiae Helescopiae), long kui (Herba Solani Nigri), bai mao xia ku cao (Herba Ajugae Decumbentis), xia ku cao (Spica Prunellae), shi jian chuan (Herba Salviae Chinensis), ban zhi lian (Scutellariae Barbatae Herba), ban bian lian (Herba Lobeliae Radicantis), chuan xin lian (Andrographis Herba), chong lou (Rhizoma Paridis), ban lan gen (Radix Isatidis), da qing ye (Folium Isatidis), hu zhang (Rhizoma Polygoni Cuspidati), zi cao (Radix Arnebiae), pu gong ying (Herba Taraxaci cum Radice), zi hua di ding (Herba Violae), huang lian (Rhizoma Coptidis), huang qin (Radix Scutellariae), huang bo (Cortex Phellodendri), ku shen (Sophorae Flavescentis Radix), long dan cao (Gentianae Radix et Rhizoma), tu fu ling (Rhizoma Smilacis Glabrae), etc. Heat-clearing and detoxification drugs are more cool and bitter, so when choosing to use it, doctors should pay attention to the number and dosage of medicine, so as to prevent bitter cold injuring the healthy qi and affecting stomach function.

（二）疏理气机法

1.2 The method of regulating qi

该法针对肝癌癌毒以气滞为主而设，对肝郁气滞、脾虚气滞较为合适。气滞是肝癌发生发展过程中最基本的病理变化。其他病理因素如血瘀、湿阻、痰凝、湿热、热毒的生成与变化无不与气滞相关，故癌毒内生与气滞密切相连。因此，理气药在肝癌的治疗中贯穿全程，必不可少，至关重要。对于肝癌，临床常用的理气药有柴胡、青皮、预知子、陈皮、枳壳、制香附、郁金、炒延胡索、川楝子、大腹皮、佛手等。理气药亦有在肝、在脾之不同，肝气郁滞宜选疏肝理气之品，脾虚气滞当重选健脾理气之药。

The method is mainly designed for liver cancer with characteristic of qi stagnation, is more suitable for liver depression and qi stagnation, spleen deficiency and qi stagnation. Qi stagnation is one of the most basic pathological changes in the generation and development of liver cancer. The generation and development of other pathological factors such as blood stasis, wet resistance, phlegm coagulation, dampness and heat, heat toxin are all related to qi stagnation, so the endogenous generation of cancer toxin are closely related to qi stagnation. Therefore, medicine for qi regulating is necessary and crucial throughout the whole treatment process of liver cancer. For liver cancer, qi regulating medicines generally used in clinical practice are: chai hu (Radix Bulpleuri), qing pi (Pericarpium Citri Reticcutatae Viride), yu zhi zi (Fructus Akebiae), chen pi (Pericarpium Citri Reticulatae), zhi qiao (Fructus Aurantii), zhi xiang fu (prepared Rhizoma Cyperi) , yu jin (Radix Curcumae), chao yan hu suo (fried Rhizoma Corydalis), chuan lian zi (Fructus Toosendan), da fu pi (Arecae Pericarpium), fo shou (Fructus Citri Sarcodactylis) and so on. Qi regulating medicines are different due to the different location of the qi stagnation either in liver or in spleen, for liver depression and qi stagnation, we should choose liver dispersing and qi regulating products; for spleen deficiency and qi stagnation, we should choose medicines of spleen reinforcing and qi regulating.

（三）活血化瘀法

1.3 The method of activating blood circulation and removing blood stasis

该法是针对癌毒以瘀血为著而设。本法不仅可对应治疗瘀血，亦是治疗肿瘤、防止肿瘤扩散与转移的一个常用方法。历代医家皆重视瘀血与有形结块的关系。肝癌与古称"癥"互参，其形成的病理机制与瘀血凝滞有密切关系，因为瘀血停滞、气行不畅、气滞血瘀经久不散。对于肝癌的治疗，临床上常用的活血化瘀药有当归尾、赤芍、川芎、丹参、郁金、虻虫、水蛭、炮山甲、全蝎、蜈蚣等。使用时需注意适应证，控制剂量，以防引起出血。

The method is designed to treat liver cancer toxin with characteristic of blood stasis. This method can not only correspond to the treatment of blood stasis, but also is a common method to treat tumors and prevent tumor spreading and metastasis. Doctors in all dynasties attach great importance to the relationship between blood stasis and tangible lumps. Liver cancer is referred to "abdominal mass" in ancient TCM, the pathological mechanism of generation has close relationship with blood stasis stagnation, because blood stasis is stagnated, qi fails to flow smoothly, qi stagnation and blood stasis lingers for long time. For liver cancer treatment, medicines generally used in clinical practice to promote blood circulation and resolve blood stasis are: dang gui wei (Radix Angelicae Sinensis), chi shao (Radix Paeoniae Rubra), chuan xiong (Rhizoma Chuanxiong), dan shen (Salviae Miltiorrhizae), yu jin (Radix Curcumae), meng chong (Tabannus Bivittatus), shui zhi (Hirudo), pao shan jia (prepared Squanma Manitis), quan xie (Scorpio), wu gong (Scolopendra), etc. When using, doctors should pay attention to the indication and control the dose to prevent bleeding.

（四）化痰除湿法
1.4 The method of phlegm resolving and dampness removing

痰凝湿聚是致使肝癌癌毒形成的基本病理之一，化痰除湿法正是针对痰湿这个病理因素而设立的。化痰除湿不仅对因，而且可以减轻临床症状，使肝癌发展转移得以控制。在肝癌治疗中，常用化痰除湿药物有山慈菇、茯苓、猪苓、泽泻、车前子、薏苡仁、木防己、大贝母、皂角刺、半夏、葶苈子、苍术、厚朴、藿香、佩兰、蚕砂、煨草果等。

Phlegm coagulation and wet cohesion is one of the basic pathologies causing the formation of liver cancer toxin. The phlegm resolving and dampness removing method is specially established for this pathological factor. Phlegm resolving and dampness removing method is not only adaptable for the cause of disease, it can also reduce clinical symptoms, make the development and metastasis of liver cancer controllable. In the treatment of liver cancer, medicines generally used for phlegm resolving and dampness removing in clinical practice are shan ci gu (Pseudobulbus Cremastrae Variabilis), fu ling (Poria), zhu ling (Polygorus Umbellatus), ze xie (Rhizoma Alismatis), che qian zi (Semen Plantaginis), yi yi ren (Semen Coisis), mu fang ji (Radix Cocculi Trilobi), da bei mu (Bulb of Thunberg Fritillary), zao jiao ci (Gleditsiae Spina), ban xia (Rhizoma Pinelliae), ting li zi (Semen Lepdii seu Descurainiae), cang zhu (Rhizoma Atractylodis), hou po (Cortex Magnoliae Officinalis), huo xiang (Herba Agastaches seu Pogostemonis), pei lan (Herba Eupatorii), can sha (Faeces Bombycis), wei cao guo (Fructus Tsaoko) and so on.

（五）清热利湿法
1.5 The method of heat clearing and dampness removing

湿热亦是致使肝癌癌毒形成的基本病理之一。清热利湿法即是针对湿热毒邪，或湿浊蕴而化热成毒设立的。在肝癌的治疗中，常用的清热化湿药有黄连、黄芩、黄柏、夏枯草、田基黄、茵陈、垂盆草、苦参、虎杖、凤尾草、鸡骨草、酢浆草、白鲜皮、地肤子、金钱草、海金沙等。

Dampness and heat is also one of the basic pathologies that cause the formation of liver cancer toxin. The method of clearing heat and dampness removing is established specially for dampness, heat and toxic evil, or accumulation of dampness and turbidity transmitted into heat and toxin. In the treatment of liver cancer, medicines generally used for heat clearing and dampness removing are: huang lian (Rhizoma Coptidis), huang qin (Radix Scutellariae), huang bo (Cortex Phellodendri), xia ku cao (Spica Prunellae), tian ji huang (Grangea Maderas Patana), yin chen hao (Cacumen Artemistae Scopariae), chui pen cao (Herba Sedi Sarmentosi), ku shen (Sophorae Flavescentis Radix), hu zhang (Rhizoma Polygoni Cuspidati), feng wei cao (Herba Pterdis Multifidae), ji gu cao (Herba Abri), cu jiang cao (Oxalis Cormiculta), bai xian pi (Cortex Dictamni Radicis), di fu zi (Kochiae Fructus), jin qian cao (Herba Lysmachiae), hai jin sha (Lygodii Spora) and so on.

（六）软坚散结法
1.6 The method of hardness softening and bind dispelling

该法是针对肝癌、结块坚硬所设，是使用软坚散结药物使肿块软化、缩小、消散的治疗方法。肿瘤古称石瘕、岩，多为有形之物，坚硬如石。在治疗肝癌时常用的软坚散结类药物有龟甲、鳖甲、牡蛎、海浮石、海藻、瓦楞子、昆布、海蛤壳、夏枯草、穿山甲、地龙、白芥子、半夏、胆南星、瓜蒌、天葵子、山慈菇等。

The method is designed for liver cancer with hard mass. It uses medicines of hardness softening and bind dispelling to soften, shrink and dissipate the mass. Tumor in ancient times is called stone mass, rock mass, is mostly tangible thing, as hard as stone. In the treatment of liver cancer, medicines generally used to soften hardness and dispel binds are: gui jia (Plastrum Testudinis), bie jia (Carapax Trionycis seu Amydae), mu li (Ostreae), hai fu shi (Os Costaziae), hai zao (Herba Sargassi), wa leng zi (Choncha Arcae), kun bu (Thallus Laminariae seu Eckloniae), hai ge qiao (Concha Cyclinae), xia ku cao (Spica Prunellae), chuan shan jia (Squanma Manitis), di long (Lumbricus), bai jie zi (Semen Sinapis Albae), ban xia (Rhizoma Pinelliae), dan nan xing (Arisaema Cum Bile), gua lou (Trichosanthis Fructus), tian kui zi (Semiaquilegiae Radix), shan ci gu (Pseudobulbus Cremastrae Variabilis) and so on.

二、扶正补虚法
2. To strengthen the healthy qi and tonify the deficiency method

扶正之法是治疗肝癌必要时的防御性姑息疗法。对于中晚期患者，对于已经或正在进行手术或介入、放疗、化疗的肝癌患者，在邪毒肆虐的同时，因已表现出正虚之征，需配合使用补虚扶正之治。肿瘤的发生与正气亏虚密切相关。

The method is a defensive palliative therapy for liver cancer when necessary. For patients in middle and advanced stages, for liver cancer patients who have finished or are undergoing surgery or intervention, radiotherapy and chemotherapy, at the same time, the pathogenic toxin is fiercely invading the body, the signs of deficiency in healthy qi has been presented, it is necessary to use the treatment of deficiency reinforcing and healthy qi strengthening. Tumor occurrence is closely related to the healthy qi deficiency.

（一）益气养血法
2.1 Qi regulating and blood nourishing method

本法为中晚期肝癌有明显气血虚弱，或化疗、放疗治疗后所致骨髓抑制及全血下降所设。常用药物有党参、黄芪、炙甘草、熟地黄、仙鹤草、鸡血藤、茜草根、当归、阿胶、白芍、黄精、何首乌等。

This method is designed for patients in middle and advanced stage of liver cancer who has obvious qi and blood weakness, or bone marrow suppression and whole blood decline after chemotherapy and radiotherapy therapy. Medicines generally used are: dang shen (Radix Codonopsitis Pilosulae), huang qi (Radix Astragali seu Hedysari), zhi gan cao (fried Radix Glycyrrhizae), shu di huang (Radix Rehmanniae Praeparatum), xian he cao (Herba Agrimoniae), ji xue teng (Caulis Spatholobi), qian cao gen (Rhizoma Rubiae), dang gui (Radix Angelicae Sinensis), e jiao (Colla Corii Asini), bai shao (Radix Paeoniae Alba), huang jing (Rhizoma Rolygonati), he shou wu (Radix Polygoni Multiflori), etc.

（二）养阴生津法

2.2 Method of generating liquid by nourishing Yin

本法为肝癌伴阴津损伤而设，常用药物有沙参、麦冬、天冬、百合、玉竹、生地黄、天花粉、西洋参、龟甲、鳖甲等。临床使用时需慎防滋阴呆胃、滋阴助湿。故可适当配伍理气助运药物。

This method is set for liver cancer with injury of Yin and liquid, medicines generally used are: sha shen (Radix Adenophorae Strictae), mai dong (Radix Ophiopogonis), tian dong (Radix Asparagi), bai he (Bulbus Lilii), yu zhu (Polygonati Odorati Rhizoma), sheng di huang (Radix Rehmanniae), tian hua fen (Radix Trichosanthis), xi yang shen (Panacis Quinquefolii Radix), gui jia (Plastrum Testudinis), bie jia (Carapax Trionycis seu Amydae) and so on. Doctors should be careful to prevent Yin nourishing from sluggishing the stomach, Yin nourishing assisting dampness in clinical application. Therefore, it can be properly matched with qi regulating and transporting promoting medicines.

（三）滋阴补肾法

2.3 Method of enriching Yin and tonifying kidney

本法为中晚期肝癌伴肝肾阴亏所设，常用药物有生地黄、熟地黄、何首乌、制黄精、龟甲、鳖甲、女贞子、枸杞子、墨旱莲、五味子、知母等。

This method is for patients in middle and advanced stage of liver cancer with Yin deficiency of liver and kidney, medicines generally used are: sheng di huang (Radix Rehmanniae), shu di huang (Radix Rehmanniae Praeparatum), he shou wu (Radix Polygoni Multiflori), zhi huang jing (Rhizoma Rolygonati), gui jia (Plastrum Testudinis), bie jia (Carapax Trionycis seu Amydae), nv zhen zi (Fructus Ligustri), gou qi zi (Lycii Fructus), mo han lian (Herba Ecliptae), wu wei zi (Fructus Schisandalis), zhi mu (Rhizoma Anemarrhennae), etc.

（四）补肾温阳法

2.4 Method of tonifying kidney by warming Yang

本法为肝癌伴肾阳虚所设，选用补肾温阳法治之，常取金匮肾气丸、右归丸、附子理中汤为基础方，加味淫羊藿、巴戟天、桂枝等。

This method is designed for patients of liver cancer with kidney Yang deficiency. Jingui Shenqi Pill, Yougui Pill, Fuzi Lizhong Decoction are usually used as basic prescriptions. Medicines for addition are: yin yang huo (Epimedii Folium), ba ji tian (Morindae Officinalis Radix), gui zhi (Cmnamomi Mmulus), etc.

（五）健脾助运法

2.5 Method of spleen reinforcing and transportation assisting

本法为肝癌伴脾胃虚弱、食积不行而设。晚期肝癌虽然呈上腹积硬而牢痛之邪实表现，但治疗仍要从本虚着手，以补脾为主。常用的健脾助运药有黄芪、党参、人参、白术、怀山药、焦山楂、炒神曲、炒谷芽、炒麦芽、神曲、鸡内金、砂仁等。

This method is designed for patients of liver cancer accompanied by the spleen and stomach weakness and dyspepsia. Although the advanced liver cancer is manifested as sthenia pathogen of abdominal hard mass with fixed pain and firm pain in the upper abdomen, the treatment should still start from the root asthenia to tonify the spleen. Medicines generally used for spleen reinforcing and transport assisting are: huang qi (Radix Astragali seu Hedysari), dang shen (Radix Codonopsitis Pilosulae), ren shen (Radix Ginseng), bai zhu (Rhizoma Atractylodis Macrocephalae), huai shan yao (Tuber Dioscoreae), jiao shan zha (fried Fructus Crataegi), chao shen qu (fried Massa Medicata Fermentata), chao gu ya (fried Setariae Fructus Germinatus), chao mai ya (fried Hordei Fructus Germinatus), shen qu (Messa Medicata Fermentata), ji nei jin (Endothlium Corneum Gigeriae Galli), sha ren (Fructus Amomi) and so on.

第四节　辨证治疗

Section 4 Treatment with Syndrome Differentiation

一般来说，肝癌初期，癌毒多以气滞、血瘀、痰凝、湿浊、湿热、火郁热毒各有偏盛，或痰瘀互结，湿浊、湿热毒瘀互结，表现为邪实壅盛，正虚不著；中期肝癌，毒势鸱张，癌毒淫溢，多因互结，耗气伤阴竭血，而邪实不减，表现为邪实正虚兼夹；肝癌晚期，癌毒毒势仍盛，流散四方，或入血动风、内陷心包，正气大虚，逐渐出现阴竭阳虚、阴阳离决。总之，肝癌癌毒暴戾，在整个病程中皆有浊毒壅盛的表现。随着病情的发展、病程的延长，病愈深，正愈虚。

Generally speaking, in the early stage of liver cancer, qi stagnation, blood stasis, phlegm coagulation, dampness turbidity, dampness heat, fire depression and heat toxin, each of them might be excessively abundant, or co-coagulation of phlegm and stasis, co-coagulation of damp and urbidity, damp and heat, toxin and stasis, presenting abundance of sthenia pathogen, deficiency of healthy qi. In the middle-stage of the liver cancer, disease toxin develops fiercely, cancerous toxin overflows in the body, combination of various pothogenic factors consumes qi, damages Yin, wears out blood, but the sthenia pathogen is not reduced, sthenia pathogen and asthenia healthy qi exist simultaneously. In late stage of liver cancer, the cancerous toxin still develops fiercely, scatters towards the whole body, or get into blood stirring wind, sink in pericardium, healthy qi is extremely deficient, and gradually Yin is exhausted and Yang is deficient, Yin and Yang separates from each other. In short, liver cancer is violent, abundance of turbid toxin is manifested in the whole course of the of the disease. Along with the development of the disease, and the extension of the disease course, the deeper the disease goes, more deficient the healthy qi turns to be.

一、肝郁脾虚证
1. Liver depression and spleen deficiency syndrome

（一）证候
1.1 Symptoms

右胁疼痛，右胁下痞块，目黄，身黄，腹胀，平时急躁易怒，嗳气，倦怠乏力，纳食减少，小便黄，舌淡苔薄，边有齿痕，脉弦细。

With pain and ruffian under the right side of abdomen, yellow eyes, yellow body, abdominal distension, irritability, belching, fatigue, poor appetite, yellow urine, light and teeth-printed tongue with thin moss, string thready pulse.

（二）治法
1.2 Treatment method

疏肝理气健脾。

To disperse the liver, regulate qi and reinforce the spleen.

（三）方药
1.3 Prescription and medicines

柴胡疏肝散加减。药用柴胡、白芍、白术、黄芪、香附、木香、枳壳、陈皮、川芎、甘草。

Addition and reduction of Chaihu Shugan Powder. Medicines: chai hu (Radix Bulpleuri), bai shao (Radix Paeoniae Alba), bai zhu (Rhizoma Atractylodis Macrocephalae), huang qi (Radix Astragali seu Hedysari), xiang fu (Rhizoma Cyperi) , mu xiang (Radix Aucklandiae), zhi qiao (Fructus Aurantii), chen pi (Pericarpium Citri Reticulatae), chuan xiong (Rhizoma Chuanxiong), gan cao (Radix Glycyrrhizae).

（四）加减
1.4 Addition and reduction

疼痛甚者加延胡索、川楝子、白芷；食滞不消加焦神曲、焦山楂。

For patients with more severe pains, add yan hu suo (Rhizoma Corydalis), chuan lian zi (Fructus Toosendan), bai zhi (Radix Angelicae Dahuricae); for symptom of dyspepsia, add jiao shen qu (fried Massa Medicata Fermentata), jiao shan zha (Fried Fructus Crataegi).

二、肝肾阴虚证
2. Syndrome of Yin deficiency of liver and kidney

（一）证候
2.1 Symptoms

腹痛隐隐，身黄，目黄，皮肤瘙痒，五心烦热，口眼干涩，形体消瘦，腰膝酸软，舌质红或绛，少苔，脉弦细。

With vague abdominal pain, yellow body, yellow eyes, itchy skin, upset heart, hands and feet, dry and astringent mouth and eyes, thin body, soft waist and knees, red or purple tongue, less moss, string thready pulse.

（二）治法
2.2 Treatment method

滋阴清热，补益肝肾。
To nourish Yin and clear heat, and tonify liver and kidney.

（三）方药
2.3 Prescription and medicines

知柏地黄丸加减。药用生地黄、熟地黄、知母、白芍、黄柏、牡丹皮、山茱萸、麦冬、陈皮、五味子、泽泻、北沙参、枸杞子。

Prescription of Zhibai Dihuang Pill with addition and reduction. Medicines: sheng di huang (Radix Rehmanniae), shu di huang (Radix Rehmanniae Praeparatum), zhi mu (Rhizoma Anemarrhennae), bai shao (Radix Paeoniae Alba), huang bo (Cortex Phellodendri), mu dan pi (Cortex Moutan), shan zhu yu (Corni Fructus), mai dong (Radix Ophiopogonis), chen pi (Pericarpium Citri Reticulatae), wu wei zi (Fructus Schisandalis), ze xie (Rhizoma Alismatis), bei sha shen (Glehniae Radix), gou qi zi (Lycii Fructus).

（四）加减
2.4 Addition and reduction

虚热时作、口渴欲饮加银柴胡、青蒿；睡眠差加酸枣仁、合欢皮、百合。

Deficiency heat, thirsty with want to drink, add yin chai hu (Radix Stellariae), qing hao (Artemisiae Annuae Herba); in case of poor sleep, add suan zao ren (Semen Ziziphi Jujubae), he huan pi (Albiziae Cortex), bai he (Bulbus Lilii).

三、气血两虚证
3. Dual deficiency of qi and blood

（一）证候
3.1 Symptoms

纳少倦怠，气短懒言，乏力，面色苍白，身日瘦而腹日大，沉困怠情，纳谷欠香，恶心呕吐，身黄，目黄，皮肤瘙痒，衄血或紫斑，心悸失眠，食后腹胀，大便干稀不调，舌质淡，舌体胖或有齿印，苔薄白，脉细弱。

Poor appetite, short of breath and lazy to speak, fatigue, pale complexion, thin body and abdominal full, sleepy, fragrant, ageusia, nausea and vomiting, yellow body, yellow eyes, itchy skin, epistaxis or purple spots, palpitations, insomnia, abdominal distension after eating, dry or loose stool, light and fat tongue with teeth-print, thin white moss, thready weak pulse.

（二）治法
3.2 Treatment method

健脾益胃，气血双补。

Strengthen the spleen and nourish the stomach, and replenish qi and blood.

（三）方药
3.3 Prescription and medicines

八珍汤加减。药用潞党参、炒白术、云茯苓、炒当归、川芎、白芍、熟地黄、炙甘草、炒山药、炒谷芽、炒麦芽。

Bazhen Decoction. Medicines: lu dang shen (Radix Codonopsitis Pilosulae), chao bai zhu (fried Rhizoma Atractylodis Macrocephalae), fu ling (Poria), dang gui (Radix Angelicae Sinensis), chuang xiong (Rhizoma Chuanxiong), bai shao (Radix Paeoniae Alba), shu di huang (Radix Rehmanniae Praeparatum), zhi gan cao (fried Radix Glycyrrhizae), chao shan yao (fried Dioscoreae Rhizoma), chao gu ya (fried Setariae Fructus Germinatus), chao mai ya (fried Hordei Fructus Germinatus).

（四）加减
3.4 Addition and reduction

脾气亏虚明显者加黄芪；血亏甚者加阿胶、枸杞子；阴虚者加石斛、天冬。

Obvious deficiency of spleen qi, add huang qi (Radix Astragali seu Hedysari); blood deficiency, add e jiao (Asini Corii Colla) and gou qi zi (Lycii Fructus); Yin deficiency, add shi hu (Dendrobii Caulis) and tian dong (Radix Asparagi).

四、瘀血阻络证
4. Resistance of collatera by blood stasis

（一）证候
4.1 Symptoms

右腹疼痛如针刺，痛处固定不移，或扪及包块，拒按，腹部胀满，肌肤甲错、爪甲不荣，舌质暗红或紫红，或夹瘀斑，脉沉涩。

The pain in the right abdomen is as being needled, the pain is fixed, or palpate the lump, refuse to be pressed, abdominal distention, scaly skin, pale claw and nails, dark red or purple tongue, or with ecchymosis, sunk astringent pulse.

（二）治法

4.2 Treatment method

活血行气，祛瘀通络。

To promote blood circulation and acitivate qi, remove blood stasis and unblock collaterals.

（三）方药

4.3 Prescription and medicines

膈下逐瘀汤加减。药用当归、川芎、桃仁、红花、赤芍、五灵脂、延胡索、香附、枳壳、厚朴、丹参。

Gexia Zhuyu Decoction with addition and reduction. Medicines: dang gui (Radix Angelicae Sinensis), chuan xiong (Rhizoma Chuanxiong), tao ren (Semen Persicae), hong hua (Flos Carthami), chi shao (Radix Paeoniae Rubra), wu ling zhi (Faeces Trogopterorum), yan hu suo (Rhizoma Corydalis), xiang fu (Rhizoma Cyperi) , zhi qiao (Fructus Aurantii), hou po (Cortex Magnoliae Officinalis), dan shen (Salviae Miltiorrhizae).

（四）加减

4.4 Addition and reduction

肝气郁结者加柴胡、郁金；纳呆、大便稀溏者加白术、白豆蔻、茯苓。

Liver qi stagnation, add chai hu (Radix Bulpleuri), yu jin (Radix Curcumae); anorexia, loose stool, add bai zhu (Rhizoma Atractylodis Macrocephalae), bai dou kou (Fructus Amomi Rotundus), fu ling (Poria).

五、浊毒内蕴证
5. The internal accumulation of turbid toxin

（一）证候

5.1 Symptoms

腹满胀痛，时有嗳气，胁下癥积进行性增大，质地坚硬，表面凹凸不平，口干口苦，面色晦暗或黧暗，衄血或紫斑或崩漏，纳呆，小便黄赤如浓茶，大便黏腻不爽，舌质暗红，苔黄厚腻，脉弦滑。

Abdominal full and distention pain, sometimes belching, hypochondria enlarging continuously, with hard texture, uneven surface, dry and bitter mouth, dark or dark black complexion, bleeding or purple spots or leakage of blood, anorexia, yellow red urine as thick tea, sticky and difficult stool, dark red tongue, yellow thick and greasy moss, string slippery pulse.

（二）治法

5.2 Treatment method

清热利湿，化浊解毒。

To clear heat and dispel dampness, resolve turbidity and remove toxin.

（三）方药

5.3 Prescription and medicines

化浊解毒方加减。药用白花蛇舌草、半边莲、半枝莲、茵陈、黄芩、黄连、陈皮、竹茹、半夏。

Prescription of turbidity resolving and toxin removing with addition or reduction. Medicines: bai hua she she cao (Herba Oldenlandiae Diffusiae), ban zhi lian (Scutellariae Barbatae Herba), ban bian lian (Herba Lobeliae Radicantis), yin chen (Herba Artemisiae Scophoriae), huang qin (Radix Scutellariae), huang lian (Rhizoma Coptidis), chen pi (Pericarpium Citri Reticulatae), zhu ru (Caulis Bambusae in Taenian), ban xia (Rhizoma Pinelliae).

（四）加减

5.4 Addition and reduction

小便量少者，加车前子、萹蓄、瞿麦；若呕吐甚者，加半夏、竹茹。

Little quantity of urine, add che qian zi (Semen Plantaginis), bian xu (Herba Polygoni Avicularis), qu mai (Herba Dianthi cum Flore); if vomiting, add ban xia (Rhizoma Pinelliae), zhu ru (Caulis Bambusae in Taenian).

第七章 溃疡性结肠炎浊毒论
Chapter 7 On Turbid Toxin of Ulcerous Colitis

第一节 病因病机
Section 1 Etiology and Pathogenesis

一、古代中医名家对本病的认识
1. The understanding of the ancient TCM masters on this disease

溃疡性结肠炎这一病名在中国古代医家文献中是没有记载的，但是根据其病因、病机以及临床表现，可以将其归属于中医学"肠澼""赤沃""大瘕泄""下利""休息痢""滞下"等范畴中。

The name of ulcerous colitis is not recorded in ancient TCM works, but according to its etiology, pathogenesis and clinical manifestations, it can be attributed to TCM "dysentery", "erthral mucous dysentery", "acute temesmus", "dysentery and diarrhea", "chronic dysentery", "dysentery" and other categories.

《素问·太阴阳明论》云："故犯贼风虚邪者，阳受之；食饮不节，起居不时者，阴受之。阳受之则入六腑，阴受之则入五脏。入六腑则身热不时卧，上为喘呼；入五脏则䐜满闭塞，下为飧泄，久为肠澼。"《诸病源候论·痢病诸候》云："休息痢者，胃脘有停饮，因痢积久，或冷气，或热气乘之，气动于饮，则饮动，而肠虚受之，故为痢也……故其痢乍发乍止，谓之休息痢也。"又云："热毒乘经络，血渗肠内，则变为脓血痢，热久不歇，肠胃转虚，故痢久不断。"《济生方·痢疾》云："今之所谓痢疾者，即古所谓滞下是也……夫人饮食起居失其宜，运动劳役失其度，则脾胃不充，大肠虚弱，而风冷暑湿之邪，得以乘间而入，故为痢疾也"。张景岳在《景岳全书·泄泻》中提出："凡《内经》有言飧泄者，有言濡泻者，皆泄泻也。有言肠澼者，即下痢也，然痢之初作，必由于泻，此泻之与痢本为同类，但泻浅而痢深，泻轻而痢重。泻由水谷不分，由于中焦，痢以脂血伤败，病在下焦……此泻痢之证治有不同，而门类亦当有辨。然病实相关，不可不兼察以为治也。"王肯堂在《证治准绳·滞下》中云："谓治诸痢，莫若以辛苦寒药而治，或微加辛热佐之。辛能开郁，苦能燥湿，寒能胜热，使气宣平而已。"《医宗必读·痢疾》中云："愚按：痢之为证，多本脾肾……然而尤有至要者，则在脾肾两脏……是知在脾者病浅，在肾者病深。肾为胃关，开窍于二阴，未有久痢而肾不损者，故治痢而知补肾，非其治也。"

Simple Conversation-Discussion on Taiyin and Yangming says: "When the pathogenic wind and asthenia evil attack human body, Yang suffers; when uncontrolled diet, and irregular dailylife affects human health, Yin suffers. When Yang suffers, the disease enters six fu-orgens, when Yin suffers, the disease enters five zang-organs. When disease enters the six fu-organs, it will lead to fever and restless sleep, and panting; when disease enters five zang-organs, it will cause distention, fullness, occlusion, Sunxie (acute diarrhea with undigested food in it), and dysentery with time passes." *Zhu Bing Yuan Hou Lun (General Treatise on Causes of Manifestations of all Diseases)-On Dysentery* says: "Chronic dysentery is caused by retained water in the stomach, the water retention accumulates for a long time because of diarrhea, either cold air, or hot air attacks on the retention of water, the retention is pushed forward into deficient intestine, thus diarrhea occurs... as the diarrhea starts and stops abruptly, it is called chronic dysentery." "Heat toxin invades meridians, blood infiltrates into the intestine, it will become pus dysentery. Heat sustains for a long time, intestines and stomach turns to be deficient, so dysentery continues for a long time." *Jisheng Fang Prescriptions-On Dysentery* says: "today's so-called dysentery is called 'zhixia' (dysentery) in ancient time... When diet and daily life are inappropriate, uneven allocation of exercising and work, the spleen and stomach are not abundant, the large intestine is weak, and the evil of wind, cold and summer dampness, get a chance to step in, so dysentery occurs." Zhang Jingyue put forward in *Complete Woks of Jingyue-On Diarrhea:*" Expressions as 'sui xie' (acute diarrhea with undigested food in it)', 'ru xie (lingering diarrhea) in *The Medical Classic of the Yellow Emperor* are all diarrhea. There is a saying of 'changbi (dysentery), it means dysentery diarrhea, but the beginning of dysentery, must be caused by diarrhea, this diarrhea and dysentery is the same category, but diarrhea is shallow, dysentery is deeper, diarrhea is light and dysentery is more severe. Diarrhea is caused by dyspepsia in middle energizer. Dysentery is caused by damage of fat and blood, the location is in the lower energizer... Although there are differences to differentiate and treat diarrhea and dysentery, the disease is really related in nature, and must be considered concurrently in treatment. Wang Kentang said in *Zheng Zhi Zhun Sheng (Standard of Medical Treatment)*-Dysentery: "To treat dysentery, it is no better than using acrid, bitter, cold medicine, or slightly adding some acrid-heat medicines for assistance. Acridness can relieve depression, bitter can dry dampness, cold can restrict heat, so as to make qi regular and smooth." *Necessary References For Medical Colleagues-Dysentery* says: "Dysentery is mostly generated from spleen or kidney... sometimes even in the spleen as well as kidney... If the disease is in the spleen, the disease is thinner, if the disease is in kidney, it is deeper. The kidney is the switch of stomach, the urethra and anus are the orifices to kidney, long-time dysentery will surely damage the kidney, so treating dysentery must tonify kidney at the same time."

总而言之，溃疡性结肠炎其症状表现，与中医学文献中"痢疾""泄泻"相似。所以可以运用古代文献中关于"痢疾""泄泻"的病因病机、治法治则的记载，来指导溃疡性结肠炎的临床诊断和治疗。

To summarize the above, the symptoms of ulcerous colitis are similar to the symptoms of "dysentery" and "diarrhea" in the ancient Chinese medical literature. Therefore, the etiology and pathogenesis, treatment method and principle of "dysentery" and "diarrhea" recorded in ancient literature can be used to guide the clinical diagnosis and treatment of ulcerous colitis.

二、基于浊毒理论对溃疡性结肠炎病因病机的认识

2. Understanding on the etiology of ulcerous colitis based on the theory of turbid toxin

溃疡性结肠炎病因多为感受外邪、饮食不节、情志失调和先天禀赋不足，病机特点为脾胃虚弱为本，浊毒内蕴、瘀血阻滞为标。主要是脾失健运，小肠无以分清泌浊，大肠传导失司，湿浊蕴结，浊聚久为热，热蕴成毒，浊毒壅滞，脂膜血络损伤，血败肉腐，壅滞成脓，日久浊毒内聚不散，肠道传导失司形成本病。浊毒既是一种致病因素，又是一种病理产物，起着致病的始动与复发加重的双重作用。浊毒极易耗伤正气，还易深入脏腑，胶着迁延，留恋不去，所以浊毒为活动期溃疡性结肠炎的发病关键，即使在溃疡性结肠炎的缓解期也是浊毒与正气相持阶段或因毒成虚、浊毒留恋不去的阶段。

The causes of ulcerous colitis are mostly external evil, uncontrolled-diet, emotional disorders and congenital deficiency, the characteristic of pathogenesis is weakness of the spleen and stomach, as the root, internal accumulation of turbid toxin and resistance of blood stasis as the tip. Mainly spleen looses normal transporting function, the small intestine can not separate lucidity and turbidity, large intestinal looses the function of conduction, wet turbidity accumulates, turbidity turns to be heat with time passes, heat then is transmitted into toxin, turbid toxin is abundantly obstructed, lipid membrane, blood collateral are damaged, blood and flesh are corrupted, and stagnated into pus. Turbid toxin cohesion can not be dispelled over time, plus dysfunction of intestinal conduction cause the generation of this disease. Turbid toxin is not only a pathogenic factor, but also a pathological product, which plays the dual role of pathogenic initiation and recurrence aggravation of this disease. Turbid toxin can easily damage the healthy qi, and penetrate into the viscera, glue-like, nostalgia, and lingers. So turbid toxin is the key pathogenic factor to the onset of ulcerous colitis in the active period, even the remission period of ulcerous colitis is stalemate stage of turbid toxin and healthy qi or the stage of healthy qi deficiency caused by toxin, turbid poison still lingers.

（一）病因

2.1 Causes

1.感受外邪　溃疡性结肠炎患者多在夏秋季节发病，此时炎暑流行，湿热当令，脾胃呆滞，外感湿热之邪，湿与热相合，如油裹面，胶结难解，首犯中焦阳明，郁蒸为患，导致运化失常，气血阻滞，浊毒壅盛，搏结于大肠，肉腐成脓而发病。

2.1.1 Attacked by external evil　Ulcerous colitis usually occurs in summer and autumn season, when there is heat epidemic, damp heat, the spleen and stomach are dull, exogenous damp heat, mixed together as oil and flour cemented, it first invades Yangming in middle energizer, steamed depression leads to abnormal transporting, qi and blood blocked, abundant turbid toxin binded in the large intestine, meat is corrupted into pus, therefore, the disease occurs.

2.饮食不节　溃疡性结肠炎的发病或复发与饮食不节或不洁关系密切，过食生冷或饮食不规律、暴饮暴食损伤脾胃，脾失健运，胃失和降，脾胃不能运化水谷，水反为湿，谷反为滞，湿浊内生，或从寒化，或从热化，导致寒浊或浊毒阻滞肠道；多食肥甘厚味，脾胃运化艰难，辛辣、肥甘厚腻之品易生湿生热，湿之甚化生浊，热之甚化生毒，浊毒下注

于肠道，热盛肉腐，损伤脂膜血络，利下脓血，发为溃疡性结肠炎。

2.1.2 Uncontrolled diet The onset or recurrence of ulcerous colitis is closely related to uncontrolled or unclean diet. Over-taking of cold and raw food, irregular diet, over-eating and drinking damages spleen and stomach, spleen cannot transport, stomach fails to harmonize and descend, spleen and stomach cannot transport water and grain, adverse flow of water generates dampness, adverse flow of grain generates stagnation, wet turbidity is generated internally, either is transformed into coldness, or transformed into heat, lead to cold turbidity or turbid toxin blocking the intestines; over-taking of fat, sweet and thick taste of food, makes spleen and stomach difficult to transport, spicy, fat, sweet, and thick greasy food will easily generate wet and heat, accumulation of dampness will be transmitted into turbidity, accumulation of heat will be transmitted into toxin. When turbid toxin enters intestines, abundant heat and corrupted meat damages lipid membrane and blood collateral, ulcerous colitis occurs.

3.情志失调　情志失调是本病发病及复发的重要诱因，患者恼怒、暴怒、郁怒，导致肝气亢盛或郁结，肝气横逆犯脾，或为精神紧张，思虑过度，忧思气结，思虑伤脾，致脾失健运，胃失和降，脾胃不能运化水湿，水反为湿，谷反为滞，水湿不化，积滞内停，湿凝成浊，蕴久化热，热极为毒。日久气血壅滞，损伤脉络而化为脓血，而便下赤白黏液。

2.1.3 Emotional disorder Emotional disorder is an important inducing cause of initiation and recurrence of the disease, anger, rage, depression of the patients, causes liver qi excessive and stagnated, the adverse liver qi affects spleen, or spiritual tension, over-thinking makes the qi stagnation and hurt spleen, spleen looses the function of normal transporting, stomach looses the function of harmonizing and descending, spleen and stomach cannot transport water and grain, adverse flow of water generates dampness, adverse flow of grain generates stagnation. When dampness of water cannot be vaporized, it will become stagnation and retention, dampness coagulates into turbidity, long time of accumulation is transmitted into heat, excessive heat generates toxin. Long time of qi and blood stagnation will damage the meridians and is transformed into pus blood, and then discharging with red white mucus.

4.先天禀赋不足　部分患者具有溃疡性结肠炎家族史，说明本病有遗传倾向。结合临床辨证发现，溃疡性结肠炎患者往往先天禀赋不足，素体脾肾亏虚。脾失健运，肾失温化，湿食内停。湿浊不化，阴火内生，浊毒积滞壅遏肠中，血败肉腐，内溃成疡。

2.1.4 Insufficient congenital endowment Some patients have a family history of ulcerous colitis, indicating that the disease has a genetic tendency. Combined with clinical syndrome differentiation, patients with ulcerous colitis often have congenital endowment deficiency, spleen and kidney are usually deficient. When spleen looses the function of normal transporting, kidney looses the function of warming, wet evil and food etention stay internally. Wet turbidity does not melt, Yin fire generates endogenously. Turbid toxin abundantly stagnates in the intestine, blood and flesh corrupts, internal corruption turns to be ulceration.

（二）病机

2.2 Pathogenesis

1.**浊毒内蕴为标**　浊毒为溃疡性结肠炎的主要病理因素，浊毒留滞于大肠，熏蒸肠道，与气血相搏结，使肠道传导失司，脂络受伤，气凝血滞，血败肉腐化脓而发为本病，久之则再伤脾胃，导致脾胃虚弱更甚，浊毒再生而成恶性循环，病情反复发作。且浊毒黏滞，发病缓慢，病程较长，难以速去，浊毒相搏，缠绵难解，故大肠浊毒留恋是溃疡性结肠炎反复发作迁延难愈的重要因素。

2.2.1 Internal accumulation of turbid toxin is the tip　Turbid toxin is the main pathological factor of ulcerous colitis, turbid toxin retains in the large intestine, fumigating the bowel, attacking qi and blood, causes dysfunction of intestinal conduction, lipid collateral injury, qi coagulation and blood stagnation, blood and septic corrupts to generate pus and causes this disease. Long course of ulcerous colitis repeatedly hurt the spleen and stomach, make spleen and stomach even more weak, turbid toxin regenerates, which forms a vicious cycle of repeated occurrence of the disease. And the turbid toxin is sticky, slow onset, with long course of disease, it is difficult to be resolved quickly. Turbidity and toxin fights against each other, lingering and difficult to be separated, so nostalgia of turbid toxin in large intestine is an important factor causing the repeated occurrences and recovering difficulty of ulcerous colitis.

2.**瘀血阻滞为标**　机体由于感受外邪，或为饮食七情所伤，浊毒、寒凝之邪壅塞肠中，气血与之相搏结，肠道传导失司，肠络受伤，终致气滞血瘀，瘀血阻滞肠络而发病。"久病入络""久病必瘀"，长期的瘀血阻滞使病情反复发作，缠绵难愈。又因瘀血不去，新血不生，局部肠络长年受损而无气血化生、滋养，难于修复，故正气不固，邪之欲凑，反复发作。

2.2.2 Blood stasis resistance is the tip of the disease　Human body suffers from external evil, or hurting by uncontrolled-diet and seven emotions, turbid toxin and cold coagulation evil obstructing in the intestine, fighting and binding with qi and blood, intestinal conduction function does not work, injuring intestinal collateral, eventually causes qi stagnation and blood stasis, blood stasis resisting in intestine collateral, and generation of this disease. "Long time of disease will get into the collateral", "long time of disease will generate stasis", long-term of stasis block makes the disease repeatedly occur, lingering and difficult to heal. And because the blood stasis does not leave, the new blood does not generate, local intestinal collateral is damaged for year and year, failing to generate and nourish qi and blood, nourish, so it is difficult to repair, so the healthy qi is not condensed, the evil can easily attack, leading to repeated occurrence of the disease.

3.**脾胃虚弱为本**　溃疡性结肠炎的发病多是在脾胃虚弱的基础上引起大肠传导失司，气机不畅，湿热瘀毒等病邪蕴结肠中；由于脾胃虚弱，或饮食、劳倦、思虑、久病等诸多因素作用，导致脾气受损，脾虚失于健运，运化无权，水谷不归正化，日久胶结，渐成下痢赤白。脾胃虚弱是溃疡性结肠炎发病及缠绵难愈的关键。《诸病源候论》指出："由脾胃大肠虚弱，风邪乘之，则泄痢。虚损不复，遂连滞涉引岁月，则为久痢也。"

2.2.3 Weak spleen and stomach is the root of the disease　The onset of ulcerous colitis is caused by dysfunction of intestinal conduction, abnormal operation of qi mechanism, pathogenic factors like dampness, evil, stasis and toxin accumulated in the intestines on the basis of weak spleen and stomach; weakness of spleen and stomach, or diet, fatigue, thinking, long course of disease and many other factors, damage spleen qi, deficient spleen looses the function of healthy transporting, or transporting without efficiency, water and grain is not properly processed, and is glue- bind with time passes, gradually transformed into red and white dysentery. The weakness of the spleen and stomach is the key factor to the onset and lingering of ulcerous colitis. It is pointed out in *General Treatise on Causes and Manifestation of All Diseases* "In case of the deficiency of spleen, stomach and large intestine, if the wind evil attacks, diarrhea occurs. If the deficiency cannot recover, or even last for months and years, then it becomes dysentery."

第二节　辨证要点
Section 2　Key Points of Syndrome Differentiation

一、辨气血
1. To distinguish qi and blood

下痢白多赤少，湿邪伤及气分；赤多白少，或以血为主者，热邪伤及血分。

If the dysentery is with more white content than red, evil of dampness injures qi; if the dysentery is with more red content than white, or mainly blood, heat evil injures blood.

二、辨虚实
2. To distinguish asthenia and sthenia

一般说来，起病急骤，病程短者属实；起病缓慢，病程长者多虚。形体强壮，脉滑实有力者属实；形体薄弱，脉虚弱无力者属虚。腹痛胀满，痛而拒按，痛时窘迫欲便，便后里急后重，暂时减轻者为实；腹痛绵绵，痛而喜按，便后里急后重不减，坠胀甚者为虚。

Generally speaking, disease with sudden onset and short course is sthenia; disease with slow onset, long course is mostly asthenia. If the patient is physically strong with slippery and solid pulse, the disease is sthenia; if the patient is physivally thin and weak with weak pulse, the disease is asthenia. If the patient is abdominal painful with distention fullness, painful but refuses to be pressed, painful and want to relieve himself at once, tenesmus feels temporarily reduced after stool discharging, the disease is sthenia; vague abdominal pain, painful but like to be pressed, tenesmus feels no reduction but even falling distention, the disease is asthenia.

三、辨寒热
3. To distinguish cold and heat

痢下脓血鲜红，或赤多白少者属热；痢下黏稠臭秽者属热；身热面赤，口渴喜饮者属热；舌红苔黄腻，脉滑数者属热。痢下白色黏冻涕状，或赤少白多者属寒；痢下清稀而不甚臭秽者属寒；面白肢冷形寒，口淡不渴者属寒；舌淡苔白，脉沉细者属寒。

If the dysentery pus blood is bright red, or with red content more than white, the disease is hot; If the dysentery is sticky and thick, the disease is hot; if the patient is hot in body with red face, thirsty and likes to drink, the disease is hot; if the patient is with red tongue, yellow greasy moss, slippery rapid pulse, the disease is hot. Patient with white sticky cold dysentery, or dysentery with red content more than white, the disease is cold; if dysentery is clear and loose, but not very foul, the disease is cold; if the patient is with white face, cold limbs and body, light taste in mouth, but not thirsty, the disease is cold; if the patient is with light tongue, white moss, sunk thready pulse, the disease is cold.

第三节　治疗原则
Section 3　Principles of Treatment

一、分清标本缓急
1. To distinguish tip and root, slow and urgent

溃疡性结肠炎病机属虚实夹杂，活动期溃疡性结肠炎以邪实为主，浊毒血瘀之象明显，当急则治其标，缓解期当缓则治其本。活动期溃疡性结肠炎浊毒血瘀之象明显，以化浊解毒、凉血活血为主，缓解期由于病程迁延日久，正气耗伤，浊毒未净；加之脾肾受损，肾阳虚衰，治宜"标本同治"，采用温肾健脾，佐以清化活血之法。

The pathogenesis of ulcerous colitis belongs to syndrome of intermingling of asthenia and sthenia, the ulcerous colitis in active period is mainly evil sthenia, the image of turbid toxin and blood stasis is obvious, for the urgent occurrence of disease, we should treat its tip with method of resolving turbidity and removing toxin, promoting the circulation of blood and cooling blood. In the remission period, for slow occurrence of the disease, we should treat its root. In the remission period, as the course of disease has lasted for a long time, the healthy qi is destructively consumed, turbid toxin has not been thoroughly removed, the spleen and kidney is damaged, kidney Yang is severely deficient, we should treat "tip and root" simultaneously, by using the method of warming the kidney and reinforce the spleen, assisted by the method of purifying and promoting blood circulation.

二、注重调气和血
2. Pay attention to qi regulating and blood harmonizing

调气和血法为本病的通用治则，湿阻肠中，易碍气机运行，热邪煎灼津液又致瘀血，热迫血溢，气血壅滞肉败血腐，随大便混杂而下，故正如刘河间所说："调气则后重自除，行血则便脓自愈。"调气和血可顺畅肠腑凝滞之气血，祛除腐败之脓血，以改善腹痛、里急后重、下痢脓血等临床症状。

Method of qi regulation and blood harmonizing is commonly used for general treatment of the disease. Resistance of dampness in intestines may easily hinder the normal operation of qi mechanism, heat evil frying and burning fluid liquid causes blood stasis, heat presses blood to overflow, blood is abundantly stagnated, corrupted flesh and rotted blood is discharged with stool. So as Liu Hejian said: "qi regulation will remove the tenesmus, blood promotion will cure pus in stool." Qi regulating and blood harmonizing can smooth the circulation of intestinal stagnated qi and blood, dispel the corrupted blood pus, so as to improve the symptoms of abdominal pain, tenesmus, dysentery with blood pus and so on.

三、扶正祛邪并重
3. Pay dual attention to strengthening the healthy qi and dispelling the evil

溃疡性结肠炎缓解期应扶正祛邪，缓解期虽然脓血便已除，邪势渐去，其病机仍以浊毒留滞、虚实夹杂为特点，因此在治疗上应注意在扶正的同时配合清化活血、疏泄导滞，不能一味使用温补收涩之品，尤其应慎用涩肠止泻之品，以防闭门留寇，加重病情。

Treatment of ulcerous colitis in remission period should be strengthening the healthy qi and dispelling the evil, although pus has been removed, evil advantage is disappearing gradually, but the pathogenesis is still characterized by turbid toxin stagnation, mingling of asthenia and sthenia, so in treatment we should pay attention to strengthening the healthy qi while cooperating with purifying and promoting blood circulation, dredging and conduction the stagnation, not blindly using tonic and astringent medicines, being especially cautious when using intestine astringent and diarrhea stopping products, in prevention of keeping the evil in closed doors and aggravating the disease.

四、整体治疗与局部治疗相结合
4. Combination of holistic treatment and local treatment

在溃疡性结肠炎的治疗中将整体脏腑辨证与局部用药相结合，内外合治，标本兼顾，在临床取得了较好的疗效。局部治疗主要为中药保留灌肠，可直接作用于局部病灶，对溃疡起到抗炎、止血、促进愈合的作用，还能避免大剂量化浊解毒药物阻碍胃气的弊端。

In treatment of ulcerous colitis, combination of the holistic viscera syndrome differentiation and medicine using in local area, internal and external treatment, tip and root treatment, has achieved good effect in clinical practice. Local treatment is mainly using traditional Chinese medicine to retain enema, which can directly act on local lesions, play a role of anti-inflammation, bleeding stopping and healing promoting of ulcers, and can also avoid the disadvantages of using high dose of turbidity resolving and toxin removing drugs hindering gastric qi.

五、顾护胃气为要
5. It is most important to protect and care stomach qi

"人以胃气为本，而治痢尤要。"这是因为活动期大量运用苦寒药物，虽善清溃疡性结肠炎之标，但过用苦寒有碍脾胃健运，长时间大剂量使用，有损伤胃气之弊，且有凉伏热毒及化燥伤阴之弊，因此临证应适量运用苦寒药物，并适当加入顾护胃气之品，并贯穿于治痢的始终。

"Stomach qi is the root of life, especially in dysentery treating." This is because in the active period, great amount of bitter cold drugs has been used, although it is good to clear the tip of ulcerous colitis, but over-taking of bitter cold medicines will affect the normal operation of spleen and stomach, long time using with big doses, has the disadvantages of damaging stomach qi, and cooling and embedding the heat toxin and transforming it into dryness which injures Yin. So throughout the whole process of dysentery treatment, bitter and cold drugs should be used with proper dosage, and appropriately some medicines should be added to protect and care stomach qi.

第四节 常用治法
Section 4 The Common Method of Treatment

一、化浊解毒法
1. Method of turbidity resolving and toxin removing

对于溃疡性结肠炎的治疗化浊解毒法要贯穿始终，并灵活应用。

The method of turbidity resolving and toxin removing should be carried out throughout the treatment process of ulcerous colitis and applied flexibly.

（一）芳香化浊解毒法
1.1 To resolve turbidity and remove toxin by using aroma medicines

脾胃失司，湿浊之邪阻于中焦，日久化生浊毒。气味芳香之品多具有醒脾运脾、化浊辟秽的作用，常用药物为藿香、佩兰、半夏、苍术、白术、砂仁、紫豆蔻、陈皮等品。

Dysfunction of spleen and stomach causes resistance of dampness evil in middle energizer, generating turbid toxin with time passes. Medicines with fragrant smell, mostly have the effect of awakening and transporting spleen, resolving turbidity and dispelling the foul. Medicines generally used are: huo xiang (Herba Agastaches seu Pogostemonis), pei lan (Herba Eupatorii), ban xia (Rhizoma Pinelliae), cang zhu (Rhizoma Atractylodis), bai zhu (Rhizoma Atractylodis Macrocephalae), sha ren (Fructus Amomi), zi dou kou (Purple Cardamom Kernel), chen pi (Pericarpium Citri Reticulatae) and other products.

（二）通腑泄浊解毒法

1.2 To discharge turbidity and remove toxin by dredging fu-organs

浊毒内停日久，可致腑气不通，邪滞壅盛。本法运用通泻药物荡涤腑气，保持腑气通畅，使浊毒之邪积从下而走，属中医学下法范畴。药用大黄、厚朴、枳实、芦荟等。

Turbid toxin stays internally for a long time, it will cause obstruction of the qi of fu-organ, and abundant stagnatino of pathogenic evil. This method uses purging medicine to clean up the qi of fu-organ, keep the stomach qi unobstructed, make the evil accumulation of turbid toxin exit with stool, it belongs to purging method of TCM. Mediciines: da huang (Radix et Rhizoma Rhei), hou po (Cortex Magnoliae Officinalis), zhi shi (Fructus Aurantii Immaturus), lu hui (Aloe), etc.

（三）淡渗利湿解毒法

1.3 To remove toxin by dispelling dampness with bland medicines

湿浊同源，湿久凝浊，久则浊毒内蕴。使用甘淡利湿之品，可使浊毒之邪从下焦排出。

Wet and turbidity share the same source, wet will be coagulated into turbidity for a long time, then turbid toxin is internally accumulated. To use sweet, light and wet-dispelling products, can discharge the turbid toxin evil from the lower energizer.

（四）清热燥湿解毒法

1.4 To remove toxin by clearing heat and drying dampness

湿久凝浊，热久生毒，凡湿热之证，缠绵不解，皆可化生浊毒。故清热燥湿法可从发病的来源上遏制浊毒的产生和传变。常用药物为黄连、黄柏、黄芩、栀子、龙胆草等。

Wet will be coalgulated into turbidity for a long time, Heat will generate toxin with time passes. Lingering of the syndrome of dampness and heat will generate turbid toxin. Therefore, the method of heat-clearing and dampness drying can curb the generation and transmission of turbid toxin from the source of disease. Medicines generally used are: huang lian (Rhizoma Coptidis), huang bo (Cortex Phellodendri), huang qin (Radix Scutellariae), zhi zi (Fructus Gardeniae), long dan cao (Gentianae Radix et Rhizoma), etc.

（五）以毒攻毒化浊法

1.5 To resolve turbidity by attacking poison with poison

浊毒结于体内，毒陷邪深，非攻不克，故常用有毒之品，借其性峻力猛以攻邪，以毒攻毒之应用，应适可而止，衰其大半而止，要根据患者的体质状况和耐攻承受能力，把握用量、用法及用药时间，方能收到预期的效果。常用的药物有：斑蝥、全蝎、水蛭、蜈蚣、蟾蜍、土鳖虫、守宫等。

Stagnation of turbid toxin in the body, sunk toxin and deep evil, cannot be resolved unless attacking, so toxic products are commonly used to attack evil by its fierce force. Application of the method of attacking poison with poison should be stopped at appropriate time when more than half of the evils are defeated. The dosage, usage method and medication time should be in accordance with the patient's physical condition and resistance ability, so as to realize the desired effect. Medicines generally used are: ban mao (Mylabris), quan xie (Scorpio), shui zhi (Leech), wu gong (Scolopendra), chan chu (Bufo), tu bie chong (Eupolyphaga Steleophaga), shou gong (Gekko) and so on.

二、健脾益气法
2. To reinforce the spleen and replenish qi

溃疡性结肠炎患者由于素体脾胃虚弱，或后天失于调摄，或本病攻伐，多有脾虚表现，脾虚亦是溃疡性结肠炎复发之根本，而以健脾益气之剂，使脾胃之气调和，升清降浊，肠络清疏，传化如常，方可达到补而不滞、脾健余邪除的治疗效果。常用药物有党参、白术、炙甘草、茯苓、山药、黄芪等，方剂常选用异功散、香砂六君子汤、参苓白术散、补中益气汤等加减。

Most of the ulcerous colitis patients have the manifestation of spleen deficiency due to usual weakness of spleen and stomach, shortness of the acquired regulation, or the disease attacking. Spleen deficiency is also the root of recurrence of ulcerous colitis, to realize the treatment effect of reinforcement without stagnation, reinforcing spleen and removing the remaining evil, prescription of strengthening spleen and nourishing qi to regulate spleen and stomach qi, ascend lucidity and descend turbidity, ensure clean and unblocking of intestinal collateral, and normal transporting and transforming as usual. Medicines generally used include: dang shen (Radix Codonopsitis Pilosulae), bai zhu (Rhizoma Atractylodis Macrocephalae), zhi gan cao (fried Radix Glycyrrhizae), fu ling (Poria), shan yao (Tuber Dioscoreae), huang qi (Radix Astragali seu Hedysari), etc. Prescriptions often choose Yigong Powder (Powder of Special Effect), Xiangsha Liujunzi Decoction, Shenling Baizhu Powder, Buzhong Yiqi Decoction, etc.

三、活血化瘀法
3. To promote blood circulation and remove blood stasis

溃疡性结肠炎病程中湿浊积滞阻滞气血，热毒入络熏蒸气血，皆可导致瘀证。另外，溃疡性结肠炎患者素体正虚，加上本病攻伐，气血阴阳皆可虚，皆可致血瘀之证。临证欲活血化瘀，要做到活血而不伤正。脾气不足、气虚血瘀者可用补中益气汤，合用活血化瘀之三七、延胡索、桃仁、红花、莪术。脾肾阳虚、寒凝血瘀者可选用失笑散温经散寒、活血化瘀，或加用炮姜、附子、肉桂温补脾肾，温通经脉。若少腹疼痛不移，则以少腹逐瘀汤加减治疗。血虚致瘀者当养血活血化瘀，可用桃红四物汤化裁。阴虚血瘀者当滋阴养血而通瘀，可用一贯煎化裁。

In the course of ulcerous colitis, stagnation wet and turbidity resists qi and blood, heat and toxin enters collateral and fumigate qi and blood, can lead to blood stasis. In addition, patients of ulcerous colitis are usually deficient in healthy qi, plus the attacking from the disease, qi, blood, Yin and Yang all can be deficient, all can cause syndrome of blood stasis. To promote blood circulation and remove blood stasis clinically should not hurt the healthy qi. People with insufficient spleen qi, qi deficiency and blood stasis can be treated by using Buzhong Yiqi Decoction (Decoction of tonifying spleen and nourishing Qi), combined with prescription of medicines promoting blood circulation and removing blood stasis: san qi (Radix Notoginseng), yan hu suo (Rhizoma Corydalis), tao ren (Semen Persicae), hong hua (Flos Carthami) and e zhu (Rhizoma Curcumae). Patients with spleen and kidney Yang deficiency, cold coagulation and blood stasis can choose Shixiao Powder, to warm meridians and dispel coldness, promoting blood circulation and resolve blood stasis, or add pao jiang (prepared Ginger), fu zi (Radix Aconiti), rou gui (Cortex Cinnamomi) to warm and tonify spleen and kidney, warm meridians. If the abdominal pain does not move, use prescription of Decoction of Shaofu Zhuyu. Patients with stasis caused by blood deficiency should be treated with method of nourishing blood, promoting blood circulation and resolving blood stasis, using Taohong Siwu Decoction. Patients of Yin deficiency and blood stasis should be treated by enriching Yin and nourishing blood and unblocking blood stasis, prescription of Yiguan Decoction can be used.

四、调肝理气法
4. Method of regulating liver and qi

溃疡性结肠炎患者常伴有心情抑郁、情绪不宁等情志障碍，可引起肝气疏泄失职，影响脾胃健运；而脾气虚衰，肝木极易乘侮。因此，临证治当在健脾的同时，还应佐以疏肝或敛肝之药。肝气疏泄太过者，敛肝常选加白芍、乌梅、木瓜等；肝气疏泄不及者，配合柴胡、香附、佛手、青皮、郁金等疏肝之品。柴胡疏肝散、逍遥散、痛泻要方是常用方剂。

Patients of ulcerous colitis are often accompanied by depression, unpeaceful mood, and other emotional disorders, which can cause dysfunction liver qi dispersing, affecting normal operation of the spleen and stomach. When spleen qi is deficient, liver wood can easily ove- restrict the spleen. Therefore, in clinical treatment, while reinforcing the spleen, liver dispersing or astringing medicines should be supplemented. If liver qi is over- dispersed, liver astringing medicines usually use bai shao (Radix Paeoniae Alba), wu mei (Fructus Mume), mu gua (Chaenomels Fructus); if the liver qi is under-dispersed, cooperating with medicines of chai hu (Radix Bulpleuri), xiang fu (Rhizoma Cyperi), fo shou (Fructus Citri Sarcodactylis), qing pi (Pericarpium Citri Reticcutatae Viride), yu jin (Radix Curcumae) and other liver soothing medicines, and prescriptions like Chaihu Shugan Powder, Xiaoyao Powder, Prescription For Pain and Diarrhea are generally used.

五、调肺化痰法
5. Method of regulating the lung and dispelling phlegm

肺与大肠相表里，大肠的传导功能依赖于肺气的宣发与肃降，溃疡性结肠炎肺气亏虚，水谷不归正化，以致痰湿下流，留滞大肠，痰湿久羁不去，势必酿热成毒，壅滞气血，损膜伤络，内溃成疡。因此，肺气失调、痰湿滞肠是溃疡性结肠炎的病机之一。临床可加用桔梗、白芷、陈皮、半夏、川贝母等调肺化痰药。

The lung and the large intestine are internal-external relation. The conduction function of the large intestine depends on the diffusing and downbearing of lung qi, patients of ulcerous colitis is usually deficient in lung qi, water and grain can not be normally transformed, so that phlegmatic hygrosis refluxes, and retains in the large intestine, retention of phlegmatic hygrosis for a long time is bound to be brewed into heat and toxin, which obstructs qi and blood, damages membrane and collateral, and causing internal ulceration. Therefore, irregular pulmonary qi, retention of phlegmatic hygrosis in intestines is one of the pathogenesis of ulcerous colitis. Clinically, jie geng (Platycodonis Radix), bai zhi (Radix Angelicae Dahuricae), chen pi (Pericarpium Citri Reticulatae), ban xia (Rhizoma Pinelliae), chuan bei mu (Fritillariae Cirrhosae Bulbus) and other phlegm drugs can be added.

六、消积导滞法
6. Method of resolving retention and removing stagnation

溃疡性结肠炎病程中积滞与湿热、瘀血、痰湿等一起阻碍腑气通降，影响肠道正常的疏泄功能。而缓解期正气亏虚，推动无力，积滞难以导下。临证常用山楂、神曲、鸡内金、莱菔子、枳实、木香、槟榔、大黄等消积导滞，使积滞去，湿热清，痰湿化，气血畅，正气得以恢复，而不易复发。

In the course of ulcerous colitis, stagnation, dampness and heat, blood stasis, and phlegm hygrosis together hinder the descending of stomach qi, affect the normal dredging function of the intestinal tract. And in the remission period, deficient healthy qi can hardly push downward the retention and stagnation. Medicines generally used for retention resolving and stagnation removing are: shan zha (Fructus Crataegi), shen qu (Messa Medicata Fermentata), ji nei jin (Endothlium Corneum Gigeriae Galli), lai fu zi (Semen Raphani), zhi shi (Aurantii Fructus Immaturus), mu xiang (Radix Aucklandiae), bing lang (Arecae Semen), da huang (Radix et Rhizoma Rhei) and other, in order to eliminate retention and stagnation, clear dampness and heat, dispel phlegmatic hygrosis, smoothen the circulation of qi and blood, restore healthy qi, avoid the recurrence of the disease.

七、益肾温肾法
7. Method of benefiting and warming kidney

由于溃疡性结肠炎患者有脾胃虚弱的基础，加上后天失于调摄及本病攻伐，缓解期有时兼见泻下不止、腰膝酸冷、畏寒怕冷、喜热饮、舌淡胖、脉沉细等，治宜温补肾阳，酌加附子、肉桂、补骨脂、益智仁、菟丝子等益肾温肾，方剂常以四神丸、真人养脏汤等加减。

As ulcerous colitis patients are usually weak in spleen and stomach, lack of acquired nourishment, suffering from the attack of the disease, in remission period of the disease, sometimes patients see diarrhea, acid and cold in waist and knees, fear of coldness, in favor of hot drink. The tongue is light in colour and fat in nature, pulse is thready sunk, etc. to treat the disease, we should appropriately warm and tonify kidney Yang, adding fu zi (Radix Aconiti), rou gui (Cortex Cinnamomi), bu gu zhi (Psoraleae Fructus), yi zhi ren (Alpiniae Oxyphyllae Fructus), tu si zi (Semen Cuscutae) to nourish and warm kidney. Prescriptions usually used are: Sishen Pill, zhenren Yangzang Decoction, etc.

八、滋阴养血法
8. Method of notifying Yin and nourishing blood

溃疡性结肠炎患者久泻久痢，伤津耗液，阴液亏耗；脾失健运，气血生化乏源，亦致阴血不足；若湿热熏蒸，下痢脓血，阴血亏损益重。临证须在健脾止泻等的基础上，选择应用滋阴养血之品，如阿胶、当归、龙眼肉、白芍、生地黄、沙参等，驻车丸合归脾汤为常用加减方剂。

Ulcerous colitis patients suffers from long - time dysentery, which hurts fluid and consumes liquid, causes deficiency of Yin liquid; besides, abnormal transporting of spleen, lack of resources of qi and blood generation, also causes Yin blood deficiency; in case of fumigation of dampness and heat, dysentery with blood pus, deficiency of Yin liquid will be more serious. Clinical treatment shoul choose the application of nourishing Yin and blood, such as e jiao (Asini Corii Colla), dang gui (Radix Angelicae Sinensis), long yan rou (longan Arillus), bai shao (Radix Paeoniae Alba), sheng di huang (Radix Rehmanniae), sha shen (Radix Adenophrae Strictae), etc. on the basis of strengthening the spleen and stopping diarrhea, prescriptions of Zhuche Pills combined with Guipi Decoction (Decoction for Invigorating the Spleen) are the generally used with addition and reduction.

九、敛疡生肌法
9. Method of astringing ulcer and generating muscle

溃疡性结肠炎肠黏膜溃疡、糜烂及隐窝脓肿之病理变化符合中医学"内痈""内疡"的特征，同时运用敛疡生肌药，可加强修复肠道损伤、维持黏膜完整的作用，临证常用地榆、白及、白蔹等。黄芪兼有健脾除湿和托毒敛疮的功效，更为常用。

The pathological changes of ulcerous colitis, ulceration of intestinal mucosa, erosion and crypt abscess are in line with the characteristics of "internal carbuncle" and "internal ulcer" in traditional Chinese medical science. At the same time, the use of medicines of ulcer astringing and muscle generating can strengthen the repairring of intestinal injury and maintain the integrity of mucosa. Medicines generally used in clinical treatment are: di yu (Radix et Rhizoma Sanguisorbae), bai ji (Bletillae Rhizoma) and bai lian (Ampelopsis Radix), etc. huang qi (Radix Astragali seu Hedysari) has the effect of spleen reinforcing and dampness removing, toxin expelling and ulcer astringing.

十、收敛固涩法
10. Method of astringing

溃疡性结肠炎患者见有腹泻不可轻易使用固涩之品，以免"闭门留寇"，反使病情加重。若症见泻下不止，选用熟附子、干姜、吴茱萸、补骨脂、益智仁等温补脾肾，柴胡、升麻、葛根等升提中气，仍未见改善者，可谨慎予以乌梅、五倍子、诃子、石榴皮、赤石脂等收敛固涩之品，方如真人养脏汤、桃花汤等。

To treat ulcerous colitis patients with diarrhea, astringents should not be used easily, so as not to "close the door before the invader leave away", making the condition aggravated. If the diarrhea does not stop, choose shu fu zi (prepared Radix Aconiti), gan jiang (Zingiberis Rhizoma), wu zhu yu (Euodiae Fructus), bu gu zhi (Psoraleae Fructus), yi zhi ren (Alpiniae Oxyphyllae Fructus), and other medicines to warm and tonify spleen and kidney, using chai hu (Radix Bulpleuri), sheng ma (Rhizoma Climicifugae), ge gen (Radix Pueriariae) and other medicine to raise up spleen qi, if still no improvement, carefully using wu mei (Fructus Mume), wu bei zi (Galla Chinensis), ke zi (Fructus Chebulae), shi liu pi (Graniti Pericarpium), chi shi zhi (Halloysitum Rubrum) and other astringent products, prescriptions such as Zhenren Yangzang Decoction, Taohua Decoction (Peach Blossom Decoction), etc.

第五节　辨证治疗
Section 5　Treatment with Syndrome Differentiation

一、气滞浊阻
1. Qi stagnation and turbidity resistance

（一）主要症状
1.1 Main symptoms

腹痛即泻，泻后痛减，常因抑郁恼怒、情绪紧张或激动而发作，大便夹脓血，黏腻不爽，胸胁胀满，烦躁易怒，嗳气纳呆，身体困重，舌淡红，苔白腻或厚腻，脉弦滑。

Abdominal pain is accompanied by diarrhea, the pain reduces after diarrhea, the symptoms usually occurs because of depression, emotional tension or excitement. Stool of the patient is sticky with pus and blood, the patient see distentional fullness in chest and hypochondrium, irritability, belching, anorexia, heavy and trapped body, with red tongue, white greasy or thick greasy moss, and string slippery pulse.

（二）治法
1.2 Treatment method

抑肝扶脾、理气化浊。

To suppress the liver and reinforce the spleen, and regulate qi and resolve turbidity.

（三）方药

1.3 Prescription and medicines

炒陈皮、白术、白芍、防风、当归、柴胡、炒枳实、茯苓、三七、炙甘草。若两胁胀痛，脉弦有力，加延胡索、郁金以疏肝止痛；便秘和腹泻交替发作，则加槟榔、沉香以疏导积滞；如腹胀腹痛者，加枳实、厚朴以行气消胀；嗳气呕恶则加旋覆花、代赭石以降逆止呕；如脾虚较重，腹泻次数增多，则加党参、升麻以升补脾气。

Chao chen pi (fried Pericarpium Citri Reticulatae), bai zhu (Rhizoma Atractylodis Macrocephalae), bai shao (Radix Paeoniae Alba), fang feng (Radix Saposhnikoviae), dang gui (Radix Angelicae Sinensis), chai hu (Radix Bulpleuri), chao zhi shi (fried Aurantii Fructus Immaturus), fu ling (Poria), san qi (Radix Notoginseng), zhi gan cao (fried Radix Glycyrrhizae). In case of hypochondrium distentional pain, powerful string pulse, add yan hu suo (Rhizoma Corydalis) and yu jin (Radix Curcumae) to soothe the liver and relieve pain. In case of constipation occurring alternatively with diarrhea, add bing lang (Arecae Semen), chen xiang (Lingnum Aquilariae Resinatum) to relieve and dredge stagnation. In case of abdominal distention and pain, add zhi shi (Aurantil Fructus Immaturus), hou po (Cortex Magnoliae Officinalis) to smoothen qi and dispel distention. In case of belching, vomitting and nausea add xuan fu hua (Flos Inulae) and dai zhe shi (Haematitum) to downbear counterflow and stop vomitting. In case of severely deficient spleen increasing the frequency of diarrhea, add dang shen (Radix Codonopsitis Pilosulae) and sheng ma (Rhizoma Climicifugae) to reinforce spleen qi.

二、浊毒内蕴
2. Internal accumulation of turbid toxin

（一）主要症状

2.1 Main symptoms

便中夹带脓血臭秽，里急后重，胃痞纳呆，身热，肛门灼热，大便黏腻不爽，小便短赤,舌暗红，苔黄厚腻，脉弦细滑。

Foul stool with pus and blood, tenesmus, gastric mass and anorexia, fever, hot anus, sticky stool, short and red urine, dark red tongue, with yellow thick greasy moss, string thin and slippery pulse.

（二）治法

2.2 Treatment method

化浊解毒，凉血宁血。

To resolve turbidity and remove toxin, cool the blood and stop bleeding.

（三）方药

2.3 Prescription and medicines

黄芩、黄连、大黄、槟榔、木香、当归、芍药、甘草、肉桂。大便脓血较多者，加侧柏炭、地榆炭、大黄炭凉血止痢；大便白冻、黏液较多者，加苍术、薏苡仁健脾燥湿；腹痛较甚者，加延胡索、乌药、枳实理气止痛；热甚者，加葛根、金银花、连翘解毒退热。

Huang qin (Radix Scutellariae), huang lian (Rhizoma Coptidis), da huang (Radix et Rhizoma Rhei), mu xiang (Radix Aucklandiae), dang gui (Radix Angelicae Sinensis), shao yao (Radix Paeoniae Alba), gan cao (Radix Glycyrrhizae), rou gui (Cortex Cinnamomi). More pus and blood in stool, add ce bai tan (Platycladi Cacumen charcoal), di yu tan (Radix et Rhizoma Sanguisorbae Carbon), da huang tan (Rhubarb Charcoal) to cool blood and stop diarrhae; jelly stool with more mucus, add cang zhu (Rhizoma Atractylodis), yi yi ren (Semen Coisis) to reinforce spleen and dry dampness; for severe abdominal pain, add yan hu suo (Rhizoma Corydalis), wu yao (Radix Linderae), zhi shi (Aurantii Fructus Immaturus) to regulate qi and relieve pain; for more severe fever, add ge gen (Radix Pueriariae), jin yin hua (Lonicerae Japonicae Flos), lian qiao (Forsythia Fructus) to remove toxin and bring down the fever.

三、浊毒壅盛
3. Abundant obstruction of turbid toxin

（一）主要症状
3.1 Main symptoms

起病急骤，壮热口渴，头痛烦躁，恶心呕吐，大便频频，痢下鲜紫脓血，腹痛剧烈，后重感特著，甚者神昏惊厥，舌质红绛，苔黄燥，脉滑数或微欲绝。

Sudden and abrupt onset, high fever and thirsty, headache and irritability, nausea and vomiting, frequent stool, dysentery with fresh purple pus and blood, severe abdominal pain, severe tenesmus, even convulsion without consciousness, red tongue, yellow dry moss, slippery string or slight and depleting pulse.

（二）治法
3.2 Treatment method

化浊解毒，凉血除积。

To resolve turbidity and remove toxin, cool the blood and eliminate the accumulation.

（三）方药
3.3 Prescription and medicines

白头翁、黄连、黄柏、秦皮、黄芩、木香、炒当归、炒白芍、生地榆、白蔹、三七、槟榔、肉桂、甘草。如热毒侵入营血，高热神昏谵语者，可加用紫雪丹或安宫牛黄丸以清解热毒，开窍安神；若高热、抽搐痉厥，加用紫雪散、全蝎、钩藤以清热息风镇痉；如呕吐频繁，胃阴耗伤，舌红绛而干，则可酌加西洋参、麦冬、石斛，扶阴养胃。

Bai tou weng (Pulsatillae Raidx), huang lian (Rhizoma Coptidis), huang bo (Cortex Phellodendri), qin pi (Cortex Fraxini Caulis), huang qin (Radix Scutellariae), mu xiang (Radix Aucklandiae), chao dang gui (fried Radix Angelicae Sinensis), chao bai shao (fried Radix Paeoniae Alba), sheng di yu (Raw Sanguisorbae Radix), bai lian (Ampelopsis Radix), san qi (Radix Notoginseng), bing lang (Arecae Semen), rou gui (Cortex Cinnamomi), gan cao (Radix Glycyrrhizae). If heat toxin gets into the nutrient-blood, patient have high fever, unconsciousness, delirium, add Purple Snow Dan or Angong Niuhuang Pill to clear heat and remove toxin, open the orifice and tranquilizing mind. For high fever with convulsions, add Purple Snow Powder, quan xie (Scorpio), gou teng (Uncariae Ramulus Cum Uncis) to clear heat, extinguish wind and release convulsion. In case of frequent vomiting, over-consumption of stomach Yin, with red and dry tongue, add xi yang shen (Panacic Quinquefolii Radix), mai dong (Radix Ophiopogonis), shi hu (Dendrobii Caulis), to reinforce Yin and nourish the stomach.

四、寒浊内阻
4. Internal resistance of coldness and turbidity

（一）主要症状
4.1 Main symptoms

腹痛拘急，痢下赤白黏冻，白多赤少，或纯为白冻，里急后重，脘胀腹满，头身困重，舌苔白腻，脉濡缓。

Abdominal pain and acute, dysentery with red white sticky jelly, or with white content more than red content, or pure white jelly, tenesmus, abdominal distension and abdomen fullness, head and body heavy and fatigue, white greasy tongue moss, slow weak pulse.

（二）治法
4.2 Treatment method

温中燥湿，调气和血。

To warm the middle energizer and dry the dampness, regulate qi and harmonize blood.

（三）方药
4.3 Prescription and medicines

藿香、苍术、厚朴、半夏、陈皮、木香、枳实、桂枝、炮姜、芍药、当归。兼有表证者，加荆芥、紫苏叶、葛根解表祛邪；夹食滞者，加山楂、神曲消食导滞；若湿邪偏重，白痢如胶冻，腰膝酸软，腹胀满，里急后重甚者，改用胃苓汤加减，以温中化湿健脾。

Huo xiang (Herba Agastaches seu Pogostemonis), cang zhu (Rhizoma Atractylodis), hou po (Cortex Magnoliae Officinalis), ban xia (Rhizoma Pinelliae), chen pi (Pericarpium Citri Reticulatae), mu xiang (Radix Aucklandiae), zhi shi (Aurantii Raidix Immaturus), gui zhi (Cmnamomi Mmulus), pao jiang (prepared Ginger), shao yao (Radix Paeoniae Alba), dang gui (Radix Angelicae Sinensis). If accompanied with exosyndrome, add jing jie (Herba Schizonepetae), zi su ye (Folium Perillae), ge gen (Radix Puerariae) to release external and dispel pathogenetic factors. With food stagnation, add shan zha (Fructus Crataegi), shen qu (Messa Medicata Fermentata) to digest food and dredge stagnation. If the wet evil is heavy, with white dysentery like glue jelly, lassitude loin and knees, abdominal distension full, tenesmus, use Wei Ling Decoction with addition or reduction, in order to warm the middle energizer, resolve the dampness and reinforce the spleen.

五、浊毒瘀阻
5. Congestion of turbid toxin

（一）主要症状
5.1 Main symptoms

面色晦暗，胁腹胀满，黏液脓血便，泻下不爽，腹痛拒按，嗳气食少，舌紫或瘀斑、瘀点，苔黄腻，脉弦涩滑。

Dark complexion, hypochondrium and abdominal distention and fullness, stool with mucus, pus and blood, uncomfortable diarrhea, with abdominal pain but refused to be pressed, belching, poor appetite, purple tongue or with ecchymosis, petechia, yellow greasy moss, string astringent and slippery pulse.

（二）治法
5.2 Treatment method

化瘀通络，止痛止血。

To remove blood stasis, unblock collaterals, relieve pain and stop bleeding.

（三）方药
5.3 Prescription and medicines

蒲黄、五灵脂、延胡索、没药、赤芍、小茴香、干姜、当归、川芎、官桂。如食滞加槟榔、山楂以消食导滞；如血热、大便暗红色较多，加三七、大黄炭以凉血止血；如气虚明显，见神疲、乏力、肢倦者，加党参、白术以益气行血。

Pu huang (Pollen Typhae), wu ling zhi (Faeces Trogopterorum), yan hu suo (Rhizoma Corydalis), mo yao (Resina Commiphorae Myrrhae), chi shao (Radix Paeoniae Rubra), xiao hui xiang (Foeniculi Fructus), gan jiang (Zingiberis Rhizoma), dang gui (Radix Angelicae Sinensis), chuan xiong (Rhizoma Chuanxiong), guan gui (Cmnamomi Mmulus). For food stagnation, add bing lang (Arecae Semen), shan zha (Fructus Crategi) to eliminate food stagnation. in case of blood fever, dark red stool, add san qi (Radix Notoginseng), da huang tan (Rhubarb Charcoal) to the above prescription, to cool the blood and stop bleeding; if qi deficiency is obvious, see fatigue, limb fatigue, add dang shen (Radix Codonopsitis Pilosulae) and bai zhu (Rhizoma Atractylodis Macrocephalae) to replenish qi and promote blood circulation.

六、浊毒伤阴
6. Turbid Toxin hurt Yin

（一）主要症状
6.1 Main symptoms

腹泻时作，腹中隐痛，腹胀不适，便血鲜红黏稠，常伴有疲乏头昏，盗汗，心烦不寐，舌质偏暗红，少苔，脉细弱。

Diarrhea, vague pain in the abdomen, abdominal distension and discomfort, sticky thick stool with fresh red blood, often accompanied by fatigue, dizziness, night sweating, upset, insomnia, dark red tongue , with little moss, thready weak pulse.

（二）治法
6.2 Treatment method

益气养阴，健脾补肾。

To replenish qi and nourish Yin, reinforce spleen and tonify kidney.

（三）方药
6.3 Prescription and medicines

黄连、阿胶（烊化）、当归、太子参、北沙参、麦冬、白芍、乌梅、山药、三七、炙甘草。如大便下血则加地榆清肠止血；如便秘与泄泻交替，可用大剂量白术（30g以上）、山药、何首乌、当归健脾益肾，养血润肠。

Huang lian (Rhizoma Coptidis), e jiao (Asini Corii Colla) (melting), dang gui (Radix Angelicae Sinensis), tai zi shen (Radix Pseudostellariae), bei sha shen (Radix Adenophrae Strictae), mai dong (Radix Ophiopogonis), bai shao (Radix Paeoniae Alba), wu mei (Fructus Mume), shan yao (Tuber Dioscoreae), san qi (Radix Notoginseng), zhi gan cao (fried Radix Glycyrrhizae). In case of stool with blood, add di yu (Radix et Rhizoma Sanguisorbae) to clear intestines to stop bleeding; in case of constipation alternates with diarrhea, use more than 30g of bai zhu (Rhizoma Atractylodis Macrocephalae), and shan yao (Tuber Dioscoreae), he shou wu (Radix Polygoni Multiflori), dang gui (Radix Angelicae Sinensis) to reinforce spleen and replenish kidney, nourish blood and lubricate intestines.

七、浊毒损阳
7. Turbid toxin damages Yang

（一）主要症状
7.1 Main symptoms

黎明之前，肠鸣腹痛腹泻，泻后则安，大便为黏液血样，遇寒即发，形寒肢冷，口淡纳少，喜热饮，腰酸乏力，面色苍白，舌淡，苔白，脉沉细无力。

Bowel sound, abdominal pain and diarrhea in early morning, feel ok after diarrhea, stool with mucus blood, occurs when coming across cold, cold body and limbs, light taste in mouth and poor appetite, in favor of hot drink, lassitude and fatigue in loin, pale face, the light tongue, white moss, and weak thready and fatigue pulse.

（二）治法

7.2 Treatment method

健脾温肾止泻。

To reinforce the spleen, warm the kidney and stop the diarrhea.

（三）方药

7.3 Prescription and medicines

党参、干姜、炒白术、甘草、补骨脂、肉豆蔻、吴茱萸、五味子、生姜、三七。如脾阳虚为主者，重用党参、白术、炮姜；肾阳虚偏重者，重用附子、肉桂、补骨脂；滑脱不禁，舌苔无滞腻者，加罂粟壳、诃子肉、赤石脂、石榴皮等。

Dang shen (Radix Codonopsitis Pilosulae), gan jiang (Zingiberis Rhizoma), chao bai zhu (fried Rhizoma Atractylodis Macrocephalae), gan cao (Radix Glycyrrhizae), bu gu zhi (Psoraleae Fructus), rou dou kou (Semen Myristicae), wu zhu yu (Euodiae Fructus), wu wei zi (Fructus Schisandalis), sheng jiang (Rhizoma Zingiberis Recens), san qi (Radix Notoginseng). If spleen Yang deficiency is the key factor, use large dosage of dang shen (Radix Codonopsitis Pilosulae), bai zhu (Rhizoma Atractylodis Macrocephalae), pao jiang (prepared Ginger); if kidney Yang deficiency is the key factor, use large amount of fu zi (Radix Aconiti), rou gui (Cortex Cinnamomi) and bu gu zhi (Psoraleae Fructus); in case of incontinence of feces, tongue moss without stagnated greasiness, add ying su ke (Papaveris Pericarpium), ke zi rou (Fructus Chebulae), chi shi zhi (Holloysitum Rubrum), shi liu pi (Granati Pericarpium), etc.

八、寒热错杂
8. Cold-heat complicated syndrome

（一）主要症状

8.1 Main symptoms

黏液血便，便下不爽，口渴不喜饮或喜热饮，腹痛绵绵，喜温喜按，倦怠怯冷，小便淡黄，舌质红或淡红，苔薄黄，脉细缓或濡软。

Difficult stool with mucus and blood, thirsty but dislike to drink or in favor of hot drink, vague abdominal pain, like to be warmed and pressed, tired and fear of cold, pale yellow urine., with red or light red tongue, thin yellow moss, and thready slow or soft weak pulse.

（二）治法

8.2 Treatment method

温中补虚，清热化湿。

To warm the middle energizer and tonify the deficiency, clear heat and dispel dampness.

（三）方药

8.3 Prescription and medicines

乌梅、黄连、黄柏、肉桂、炮姜、党参、炒当归、三七、炙甘草。大便伴脓血者，去川椒、细辛，加秦皮、地榆；腹痛甚者，加徐长卿、延胡索。

Wu mei (Fructus Mume), huang lian (Rhizoma Coptidis), huang bo (Cortex Phellodendri), rou gui (Cortex Cinnamomi), pao jiang (prepared Ginger), dang shen (Radix Codonopsitis Pilosulae), chao dang gui (fried Radix Angelicae Sinensis), san qi (Radix Notoginseng), zhi gan cao (fried Radix Glycyrrhizae). Stool with pus and blood, reduce chuan jiao (Zanthoxuli Pericarpium), xi xin (Herba Asari cum Radice), add qin pi (Cortex Fraxini Caulis), di yu (Radix et Rhizoma Sanguisorbae); more severe abdominal pain, add xu chang qing (Cynanchi Paniculati Radix et Rhizoma), yan hu suo (Rhizoma Corydalis).

第八章 结肠癌浊毒论
Chapter 8 On Turbid Toxin Of Colon Cancer

第一节 病因病机
Section 1 Etiology and Pathogenesis

一、古代中医名家对结肠癌的认识
1. The understanding of colon cancer by the ancient traditional Chinese medicine masters

古代中医认为结肠癌属于"肠蕈""积聚"等范畴，除古医籍之外，古典文学、历史、地理等对此均有论述，如《说文解字》《尔雅》《周礼》，甚至殷墟甲骨文中也有关于肿瘤症状、治法的描述。

Ancient TCM believes that colon cancer belongs to the category of "abdominal mass" and "accumulated mass". In addition to ancient medical records, ancient classical literature, history and geography such as *Shuo Wen Jie Zi, Er Ya, Rites of Zhou Dynasty*, and even in the oracle bone inscriptions in Yin ruins have discussions about the disease.

（一）秦——西汉时期（公元前221—公元25年）
1.1 From Qin to Western Han dynasty (221 BC – 25 AD)

《黄帝内经》作为我国现存较早的医学书籍，对肿瘤有相当丰富的记载，其因"邪居其间，久而内着"而成，有"肠蕈""石瘕""肠风""脏毒"等诸多之证。

The Medical Classic of Yellow Emperor as an earlier existing medical book in China, has rich records of tumors, it is generated because "evil lives internally over time", there are "abdominal mass", "stone mass", "bloody defecation", "evil in zang -organs" and many other syndromes.

《灵枢·水胀》曰："肠覃何如？岐伯曰：寒气客于肠外，与卫气相搏，气不得荣，因有所系，癖而内著，恶气乃起，瘜肉内生。其始生也，大如鸡卵。"《灵枢·刺节真邪》云："有所结，气归之，卫气留之，不得反，津液久留，合而为肠瘤，久者数岁乃成……"

Spiritual Pivot-Edema says: "How about abdominal mass? Qibo said, 'the cold evil from outside the intestines, combats with defensive qi, prevents the qi from nourishing the body, as it lingers long, dyspeptic disease occurs, generating morbid qi and polyp, at the initial period, it appears as big as an chicken egg." *Spiritual Pivot-Cijie Zhenxie: Discussion on the Five Sections in Needling and Comments on the Genuine-Qi and Pathogenic Factors* says: "When pathogenic factor is stagnated, evil qi enters, which cannot leave due to prevention of defensive qi, combined with retained fluid and liquid, intestinal tumor is generated, under chronic condition, the tumor may be formed in several years…"

（二）东汉——三国时期（公元25—265年）

1.2 In the period from Eastern Han dynasty to Three Kingdoms Times (25 AD – 265 AD)

汉代王充云："欲得长生，肠中常清；欲得不死，肠中无渣。"

The Han dynasty Wang Chong said: "If you want to live longer, intestines should often be cleared; if you want to never die, do not leave residue in the intestines."

（三）晋南北朝、隋代时期（公元265—618年）

1.3 In the period from Jin dynasty, Southern and Northern dynasties to Sui dynasty (265 AD – 618 AD)

晋代葛洪在《肘后备急方》卷四"治卒心腹癥坚方第二十六"中说："凡癥坚之起，多以渐生，如有卒觉，便牢大，自难治也。腹中癥有结积，便害饮食，转羸瘦。"其认识到肿瘤的发生发展是逐渐发展的过程，往往自我发觉异常时多属晚期，并认识到"长生要清肠，不老须通便"。

Ge Hong of the Jin dynasty said in "Prescription 26 of Sudden Occurrence of Abdominal Mass", the fourth volume of *Zhouhou Beiji Fang (Elbow Reserve Emergency Prescriptions),* "All diseases like abdominal mass generates gradually at the beginning, when patient feels it suddenly, it becomes large and firm, thus it is difficult to cure. As abdominal mass has accumulation, it harms patient's appetite, patients will turn thin physically." It is realized that generation and development of tumor is a gradual process, once it is felt and found by patients, the disease usually enters late stage. And it is also realized that "longlife requires regular clearing of the intestine, immortality requires normal defecation".

（四）唐代时期（公元618—907年）

1.4 In Tang dynasty (618 AD – 907 AD)

唐代孙思邈指出："便难之人其面多晦，面晦者必难便。"唐代王焘《外台秘要·卷十二·积聚方五首》云："积者阴气，五脏所生，始发不离其部，故上下有所穷；聚者阳气，六腑所成，故无根本，上下无所留止。其痛无常处……疗腹内积聚，癖气冲心，肋急满，时吐水，不能食。"

Sun Simiao pointed out that patients with difficult stool is usually gloomy in complexion, and the patient with gloomy complexion is usually difficult to discharge stool. Wang Tao of the Tang dynasty said in *Waitai Miyao Prescription (Arcane Essentials From The Imperial Library)-Five Prescriptions for Abdominal Mass:* "Fixed Mass is accumulation of Yin qi, generated in five zang-organs, at the very beginning, it is fixed in local area, with upper and down margin; movable mass is the gathering of Yang qi, generated in six fu-organs, so it is not fixed, often moving up and down without margin, the pain is movable without certain location… to heal abdominal mass either fixed or movable, symptoms as dyspeptic qi, hypochondrium fullness, vomiting of liquid, poor appetite should be cared."

（五）宋代时期（公元960—1279年）
1.5 Song Dynasty (960 AD – 1279 AD)

《卫济宝书》第一次使用"癌"字，所谓"癌疾初发，却无头绪，只是肉热痛，过一七或二七，忽然紫赤微肿，渐不疼痛，逶迤软熟紫赤色，只是不破。宜下大车螯散取之，然后服排脓、败毒、托里、内外等散，然后用藿香膏贴之"。其后，宋元两代医家论述"乳岩"，均以岩字代替癌字。

Wei Ji Treasure Book first uses the word "cancer", it said "at the beginning of cancer disease, no threads can be gathered up, nothing different from muscular fever and pain, after 7 or 14 days, suddenly purple red micro swelling occurs, it develops gradually with no pain, meandering soft ripe of purple red colour, but not broken. It is appropriate to use prescription of Dache Ao Powder to treat it, and then use prescription of Pai Nong Powder, Bai Du Powder, Tuo li Powder, Nei Wai Powder, and then use patchouli paste to bind on it". Later, the two dynasties of Song and Yuan doctors discussed "mastrocarcinoma (rock breast)", with the word "rock"replacing the word "cancer".

《圣济总录》一书记载的肿瘤病概念为："瘤之为义，留滞而不去也。气血流行不失其常，则形体和平，无或余赘。及郁结壅塞，则乘虚投隙，病所由生。"

The concept of cancer disease recorded in *The General Record of Shengji* is: "The word Tumor (reading 'liu' in Chinese) indicates 'staying without leaving away'. When circulation of qi and blood is normal, the body is peaceful with no redundant. When depression and stagnation obstructs the circulation of qi and blood, pathogenic factor of tumor invades, the disease occurs."

（六）元代时期（公元1279—1368年）
1.6 In the Yuan dynasty (1279AD – 1368AD)

朱丹溪提出了"阳常有余，阴常不足"及"相火论"等学说，强调"凡人身上中下有块者，多是痰"。《丹溪手镜·积聚六》云："肠胃不虚，邪气无从而入。人惟坐卧风湿，醉饱房劳，生冷停寒，酒面积热，以致营血失道，渗入大肠，此肠风脏毒之所由也。"提出"痰在肠胃间者，可下而愈"，以二陈汤为治痰基本方。

Zhu Danxi put forward the theories of "Yang is often surplus, Yin is often insufficient" and "Minister - Fire theory", emphasizing that "most of the mass in upper, middle and lower-energizer of human body are phlegm." *Danxi Hand Mirror-On Abdominal Mass Six* said: "If the stomach is not deficient, evil cannot get in. People only sit and ly down in rheumatic atmosphere, over drinking and eating, excessive sexual intercourse, raw and cold substances will make the coldness stay in stomach, while wine and cooked wheaten food accumulates heat, so that nutrient-blood looses channel to circulate, infiltrates into the large intestine, this is the cause of bloody defecation and intestinal toxin." It Pointed out that "phlegm in the stomach and intestines can be purged and cured", with Erchen Decoction as the basic prescription of phlegm resolving.

（七）明清时期（公元1368—1840年）

1.7 Ming and Qing dynasties (1368AD – 1840AD)

《外科正宗·脏毒》说："蕴毒结于脏腑，火热流注肛门，结而为肿，其患痛连小腹，肛门坠重，二便乖违，或泻或秘，肛门内蚀，串烂经络，污水流通大孔，无奈饮食不餐，作渴之甚，凡此未得见其生。"

Surgical Authentic-Toxin in Zang-organs says: "Accumulated toxin is stagnated in the viscera, fire heat flows into anus. Knot and swollen, its pain is connected with lower abdomen, anus is dropping heavy, feces are abnormal, either diarrhea or constipation, anal erosion develops along with meridians, foul water flows through large hole, but patients can not eat, very thirsty, this disease has never been cured."

《外科大成·论痔漏》说："锁肛痔，肛门内外犹如竹节锁紧，形如海蜇，里急后重，便粪细而带扁，时流臭水，此无治法。"

Surgical Dacheng-On Hemorrhoids Leakage says: "Anus locking hemorrhoids, indicates that anus seems to be locked by bamboo lock from inside and outside, the form is like jellyfish, tenesmus, the stool is thready and flat, sometimes discharging foul water, this syndrome can not be cured."

张从正认为："夫病一物，非人体素有之也，或从外而来，或由内生，皆邪气也。"其提出了"病由邪生，攻邪已病"的学说，创立了"攻邪论"。"汴梁曹大使女……病血瘕数年……戴人曰：小肠遗热于大肠，为伏瘕，故结硬如块，面黄不月。乃用涌泄之法，数年之疾，不再旬而效"，"积之成也，或因暴怒喜悲思恐之气"。

Zhang Congzheng believes: "Disease is not originally born in human body, it is generated by pathogenic qi either from the outside, or from the endogenous." He Put forward that "disease arises from evil, and can be cured through purging", and founded the theory "evil attacking". "Daughter of Bianliang Ambassador Cao... with disease of blood mass for several years...Congzheng said: the small intestine transforms heat to the large intestine, generates abdominal mass, hard and dull, the patient if with yellow complexion and irregular menses. It makes effect to treat the disease of several years by using the method of purging within 10 days", "the disease is evil accumulation due to anger, joy, sorrow, thinking and fear."

二、现代中医名家对结肠癌的论述

2. Discussions of modern masters of TCM on colon cancer

中医学从整体观念出发，认为肿瘤是"全身为虚，局部为实"的全身性疾病。肿瘤的发生在于脏腑功能的紊乱，故中医药治疗不只是局限在缩小肿块，消灭肿瘤细胞本身，更是从调整人体脏腑功能相协调的全身情况来考虑。40余年来，不少学者撰写了中医、中西医的肿瘤专著。

According to the wholistic sense, traditional Chinese medicine believes that the tumor is a systemic disease that "the whole body is asthenia but the local part is sthenia". The occurrence of tumors lies in the function disorder of the viscera, so TCM treatment is not limited to reducing the size of the mass and eliminating the tumor cells themselves, but also consider to regulate the viscera function in coordination with the systemic situation of the human body. Many scholars have written TCM and ITCWM monographs on tumors in last 40 years.

（一）发病机制
2.1 Pathogenesis

主要有以下几种学说：①内虚学说；②湿聚学说；③热毒学说；④气滞血瘀学说。

About the pathogenesis there are a few kind of theories as follows. a. internal deficiency theory; b. wet aggregation theory; c. heat toxin theory; d. qi stagnation and blood stasis theory.

（二）辨证思路的研究
2.2 Research on syndrome differentiation thinking

1.按湿热瘀毒论治　大肠癌的发生主要是湿热瘀毒蕴结而致，治疗时常用清热利湿、化瘀解毒的药物。《中医肿瘤学》的作者郁仁存将大肠癌分为脾虚湿热型、湿热瘀毒型、脾肾寒湿型，主张在辨证的基础上加用解毒抗癌药。王绪鳌认为本病为肠道湿热所致，治疗以清热利湿、抗癌解毒为主，在此基础上依辨证加减用药。

2.2.1 Treatment according to obstruction of heat, dampness, stasis and toxin　The occurrence of colorectal cancer is mainly caused by the accumulation of heat, dampness, stasis and toxin, medicines of heat clearing and dampness eliminating, stasis resolving and toxin removing are generally used in clinical treatment. Yu Rencun, the author of *Oncology in Chinese Medicine*, divided colorectal cancer into pattern of spleen deficiency and humid heat, pattern of dampness, heat, stasis, toxin, pattern of cold and dampness of kidney and spleen, and advocated to use toxin-removing and anti-cancer medicines on the basis of syndrome differentiation. Wang Xuao believes that this disease is caused by intestinal dampness and heat, and the treatment should focus on clearing heat and eliminating dampness, resisting cancer and removing toxin. On this basis, drugs are added and reduced according to syndrome differentiation.

2.按脏腑虚损论治　许多学者认为大肠癌的发生与正气虚弱关系密切，正气不足，而后邪踞之，晚期患者正虚尤为明显，因而主张补益脏腑虚损，扶助正气，以提高患者抵抗力，延长患者生存期。刘树农治疗肿瘤"一正避三邪"，根据疾病不同的性质，分别补益气、血、阴、阳，使正胜邪退，病情朝好的方向转化。

2.2.2 Treatment according to deficiency of the viscera　Many scholars believe that the occurrence of colorectal cancer is closely related to the weakness of the healthy qi, as healthy qi is insufficient, the evil qi takes the place to supplement. For patients in in advanced stage the deficiency of healthy qi is even more obvious. Therefore, it is advocated to tonify the deficiency of the viscera and reinforce the healthy qi to improve patients' ability of resistance and prolong the survival of patients. Liu Shunong treats the tumor "one healthy qi avoiding three evils", according to the different nature of the disease, respectively reinforcing qi, blood, Yin, Yang, so that the healthy qi can defeat and evil qi retreat, the disease is transformed towards a better direction.

3.按癥瘕积聚论治　大肠癌即是大肠的癌肿，符合中医"肠积""癥瘕"的范畴，有些学者将肿块分型，例如热毒肿块型、脾虚肿块型等，治疗采用传统的软坚散结、破瘀消癥法。

2.2.3 Treatment according to abdominal mass　Colorectal cancer is the tumor of the large intestine, which conforms to the category of "intestinal accumulation" and "mass" in traditional Chinese medicine. Some scholars classify masses into different categories, such as heat toxin mass and spleen deficiency mass, to treat them, traditional methods of soften the hardness and dissipate binds, break stasis and resolve abdominal mass are suggested.

4.按癌毒侵袭论治　孙秉严认为"癌毒"是肿瘤致病的重要因子，只有"癌毒"与体内气血痰食等聚结，才能发生肿瘤，用药上主张以毒攻毒，散寒驱毒。实验研究证明，中药中以毒攻毒的药物，大多对癌细胞有直接的细胞毒作用。

2.2.4 Treatment according to the invasion of cancer toxin　Sun Bingyan believes that "cancer toxin" is an important factor of tumor disease. Only the aggregation of "cancer toxin" and qi, blood, phlegm and food in the body can generate tumors. Treatment method is advocated to use attacking poison with poison, dispersing coldness and removing toxin. Experimental studies have proved that most of the drugs of attacking poison with poison in traditional Chinese medicine have a direct cytotoxic effect on cancer cells.

（三）名家经验

2.3 Experiences of well-known masters

1.黄玉洁经验　黄玉洁治疗结肠癌提倡早期治疗应以攻削"瘤邪"为主，采用先攻后补或攻补兼施方法。例如以气滞为主，治以理气，散结降逆；以血瘀为主，治以活血化瘀，佐以理气；如以痰结湿聚为主，当以化痰软坚、芳香化湿，佐以健脾；以热毒蕴结为主，则泻火解毒，消肿利湿。中晚期当以培本扶正祛邪，并以补肾健脾、滋阴益气为主。

2.3.1 Huang Yujie's experience　Huang Yujie's treatment of colon cancer advocates that early treatment should mainly attack the "tumor evil", and adopt the methods of attacking first, and tonifying later, or attacking and tonifying simultaneously. For example, if qi stagnation is the main symptom, regulate qi, dissipate binds and descend the counterflow; if blood stasis is the main symptom, dominantly promote the blood circulation and resolve blood stasis, regulating qi as assistance; if the main symptom is binding of phlegm and aggregation of dampness, dominantly resolve the phlegm and soften the hardness, resolve the dampness with aroma, and reinforcing the spleen as assistance; if the accumulation of heat and toxin is the main symptom, purge the fire and remove the toxin, dissipate the swelling and resolve the dampness. In the middle and late stages of the disease, we should cultivate the root, reinforce the healthy qi and dispel evil, and tonify the kidney and reinforce the spleen, nourish Yin and replenish qi.

2.王绪鳌经验　王绪鳌治疗上采用辨证和辨病相结合的方法，以清热解毒、化瘀消肿为主，加用抗癌解毒药物，病久加用升提固涩药物。辨证精当，病证结合，遣药有序，且守方长服，故取效较捷。治疗结肠癌的基本方药为藤梨根、猫人参、白花蛇舌草、苦参、水杨梅根、生薏苡仁、凤尾草、野葡萄根、白茅根、槐角、重楼、丹参。

2.3.2 Wang Xuao's experience　Wang Xuao's treatment combines syndrome differentiation and disease differentiation, to clear heat and remove toxin, resolve blood stasis and disperse swelling dominantly, add anti-cancer and detoxification medicines, for long-time disease add ascending and astringent securing medicines. Appropriate syndrome differentiation, and combination of disease and syndrome, orderly medication, and concentrate the prescription for a long time, so the effect is quicker. The basic prescription and medicines for the treatment of colon cancer are: teng li gen (Radix Actinidae Chinensis), mao ren shen (Radix Actinidiae Valvatae), bai hua she she cao (Herba Oldenlandiae Diffusae), ku shen (Sophorae Flavescentis Radix), shui yang mei gen (Fructus Adinae Radix), sheng yi yi ren (Semen Coicis), feng wei cao (Herba Multifidae Pteridis), ye pu tao gen (Raidx Vitis Wilsonae), bai mao gen (Rhizoma Imperatae), huai jiao (Fructus Sophorae), chong lou (Rhizoma Paridis), dan shen (Salviae Miltiorrhizae).

3.周维顺经验　周维顺提出大肠癌确诊后在早期应尽快争取手术机会，中晚期可结合化疗、放疗、免疫等治疗手段。其认为该病临床各期均宜结合中医药治疗。他认为本病早期属邪实，治当清热利湿解毒，活血化瘀消积；中晚期属虚，应注重扶正，健脾益肾，滋阴养血，扶正以驱邪。

2.3.3 Zhou Weishun's experience　Zhou Weishun proposed that surgery should be obtained as soon as possible in the early stage, and combine chemotherapy, radiotherapy, immunization and other treatments in the middle and advanced stages. It is believed in all treatment solutions in each clinical stages of the disease should be combined with TCM. He believes that in the early stage, the disease is evil sthenia, it should be treated with clearing heat, disinhibit dampness and detoxification, promoting blood circulation, resolving blood stasis and dispersing accumulation. In the middle and late stagethe disease belongs to asthenia, we should pay more attention to reinforce healthy qi, invigorating the spleen and replenish kidney, enrich Yin and nourish blood, and reinforce the healthy qi to expel evilness.

4.张梦依经验　张梦依认为直肠癌多为湿热蕴结，邪毒滞留，气滞不畅所致，治疗上以清热利湿、解毒消肿为法，辅以凉血清肠。方药以白花蛇舌草、白茅根、夏枯草、仙鹤草四味药为主药，辨证施治，随症加减。

2.3.4 Zhang Mengyi's experience　Zhang Mengyi believes that rectal cancer is mostly caused by accumulation of dampness and heat, retention of evil toxin, and qi stagnation. The treatment should use the method of clearing heat and disinhibit dampness, detoxification and dispersing swelling, supplemented by cooling blood and clearing intestine. bai hua she she cao (Herba Oldenlandiae Diffusae), bai mao gen (Rhizoma Imperatae), xia ku cao (Spica Prunellae), xian he cao (Herba Agrimoniae) four drugs as the main medicines, treat with addition and reduction according to syndrome differentiation.

三、基于浊毒理论对结肠癌病因病机的认识
3. Understanding of the etiology of colon cancer based on the theory of turbid toxin

（一）病因

3.1 The etiology

1.浊毒内蕴，浊、毒、瘀互结乃本病之标　大肠主运化糟粕，《素问·灵兰秘典论》说："大肠者，传道之官，变化出焉。"大肠的传导变化作用，是胃的降浊功能的延伸，脾虚则不足以运化水湿，脾之升降功能失调，大肠传导功能失司，糟粕不能运化，顽痰宿湿阻滞肠间，缠绵难愈。痰湿久羁大肠而不去，水湿内蕴化为浊，郁热内生，浊热弥散入血而为毒。浊毒滞于脾胃，久蕴于肠腑，与气血胶结，所谓"久病必瘀""久病入络"。肠道脂络瘀阻，气血不能充养，然浊毒与瘀又合而为病，互为因果，浊毒阻于脉络久必致瘀，瘀滞于肠道久必生浊，浊瘀相干终致疾病缠绵难愈，正常黏膜逐渐演变为上皮增生，日久可致腺体上皮内瘤变甚至恶变。

3.1.1 The accumulation of turbid toxin: Inter-binding of turbidity, toxin and blood stasis is the tip of this disease　The large intestine mainly controls dross transporting, *Simple Conversation-Discussion on the Secret Canons Stored in the Royal Library* says: "The large intestine as the organ in charge of transportation, is responsible for discharging the changed substances (dross) out." The dross conduction function of the large intestine, is the extension of the turbidity downbearing function of the stomach. Deficient spleen is not capable to transport water and dampness. Dysfunction in ascending and descending of the spleen, and dysfunction in transportation of the large intestine, cause the phenomenon that the dross cannot be transported, the stubborn sputum and dampness retention resisted in the intestines, lingering and difficult to recover. Phlegmatic hygrosis stays long in large intestine and does not leave, wet water accumulates into turbidity, depressed heat is generated endogenously, the turbid heat is diffused into blood and turns to be toxin. Turbid toxin is stagnated in the spleen and stomach, long accumulated in the intestines, interbinds with qi and blood, so-called "long disease will generate blood stasis", "long disease will get into the collateral". Intestinal lipid is congested, qi and blood can not be nourished. However, turbid toxin and stasis have the relation of reciprocal causation, can combine and generate disease. Turbid toxin blocked in the vein for a long time will cause blood stasis, and stasis stagnated in the intestinal tract for a long time will generate turbidity. Turbidity and blood stasis coherence eventually cause disease which is lingering and difficult to heal. Normal mucosa has gradually evolved into epithelial hyperplasia, over time it can cause glandular intraepithelial neoplasia or even malignant change.

2.本病源于脾胃本虚　古代医家认为，先天不足，脏腑亏虚，是大肠癌发生的根本原因。《灵枢·百病始生》云："风雨寒热不得虚，邪不能独伤人……此必因虚邪之风，与其身形，两虚相得，乃客其形……是故虚邪之中人也……留而不去，传舍于肠胃之外、募原之间，留著于脉，稽留而不去，息而成积。"

3.1.2 This disease is originated from the deficiency of spleen and stomach　Ancient doctors believed that congenital deficiency and deficiency of viscera were the root cause of colorectal cancer.

Spiritual Pivot-The Occurrence of All Diseases says: "No matter wind, rain, cold and heat, without deficiency in human body, evil can not alone hurt people... it must be because the wind of deficient evil, plus the deficient body of the patient, combination of the two deficiency, get into the body of the patient. Thus when the deficient evil attacks people... it will stay but not go away, transmits from the region outside the intestines and stomach to the Muyuan (mesentery), retains in the pulse, if it keep staying but does not go, it will accumulate into mass."

3.饮食失调　常见于饮食不节或不洁、恣食生冷、饮食过饱、肥甘厚味等，多种原因伤及脾胃，脾胃运化失司，日久痰湿内生，毒邪蕴结，大肠络脉受阻，结而成积。

3.1.3 Irregular diet　It occurs generally because of uncontrolled and unclean diet, eating of raw and cold food, over-taking of food especially fat, sweet, thick taste of food. Various reasons hurt the spleen and stomach, causes transportation dysfunction of spleen and stomach, with time passes, phlegmatic hygrosis is generated endogenously, toxic evil is accumulated, collateral pulse of the large intestinal is blocked, and accumulated into abdominal mass.

4.感受外邪　也是导致大肠癌的重要原因之一。如《素问·风论》曰："久风入中，则为肠风飧泄。"认为感受风邪是肠风的主要致病原因。

3.1.4 Attacked by external evil　It is also one of the important causes of colorectal cancer. For example, *Simple Conversation-Discussion on Wind* says: "When prolonged attack of exogenous wind gets into middle energizer, blood defecation and Sunxie (diarrhea with undigested food) occur." Attacking of wind evil is the main cause of blood defecation.

5.起居不节　如《灵枢·百病始生》曰："起居不节，用力过度，则脉络伤……阴络伤则血内溢，血内溢则后血。肠胃之络伤，则血溢于肠外，肠外有寒，汁沫与血相抟，则并合凝聚不得散而积成矣。"

3.1.5 Irregular daily life　As *Spiritual Pivot -The Occurrence of All Diseases* says: "Irregular daily life and overstrain will damage the collateral... when Yin collateral are damaged, it will cause internal hemorrage, blood stool follows. When gastrointestinal collateral are damaged, hemorrage will occur outside the intestine, if there is cold, juice froth to mix up with hemorrage outside the intestines, the mixture coagulates and is unable to disperse, finally causing mass."

6.情志因素　忧思抑郁等是导致大肠癌类疾病的重要原因。如张子和《儒门事亲》曰："积之成也，或因暴怒喜悲思恐之气。"说明七情不适，人体气血瘀滞不通，可导致积聚的发生和发展。

3.1.6 Emotional factors　Anxiety and depression is an important cause of colorectal cancer. As Zhang Zi he said in his book *Confucian's Duty to Their Parents*: "The beginning of accumulation, maybe because of violent anger, joy, sorrow, thinking and fear." It indicates that discomfort of seven feelings, plus qi stagnation and blood stasis, can lead to the occurrence and development of abdominal mass.

（二）病机

3.2 Pathogenesis

1.浊毒内蕴　浊毒是一种致病因素，同时也是一种病理产物。浊毒侵犯人体而出现一系列浊毒内蕴的病证，结肠癌即为浊毒证之一，病机主要是浊毒内蕴，浊毒下注肠道，肠道传化失司，脂膜血络受损腐败化为脓血，坏血伤形，发为癌病。

3.2.1 Internal accumulation of turbid toxin Turbid toxin is a pathogenic factor as well as a pathological product. Colon cancer is one of turbid toxin syndromes occurred due to internal accumulation of turbid toxin resulting from the invasion of turbid toxin in human body. Pathogenesis is mainly internal accumulation of turbid toxin, which is transmitted into intestinal tract, causing transportation dysfunction of intestines, lipid membrane and blood collateral are damaged and corrupted into pus blood, affects blood and damages body, causing cancer at last.

2.正虚邪伏　正虚是指正气虚弱，不能抵御外邪侵犯机体，则疾病丛生，肿瘤的发生与正虚有着密切的关系。

3.2.2 Healthy qi is deficient and pathogenic factor is hidden Healthy qi is deficient refers to the weakness of healthy qi, which cannot resist the invasion of the external evil, then various kind of diseases occur, the occurrence of tumor is closely related to deficient healthy qi.

3.脏腑失调　若脏腑失调，则引起气血紊乱，或先天脏腑禀赋不足，皆为肿瘤发生的内在因素。由于患者素体不足，或后天失养，或长期患慢性肠道疾病，久治不愈，脾胃损伤，运化失司，正气虚弱，火毒、湿邪、瘀血、气滞等邪气相互交结，留而不化，日久成为肠癌。调整脏腑功能，重建机体的阴阳平衡，对于治疗肿瘤具有十分重要的意义。

3.2.3 Irregular Viscera The irregular viscera which causes qi and blood disorder, and congenital deficiency of the viscera endowment, are all the internal factors of tumor occurrence. Due to the usual weakness of patient's body, or lack of acquired nourishment, or chronic intestinal diseases for a long time, which has not been cured, spleen and stomach are damaged, leading to dysfunction of transporting and digesting. Weakness of healthy qi, fire toxin, dampness evil, blood stasis, qi stagnation and other evil intersection, stay long bun cannot be resolved, become intestinal cancer with time passes. It is of great significance for the treatment of tumors to regulate the function of viscera and rebuild the balance of Yin and Yang of the body.

（三）病理

3.3 Pathogenesis

气滞、血瘀、食伤、湿聚、痰结、毒踞、正虚、浊毒内蕴，这些病机在饮食不节、情志失调、过度劳伤或感受外来邪毒引起机体阴阳平衡失调、脏腑经络功能失司等内因、外因的作用下，机体逐渐出现气滞、血瘀、食伤、湿聚、痰结、浊毒内蕴等一系列病理性改变，最终酿成各种类型的结肠癌。这也是结肠癌形成的主要病机，正如《中藏经·积聚癥瘕杂虫论》说："积聚癥瘕……皆五脏六腑真气失，而邪气并，遂乃生焉。"

Qi stagnation, blood stasis, dyspepsia, wet aggregation, phlegmatic retention, sitting of toxin, deficiency of healthy qi, internal accumulation of turbid toxin, these pathogenesis influenced by internal and external etiology factors including uncontrolled- diet, disorder of emotion, damage of excessive strain or attacking of the external evil, which cause body imbalance of Yin and Yang, dysfunction of viscera, make a series of pathological changes like qi stagnation, blood stasis, dyspepsia, wet aggregation, phlegmatic binding, internal accumulation of turbid toxin, eventually lead to various types of colon cancer. This is also the main pathogenesis of colon cancer, as the book *Zhongzang Jing-Discussion on Accumulation, Aggregation, Abdominal mass, and Insects* says: "Abdominal mass...are all generated because healthy qi is deficient, evil takes the place."

第二节 治疗原则
Section 2 Principles of Treatment

一、以人为本，人瘤共存
1. People-oriented, life and tumors coexist

中医学认为癌瘤的病机是"毒发五脏"（全身性疾病），"毒根深茂藏"（病灶由里及表、隐蔽而广泛）。治疗特色是整体观念和辨证论治，治疗方法或祛邪消瘤，或扶正培本，目的是治病救人。

Traditional Chinese medicine believes that the pathogenesis of cancer tumor is "toxin occurs in five zang-organs"(wholistic diseases), "the root of toxin is deep, flourishing in each viscera" (lesions are hidden and scattered from the inside to surface). Treatment characteristic is the wholistic concept and syndrome differentiation treatment, treatment methods are expelling evil and eliminating cancer, or strengthening the healthy qi and cultivating the root, the purpose is to cure diseases and protect patient's life.

二、治未病原则
2. The principle of curing future disease

西医重微观，而中医强调整体治疗的观念，关注的是患者的整个身体，而不只是局限在病灶上。中医学认为病灶是全身疾病的局部表现，虽然很多时候只发生在局部，但是与整体有不可分割的联系。中医通过对整个身体的调理，可以有效地改善身体的内部环境，特别是能更有效地消除残癌，抑制复发转移，这是西医很难做到的。

Western medicine emphasizes on micro treatment, while Chinese medicine emphasizes on the concept of wholistic treatment, focusing on the whole body of the patient, not just limited to the lesion. TCM believes that the lesion is the local manifestation of wholistic diseases. Although it only occurs in the local region, it is inseparable with the wholistic body. Through the regulation of the whole body, TCM can effectively improve the internal environment of the body, especially to eliminate residual cancer and inhibit recurrence and metastasis more effectively, which is difficult for western medicine.

三、扶正祛邪并重
3. Pay equal attention to strengthening the healthy qi and dispelling the evil

虽然各医家的辨证很少是完全一致的，但是大都认同顾护脾胃在大肠癌整个治疗过程中的重要性。脾虚为大肠癌之本，治疗大肠癌，尤其是对于具有虚证表现的患者，健脾益气是其主要的治疗方法。健脾益气法通过扶正固本在改善患者生存质量方面体现出了其独特的优势。同时邪毒内蕴是其发病的重要条件，因此扶正之外尚需注重解毒。

Although the syndrome differentiation of various doctors is rarely completely consistent, most people agree with the importance of caring and protecting the spleen and stomach in the whole treatment process of colorectal cancer. Spleen deficiency is the foundational factor of colorectal cancer, so the treatment of colorectal cancer, especially for patients with manifestation of deficiency syndrome, to reinforce the spleen and replenish qi is the main treatment method. The spleen strengthening and qi replenishing method reflects its unique advantages in improving the quality of life of patients by reinforcing the healthy qi and strengthening the root. At the same time, the internal accumulation of evil toxin is an important condition for its onset, so it still needs to pay attention to detoxification.

四、局部与全身并重
4. Pay equal attention to local lesions and the disease of the whole body

中医能够延长患者生命：中医一方面从整体调理，调理结肠癌患者的身体功能，增强患者的元气、抵抗力和免疫力；另一方面，中医重点作用于局部肿瘤和全身范围内的癌细胞。中药中有大量的强力抗癌药，这些抗癌药同时作用于局部的病灶和全身范围内的癌细胞，有效地作用于肿瘤和阻止癌细胞的复发和转移，使患者最终恢复健康。

TCM can prolong the life of patients: on the one hand, TCM regulates the body function of colon cancer patients and enhances their vitality, ability of resistance and immunity; on the other hand, TCM focuses on local tumors and cancer cells throughout the whole body. There are a large number of strong anti-cancer drugs in traditional Chinese medicine, which act simultaneously on both local lesions and cancer cells in the whole body, effectively acting on tumors and preventing the recurrence and metastasis of cancer cells, so that patients can finally recover.

五、分期治疗
5. Treatment in different stages

结肠癌病位在肠，但与脾、胃、肝、肾的关系尤为密切。其病性早期以湿热、瘀毒邪实为主，晚期则多为正虚邪实，正虚又以脾肾（气）阳虚、气血两虚、肝肾阴虚多见。

Colon cancer is located in the intestine, but it is closely related to the spleen, stomach, liver and kidney. In the early stage of the disease, dampness and heat, blood stasis and evil sthenia are the main syndrome. In the late stage, the syndrome is mostly asthenia in healthy qi, but sthenia in evil, and the asthenia healthy qi mostly see spleen and kidney (qi) Yang deficiency, qi and blood deficiency, liver and kidney Yin deficiency.

六、中西医结合治疗
6. Integrated Traditional Chinese Medicine and Western medicine treatment

根据临床调查发现，早期结肠癌的综合治疗主要以手术治疗结合中医药物治疗为主，除此之外早期结肠癌常见的综合治疗措施还有中医治疗联合放、化疗，而中医治疗辅助结肠癌治疗，能够抑制或解除手术放、化疗遗留下来的不良反应。晚期结肠癌综合治疗，则多是以中医药物联合为主。

It is found from clinical investigation that comprehensive treatment in early-stage of colon cancer mainly combines surgical treatment with traditional Chinese medicine, in addition to the above, combination of TCM treatment and radiotherapy and chemotherapy. Chinese medicine treatment as assisting solution to colon cancer treatment, can inhibit or remove the adverse reactions of surgical, radiotherapy and chemotherapy. Comprehensive treatment of advanced colon cancer is mainly based on traditional Chinese medicine.

七、治养并举
7. To promote treatment and maintenance at the same time

俗语云："三分治疗，七分调养。"任何疾病的彻底治愈和患者的心身康复不仅与治疗手段有关，而且在很大程度上取决于患者的调养。科学调养有利于机体功能的恢复与体质的改善，促进疾病的治愈。肿瘤对人体的危害极大，各种肿瘤的治疗方法和手段尤其是化疗、放疗、手术对机体的破坏十分明显，因此，坚持治养并举，加强调养是肿瘤康复的关键所在。肿瘤康复过程中的调养主要有心理、饮食、体育锻炼。

As the saying goes: "thirty percent of treatment, seventy percent of recuperation". The complete cure of any disease and the patient's psychosomatic rehabilitation are not only related to the treatment means, but also depend in certain degree on the patient's recuperation. Scientific recuperation is conducive to the recovery of body function and physical improvement, and promote the curing of disease. Tumor makes great harm to human body. Various treatment methods and means of tumors, especially chemotherapy, radiotherapy and surgery, make obvious damages to the body. Therefore, recuperation is the key to tumor rehabilitation. The recuperation in the process of tumor rehabilitation mainly includes psychological, diet and physical exercise.

第三节 常用治法
Section 3 The Common Method of Treatment

结肠癌浊毒证的治疗中以化浊解毒通络为主法，辅以其他的治疗方法。常用的治疗方法有以下几种。

Treatment of colon cancer mainly depends on the method of turbidity resolving, toxin removing and collateral unblocking, with other treatment methods as supplementation. Treatment methods generally used are as follows.

一、化浊解毒法
1. Method of turbidity resolving and toxin removing

（一）宣瘀泄浊
1.1 To diffuse stasis and discharge turbidity

鉴于其浊瘀互阻的特殊病机，浊与瘀需要并重治疗，徒泄浊则瘀难去，徒化瘀则浊难除，故临床上两者同治，以清热利湿、通腑泄浊加用活血化瘀的药物。临床常用大黄以荡涤肠腑，通腑泄浊。大黄味苦寒，泻下攻积，活血化瘀，浊瘀同治。此外，酌加利湿利尿的药物，通利二便使浊邪从二便而去。但同时尚需注意，大黄为苦寒之品，易伤胃气，对辨证为脾胃虚寒者还需慎用，应中病即止。

Considering the special pathogenesis of inter-resistance of turbidity and stasis, stasis will be difficult to be diffused if only resolving turbidity, turbidity will be difficult to be resolved if only diffusing stasis. Thus dual effort should be made on turbidity and stasis in clinical treatment, in order to clear heat and disinhibit dampness and unblock the fu-organ and discharge the turbidity cooperating with medicines of blood circulation promotion and stasis resolving. Da huang (Radix et Rhizoma Rhei) is generally used clinically to cleanse intestines, unblock the fu-organ and discharge turbidity. Da huang (Radix et Rhizoma Rhei) tastes bitter with cold nature, can purge and eliminate accumulation, promote blood circulation and resolve blood stasis, treating turbidity and stasis simultaneously. In addition, medicines of dampness and urine dissipating can be properly added, so as to unblock two feces and discharge turbidity and stasis along with stool and urine. But at the same time, attention should be paid that da huang (Radix et Rhizoma Rhei) is a bitter cold product, which is easy to hurt stomach qi, for patients syndrome differentiated as deficiency and cold of spleen and stomach, rhubarb still need to be used with caution, the usage should be stopped as soon as the disease is controlled.

（二）化浊解毒
1.2 Turbidity resolving and toxin removing

浊毒实为疾病过程中产生的病理产物，然而浊毒一旦生成便可作为一种致病因素损伤人体。浊毒的致病多有顽固、多发、内损的特点，易阻滞气机、耗伤气血；其致病多凶险、复杂、难愈，病势缠绵，病程较长。基于此种特点，李佃贵以化浊解毒为要务，使浊毒速去，以免日久耗伤人体津液。

Turbid toxin is actually a pathological product generated in the process of disease, but once generated, it can be used as a pathogenic factor to damage the human body. The disease caused by turbid toxin is usually stubborn, frequently encountering and with internal damages, which is easy to block energy mechanism and consume qi and blood; more dangerous, complex, difficult to cure and with long disease course. Basing on this characteristic, Li Diangui takes turbidity resolving and toxin removing as the most important task, so as to quickly eliminate the turbid toxin to avoid wearing out the human body fluid over time.

（三）健脾化浊

1.3 To resolve the turbidity by reinforcing the spleen

脾胃为气血生化之源，而浊邪究其根本也由脾胃运化失常而来，健运脾胃可使生浊无源，脾胃运化功能失常为浊、毒与瘀的源头，可谓是"一源三歧"，因此健脾化浊可以同样可使浊毒除、瘀滞化。

The spleen and stomach is the source of qi and blood, and the root of turbidity evil is caused by abnormal operation of the spleen and stomach. The normal operation of the spleen and stomach can dispel the source of turbidity, and the abnormal operation of the spleen and stomach is the source of turbidity, toxin and stasis, so-called "one source generates three branches". Therefore, reinforcing spleen can also remove turbid toxin and resolve stasis and stagnation.

（四）行气导浊

1.4 To move qi and conduct turbidity

浊、毒、瘀虽为病理产物，一旦生成便阻滞脉络，为有形之邪，成为新的病因，而致百病由生。"六腑以传化物而不藏"，肠腑应以通降为顺，浊、瘀之邪必阻碍其通降，因此对于有形之邪应根据病情、病位之不同顺势引导，行气导浊宜重用枳实、厚朴、槟榔、莱菔子、三棱、莪术等消积导滞之品气血双调，使胃为和降，脾不瘀滞；同时"气行则血行"，也可使气血流通顺畅以防瘀滞内生，正如《寿世保元》所说："气有一息之不运，则血有一息之不行。"导浊的同时应配合黄连、大黄、芦荟、龙胆草等苦寒燥湿之品，解毒化浊，以利浊疾之速除，以防行气之燥烈伤津耗血。

Although turbidity, toxin, blood stasis are pathological products, once generated, they will block the vein, turn to be tangible evil and new etiology to generate various diseases. "Six fu-organs are in charge of transportation but not storing", the smooth operation of intestines should be unblocked and easy to descend. Turbidity and stasis evil will hinder its unblocking and descending, so the tangible evil should be conducted according to the condition, location of the disease. To move qi and conduct turbidity should use big dosage of medicines of accumulation dispersing and stagnation conducting like zhi shi (Aurantii Fructus Immaturus), hou po (Cortex Magnoliae Officinalis), bing lang (Arecae Semen), lai fu zi (Semen Raphani), san leng (Rhizoma Sparganii), e zhu (Rhizoma Curcumae), to dually regulate qi and blood, harmonize the descending of the stomach, and avoid stasis and stagnation of the spleen. At the same time, "to move qi is to promote blood circulation", so to move qi can also make qi and blood flow smoothly to prevent endogenous stasis, as *Shoushi Baoyuan (To Protect Renal Qi in the Times of Long Life)* said: "The blood circulation stops as soon as qi stops moving". At the same time of turbidity conducting, bitter cold and dampness drying products like huang lian (Rhizoma Coptidis), da huang (Radix et Rhizoma Rhei), lu hui (Aloe), long dan cao (Gentianae Radix et Rhizoma) and other, should be cooperatively used to remove toxin and resolve turbidity, in order to expel turbidity disease quickly, and prevent the dryness and fierce of qi moving to damage fluid and consume blood.

二、扶正补虚法
2. Method to strengthen the healthy qi and complement the deficiency

正虚毒盛不能托毒外达者，可用补益气血和透脓的药物扶助正气托毒外出，以免毒邪内陷，即为补托法，如托里消毒饮；缓解期毒势已去，元气虚弱可用补养的药物以恢复其正气，助养其新生，使疮口早日愈合。扶正培本治则所属治法较多，包括补气养血、健脾益胃、补肾益精等。

Patients deficient in healthy qi and abundant in evilness cannot expel toxin and outthrust pathogenic factors, should be treated with medicines of qi and blood tonifying and pus outthrusting to help healthy qi outthrust toxin in avoidance of the internal sinking toxic evil, that is, the method of tonifying and outthrusting, with prescription as Tuoli Xiaodu Yin (Decoction of internal expelling and toxin sterilization). In remission stage, the development of toxin is controlled, Patients weak in renal qi can use some tonic drugs to restore its healthy qi, nourish the acquired vitality, to heal the ulcer as quick as possible. The principle of reinforcing the healthy qi and cultivating the root includes a few methods such as tonifying qi and nourishing blood, invigorating spleen and replenishing stomach, tonifying kidney and replenishing essence, etc.

三、以毒攻毒法
3. Method of attacking poison with poison

以毒攻毒中药直接抗击癌毒瘤之所成。不论是由于气滞血瘀或痰凝湿聚或热毒内蕴或正气亏虚，久之均能瘀积成毒，毒结体内是肿瘤的根本病因之一。由于肿瘤形成缓慢，毒邪深居，非攻不克，所以临床常用有毒之品，性峻力猛，即所谓"以毒攻毒"。

To attack poison with poison, Traditional Chinese medicine uses toxic agent to directly fight against cancer. No matter due to qi stagnation and blood stasis or phlegm coagulation and dampness aggregation, or internal accumulation of heat toxin, or deficiency of healthy qi, with time passes, toxin binded in body is one of the fundamental causes of tumor. Because the tumor formation is slow, toxic evil is deeply resided, it cannot be overcome unless attacking, so toxic products with fierce power are generally used in clinical treatment, so-called "attacking poison with poison".

四、调气和血法
4. Method of qi regulating and blood harmonizing

正如刘河间所说："调气则后重自除，行血则便脓自愈。"为顺畅肠腑凝滞之气血，祛除腐败之脓血，恢复肠道之传送功能，促进损伤之肠道尽早修复，以改善腹痛、里急后重、下痢脓血等临床症状临床，常采用疏肝理气、活血化瘀、凉血止血、收湿敛疮等治法。

As Liu Hejian said: "Tenesmus will disappear when qi is regulated, pus will recover itself when blood circulation is promoted." Methods of liver dispersing and qi regulating, blood circulation promoting and stasis removing, blood cooling and bleeding stopping, dampness eliminating and astringing sores are generally used in clinical treatment, in order to smoothen the circulation of qi and blood coagulated and stagnated in the intestines, remove the corrupted pus and blood, restore the transmission function of the intestines, promote the recovering of the damages in intestines as soon as possible, so as to relieve abdominal pain, tenesmus, dysentery pus and blood, and other clinical symptoms. Fourth, method of qi regulating and blood harmonizing.

五、养肝和胃法
5. Method of nourishing the liver and harmonizing the stomach

人有胃气则生，而治肠癌尤要。由于治疗实证初期化浊解毒方药之中，苦寒之品较多，长时间大剂量使用，有损伤胃气之弊。因此，应注意顾护胃气，并贯穿于治疗的始终。常采用养肝和胃法。

Survival of life depends on stomach qi, it is especially important in treating intestinal cancer. As long time using of large dose of bitter cold products in prescriptions of turbidity resolving and toxin re moving in the initial stage of disease treatment will in certain degree bring damages to gastric qi, therefore, attention should be paid to care and protect gastric qi Liver-nourishing and stomach harmonizing method is usually used.

总之，结肠癌的治疗，热则清之，寒则温之，初则通之，久虚则补之。寒热交错者，清温并用；虚实夹杂者，通涩兼施。始终把握祛邪与扶正的辨证关系、顾护胃气贯穿于治疗的全过程。

In short, the strategy of treating colon cancer is, treating heat with clearing medicine, treating coldness with warming medicine, treating the initial disease with unblocking medicine, treating long- time deficiency with tonifying medicine, treating alterative occurrence of cold and fever with clearing and warming medicine, treating mixture of sthenia and asthenia syndrome with medicines of unblocking and astringing. To grasp the syndrome differentiation relationship between removing evil and strengthening the healthy qi, care and protect the stomach qi throughout the whole process of treatment.

第四节 辨证治疗
Section 4 Treatment with Syndrome Differentiation

一、浊毒壅滞型
1. The turbid poison obstruction type

（一）证候
1.1 Symptoms

腹部疼痛阵作，大便次数增多，下脓血和黏便，里急后重，寒热腹痛，舌苔黄腻，脉滑数。

Paroxysmal abdominal pain, increased times of stool, pus and sticky stool, tenesmus, cold and hot abdominal pain, yellow greasy tongue moss, slippery rapid pulse.

（二）病机
1.2 Pathogenesis

浊毒壅滞，气血瘀滞。

Abundant stagnation of turbid toxin, stagnation of qi and blood stasis.

（三）治则
1.3 Treatment principle

清热解毒，理气化滞。

Clearing heat and removing toxin, regulating qi and resolve stagnation.

（四）方药
1.4 Prescription and medicines

白花舌蛇草30g，半枝莲30g，莪术10g，川楝子10g，木香10g，土茯苓30g，薏苡仁20g，红藤30g，败酱草30g，地榆10g，藤梨根30g，马齿苋30g。

Bai hua she she cao (herba Oldenlandiae Diffusiae) 30g, ban zhi lian (Scutellariae Barbatae Herba) 30g, e zhu (Rhizoma Curcumae) 10g, chuan lian zi (Fructus Toosendan) 10g, mu xiang (Radix Aucklandiae) 10g, tu fu ling (Rhizoma Smilacis Glabrae) 30g, yi yi ren (Semen Coisis) 20g, hong teng (Caulis Sargentodoxae) 30g, bai jiang cao (Herba Patriniae) 30g, di yu (Radix et Rhizoma Sanguisorbae) 10g, teng li gen (Radix Actinidae Chinensis) 30g, ma chi xian (Herba Portulacae) 30g.

（五）加减运用
1.5 Addition and reduction

腹痛剧烈加延胡索、白芷；便血加仙鹤草等。

In case of severe abdominal pain, add yan hu suo (Rhizoma Corydalis), bai zhi (Radix Angelicae Dahuricae); with blood stool, add xian he cao (Herba Agrimoniae), etc.

二、痰瘀互结型
2. Binding of phlegm and blood stasis

（一）证候
2.1 Symptoms

胸闷膈满，面黄虚胖，呕吐痰涎，腹胀便溏，腹部可扪及包块，质地坚硬，固定不移，舌边暗紫，或质紫，或见瘀斑，脉细涩。

Chest distress, full diaphragm, yellow complexion, deficient fat, vomiting phlegm and saliva, abdominal distension with loose stool, abdominal palpable mass, hard and fixed, dark tongue side, or purple in nature, or with ecchymosis, astringent thready veins.

（二）病机

2.2 Pathogenesis

痰瘀交阻，坏血伤形。

Resistance of phlegm and blood stasis, bad blood damages physical shape.

（三）治则

2.3 Treatment principles

化痰散结，活血化瘀。

To resolve phlegm and disperse bind, promote blood circulation and remove blood stasis.

（四）方药

2.4 Prescription and medicines

夏枯草30g，牡蛎30g，菝葜15g，山慈菇15g，穿山甲10g，三棱10g，莪术10g，半夏10g。

Xia ku cao (Spica Prunellae)30g, mu li (Ostireae Concha) 30g, ba qia (Smilacis Chinae Rhizoma) 15g, shan ci gu (Pseudobulbus Cremastrae Variabilis) 15g, chuan shan jia (Squanma Manitis) 10g, san leng (Rhizoma Sparganii) 10g, e zhu (Rhizoma Curcumae) 10g, ban xia (Rhizoma Pinelliae) 10g.

（五）加减运用

2.5 Addition and reduction

黏液血便加地榆炭、马齿苋、仙鹤草、茜草炭、大黄炭等。

Mucus and blood stool, add di yu tan (Radix et Rhizoma Sanguisorbae Carbon), ma chi xian (Herba Portulacae), xian he cao (Herba Agrimoniae), qian cao tan (Robiae Radix et Rhizoma charcoal), da huang tan (Rhubarb Charcoal), etc.

三、脾虚湿盛型
3. Spleen deficiency and wet abundance

（一）证候

3.1 Symptoms

腹部胀满作痛，大便带黏液或脓血，胃纳不佳，形体消瘦，腹部可扪及包块，苔白或腻，脉细。

Abdominal pain and fullness, stool with mucus or pus blood, poor appetite, thin body, abdominal palpable lump, white or greasy moss, thready pulse.

（二）病机
3.2 Pathogenesis

脾气虚弱，湿邪凝聚。

Weak spleen qi, coalgulated aggregation of wet and evil.

（三）治则
3.3 Treatment principle

温补脾肾，健脾化湿。

To warm and tonify the spleen and kidney, strengthen the spleen and resolve dampness.

（四）方药
3.4 Prescription and medicines

黄芪30g，白术10g，茯苓15g，山药10g，生薏苡仁20g，熟薏苡仁20g，白花舌蛇草30g，焦山楂15g，焦神曲15g，炒谷芽15g，炒麦芽15g，炙鸡内金10g，炙甘草5g。

Huang qi (Radix Astragali seu Hedysari) 30g, bai zhu (Rhizoma Atractylodis Macrocephalae) 10g, fu ling (Poria) 15g, shan yao (Dioscoreae Rhizoma) 10g, sheng yi yi ren (raw Semen Coicis) 20g, shu yi yi ren (ripe Semen Coicis) 20g, bai hua she she cao (Herba Oldenlandiae Diffusae) 30g, jiao shan zha (fried Fructus Crategi) 15g, jiao shen qu (fried Messa Medicata Fermentata) 15g, chao gu ya (fried Setariae Fructus Germinatus) 15g, chao mai ya (fried Hordei Fructus Germiatus) 15g, zhi ji nei jin (fried Endothlium Corneum Gigeriae Galli) 10g, zhi gan cao (fried Radix Glycyrrhizae) 5g.

（五）加减运用
3.5 Addition and reduction

腹水加土茯苓、大腹皮、茯苓皮、车前子、泽泻等；疼痛酸胀，加川楝子、延胡索、乌药、白芍、甘草、炮姜。

Patients with ascites, add tu fu ling (Rhizoma Smilacis Glabrae), da fu pi (Arecae Pericarpium), fu ling pi (Poria Cocos Pericarpium), che qian zi (Semen Plantaginis), ze xie (Rhizoma Alismatis), etc; pain with sour distension, add chuan lian zi (Fructus Toosendan), yan hu suo (Rhizoma Corydalis), wu yao (Radix Linderae), bai shao (Radix Paeoniae Alba), gan cao (Radix Glycyrrhizae), pao jiang (prepared Ginger).

四、气血两虚型
4. Dual deficiency of qi and blood

（一）证候
4.1 Symptoms

全身乏力，心悸气短，头晕目眩，面色无华，虚烦不寐，自汗盗汗，舌质淡，苔薄白，边有齿痕，脉细。

Full body fatigue, palpitations, short of breath, dizziness, dull complexion, restless insomnia, sweating and night sweating, light tongue, thin white moss, teeth marks, fine pulse.

（二）病机

4.2 Pathogenesis

气血两虚。

Dual deficiency of qi and blood.

（三）治则

4.3 Treatment principle

益气养血。

Replenish qi and nourish blood.

（四）方药

4.4 Prescription and medicines

黄芪30g，白术10g，茯苓15g，当归10g，白芍10g，熟地黄10g，阿胶10g，茜草10g，鸡内金10g，甘草5g。

Huang qi (Radix Astragali seu Hedysari) 30g, bai zhu (Rhizoma Atractylodis Macrocephalae)10g, fu ling (Poria) 15g, dang gui (Radix Angelicae Sinensis) 15g, bai shao (Radix Paeoniae Alba) 10g, shu di huang (Radix Rehmanniae Praeparatum) 10g, e jiao (Asini Corii Colla) 10g, qian cao (Robiae Radix et Rhizoma) 10g, ji nei jin (Endothlium Corneum Gigeriae Galli) 10g, gan cao (Radix Glycyrrhizae) 5g.

（五）加减运用

4.5 Addition and reduction

舌红光嫩，加西洋参；肛门下坠，加黄芪、葛根、升麻、炙甘草。

Red bright and tender tongue, add xi yang shen (Panacic Quinquefoli Radix); anal straining, add huang qi (Radix Astragali seu Hedysari), ge gen (Radix Puerariae), sheng ma (Rhizoma Climicifugae), zhi gan cao (fried Radix Glycyrrhizae).

第九章　肾病浊毒论
Chapter 9　On Turbid Toxin of Nephropathy

第一节　慢性肾衰竭浊毒论
Section 1　On Turbid Toxin of Chronic Renal Failure

一、慢性肾衰竭的中医学概述
1. Overview of chronic kidney failure in Traditional Chinese medicine

慢性肾衰竭，中医学将其归属"癃闭""关格""水肿""虚劳"等范畴，现据此总结如下。

Chronic kidney failure, is classified by TCM as category of "urochesis", "frequent vomiting and dysruria", "edema", "consumptive disease" and other diseases, which is summarized as follows.

（一）癃闭

1.1 Long Bi (urochesis)

《证治准绳》指出癃和闭均为排尿困难，尿量减少，只有轻重程度和病程长短的不同。慢性肾衰竭症见排尿困难或尿少而无明显水肿者，常以癃闭辨治。

ZhengZhi ZhunSheng (Criterion of Medical Treatment) points out that both Long (dysuria) and Bi (constipation or disuria) indicate dysuria, urine volume reduction, different only in the severity and the length of the course of the disease. Chronic renal failure with dysuria or oliguria without obvious edema are generally differentiation treated as urochesis.

（二）关格

1.2 Frequent Vomiting and Dysuna

《证治汇补·关格》曰："既关且格，必小便不通，旦夕之间，徒增呕恶；次因浊邪壅塞三焦，正气不得升降。所以关应下而小便闭，格应上而生呕吐，阴阳闭绝，一日即死，最为危候。"古代医家已认识到本病是由于脾肾衰败，湿浊之邪壅塞三焦，气机逆乱所致，为急危重证候。治疗应遵循《证治准绳》"治主当缓，治客当急"的原则。

Replenishment To Syndrome Treatment-Frequent Vomiting and Dysuna says: "Both frequent vomiting and dysuna, there must be difficulty in urination, day and night, nausea and vomiting occur; as turbidity evil abundantly obstructs triple energizer, healthy qi can not ascend and descend, so Guan reacts representing the lower energizer, the urination is closed, Ge reacts representing the upper energizer, vomiting occurs, when Yin and Yang is totally closed, patient will die in one day, it is most dangerous." Ancient doctors have realized that this disease is due to decline of the spleen and kidney, wet and turbidity evil is obstructed in triple energizer, energy mechanism is in disorder, it belongs to urgent and critical syndrome. Treatment should follow the principle of *Zhengzhi Zhunsheng (Criterion of Medical Treatment)* "Treatment of host disease should be slow, treatment of guest disease should be urgent".

（三）虚劳

1.3 Consumptive Disease

《素问》"精气夺则虚"可视为虚证的提纲。治疗：张仲景重在温补脾肾并提出扶正祛邪，祛瘀生新等治法，首倡补虚不忘治实的治疗要点。李东垣重视补益脾胃。朱丹溪重视肝肾，善于滋阴降火。所以，虚劳的治疗强调重视脾肾，有实邪者攻补兼施，辨病与辨证相结合。

Simple Conversation "When essence qi is worn out, deficiency occurs" can be regarded as the outline of false evidence. Treatment: Zhang Zhongjing emphasises on the methods of warming the spleen and kidney, strengthening healthy qi and removing evil, removing blood stasis and generating new blood, and first advocated the treatment points of tonifying deficiency without forgetting treating sthenia. Li Dongyuan attaches great importance to tonifying the spleen and replenishing stomach. Zhu Danxi attaches great importance to liver and kidney, and is good at nourishing Yin and reducing fire. Therefore, the treatment of consumptive disease should emphasize the spleen and kidney, treat the syndrome with sthenia evil with both elimination and reinforcement, combining disease differentiation with syndrome differentiation.

目前中医学多认为慢性肾衰竭为本虚标实之证，本虚以脾肾两虚为主，标实以湿浊瘀血为主。其病位在脾肾。其基本病理变化为脾肾功能失常，水液代谢障碍，湿浊氮质潴留而呈现虚实夹杂，寒热交错之证候。

At present, traditional Chinese medicine believes that chronic kidney failure is the syndrome of root deficiency and tip sthenia, root deficiency mainly indicate spleen and kidney deficiency, and tip stenia is mainly wet turbidity and blood stasis. The location of the disease is in the spleen and kidney. The basic pathological changes are abnormal operation of spleen and renal function, dysfunction of water and liquid metabolism, wet and nitrogen retention, and inter-mixture of sthenia and asthenia, alternating of cold and heat.

二、慢性肾衰竭浊毒证的病因病机

2. The etiology and pathogenesis of turbid toxin syndrome of chronic kidney failure

（一）病因

2.1 The etiology

1.外邪侵袭　肾病久治不愈，气血阴阳虚衰，易遭外邪侵袭。或为风邪所伤，或因居处潮湿，损伤脾肾，致脾肾阳虚，水湿浊邪不得运化，阻滞气机变生诸证。

2.1.1 Invasion of external evil   If kidney disease cannot be cured for a long time, qi, blood, Yin and Yang deficiency will decline, patients will be easy to be attacked by external evil, or hurt by wind evil, or by damp residence, the spleen and kidney will be damaged and deficient in Yang, water wet turbidity evil which can not be transported, block the energy mechanism and generate the said diseases.

2.烦劳过度　长期从事重体力劳动，疲劳过度，则损伤脾肾；酒色过度，损伤肾气，肾阳不足，命门火衰，火不暖土，脾肾两虚。

2.1.2 Excessive physical labour   Excessive fatigue due to long time involving in heavy physical labour, damages the spleen and kidney; excessive wine and sexual intercourse, damages kidney qi, lack of kidney Yang, decline of kidney fire, fire can not warm soil, dual deficiency in spleen and kidney.

3.饮食不节　包括暴饮暴食、饮酒过度等，损伤脾胃。长期如此，则致肾脏亦损。肾伤则腰府失养，水之气化不利，故见腰痛、水肿。另外，脾胃虚损，饮食不化精微，反为湿浊。

2.1.3 Uncontrolled diet   It includes over-taking of food and drink, over-drunk of wine, etc. which damage the spleen and stomach, and in a long time, damage kidney organ also. When kidney is damaged, waist fails to be nourished, water vaporization is abnormal, thus back pain, edema occur. Besides, as spleen and stomach is deficient, diet cannot be transmitted into essence, but into damp turbidity.

4.情志所伤　长期情志不舒，肝气郁结，三焦气机不畅，一则横逆而克脾土，肝脾不和，脾失健运，水湿泛滥；一则气机阻滞，气血运行不利，可发生气滞血瘀，或肝郁日久，郁而化火，肝火灼伤肾阴，导致肝肾阴虚。

2.1.4 Emotional damage   Long-term discomfort in emotion causes depression of liver qi stagnation, abnormal operation of qi mechanism of triple energizer. As adverse liver qi restricts spleen soil, liver and spleen discord, spleen looses normal function of transportation. Affected by resistance of energy mechanism, qi and blood circulation is unsmooth, possibly lead to qi stagnation and blood stasis, or liver depression, which will be transformed into fire in a long time, liver fire will burn kidney Yin resulting in liver and kidney Yin deficiency.

5.失治误治　如在原发病治疗中治不得当，或妄投苦寒败胃之品，伤及脾肾；或妄投辛热，伤津耗阴，进一步导致气阴不足；或只注意肾外疾病的治疗，而忽视了对肾脏的调理，造成肾气损伤；或用有毒药物伤及脾肾，致使脾失健运，肾失气化，水湿阻滞，浊毒内生。

2.1.5 Delayed treatment or mistreatment   If the treatment in the original onset of the disease is improper, or incorrectly using bitter cold and stomach-affecting medicines, which hurt spleen and kidney; or incorrectly using acrid hot medicines, which damage fluid and consume Yin, lead to further insufficiency of qi Yin; or only pay attention to the treatment of disease in exception of kidney, ignoring the regulation of kidney, which causes damage of kidney qi; or toxic drugs used in treatment hurt spleen and kidney, causes transporting dysfunction of spleen and vaporizing dysfunction of kidney, resulting in resistance of moisture and internal generation of turbid toxin.

（二）病机

2.2 Pathogenesis

1.病机特点　可概括为"虚、浊、瘀、毒"，其中正虚邪实贯穿始终，正虚包括脏腑气血阴阳的虚损，邪实则有水湿、湿热、瘀血等诸种变化。正虚为本，邪实为标，虚实寒热之间呈动态变化。

2.2.1 The characteristics of the pathogenesis　It can be summarized as "deficiency, turbidity, blood stasis and toxin", in which asthenia of healthy qi and sthenia of evil is manifested throughout the whole process, asthenia healthy qi include the deficiency of qi and blood, Yin and Yang; evil shtenia actually includes pathological changes as water dampness, dampness and heat, blood stasis. Deficiency of healthy qi is the root, evil sthenia is the tip, asthenia and sthenia make dynamic changes between coldness and heat.

2.主要病机

2.2.2 The main pathogenesis

（1）气虚：慢性肾衰病变可涉及心、肝、肺、脾、肾五脏及胃、肠、膀胱等脏腑，但始终以脾肾气虚为关键，而且贯穿于整个病程。临床多见神疲乏力、气短懒言、纳差腹胀等脾气虚证及腰酸膝软、耳鸣眼花、夜尿频多等肾气虚证。

2.2.2.1 Qi deficiency: chronic renal failure lesions can involve five zang-organs of heart, liver, lung, spleen, kidney, and fu-organs of stomach, intestines, and bladder, but deficiency of spleen and kidney qi is always the key and runs throughout the whole course of the disease. Clinically we usually see fatigue, short of breath and lazy to speak, poor appetite and abdominal distension and other syndrome of spleen qi deficiency, lassitude loin and knees, tinnitus dizziness, nocturia and other syndrome kidney qi deficiency.

（2）血瘀：由于气虚、水湿、湿毒均可致瘀，故慢性肾衰患者病程日久，均可出现不同程度的血瘀症状，如面色晦暗，腰痛有定处，唇甲紫暗，舌质淡紫或有瘀斑、瘀点，舌底脉络迂曲，脉细涩。

2.2.2.2 Blood stasis: due to qi deficiency, wet water, dampness toxin can cause blood stasis, so chronic renal failure patients with long course of disease, will present different degrees of blood stasis symptoms, such as dark complexion, fixed lumbar pain, dark purple of lips and nails, light purple tongue or with ecchymosis and petechia, circuitous vein in bottom of tongue, fine and astringent pulse.

（3）浊毒："毒"指慢性肾衰中的尿毒，为脏腑衰竭代谢障碍产生的内生之毒。慢性肾衰竭患者脾肾功能衰败，久生浊毒、溺毒、热毒；或化瘀成痰，蒙神蔽窍；或浊瘀互结，导致肾衰竭。患者常见面色晦浊，舌苔浊腻；若浊犯上焦，心肺气机不利则胸闷、烦躁，甚则气短心悸；浊阻中焦，犯及脾胃，则恶心呕吐，纳呆厌食，便秘或腹胀便溏；浊阻下焦，肾失气化，开阖失司，则见尿少或尿闭，或小便清长，夜尿频多。

2.2.2.3 Turbid toxin: "Toxin" refers to the urinary toxin in chronic renal failure, which is the endogenous toxin produced by metabolic dysfunction due to viscera decline. Patients with chronic renal failure will generate turbid toxin, urinary toxin and heat toxin because of decline of spleen and kidney function. Blood stasis will be transmitted into phlegm, confusing mind and orifice. Turbidity and blood stasis agglutinate, resulting in renal failure. Patients often see dark complexion and turbid greasy tongue moss; If turbidity attacks upper energizer, chest distress, irritability, or even shortness of breath, palpitation will occur. If turbidity obstructs middle energizer, affecting spleen and stomach, nausea, vomiting, anorexia, constipation or abdominal distension and loose stool occur. If turbidity obstructs lower energizer, kidney looses the function of gasification, opening and closing, patients will have little urine or urine closure, or long and lucid urine, frequent nocturia.

三、慢性肾衰竭的浊毒证辨证论治
3. Syndrome differentiation treatment of chronic kidney failure caused by turbid toxin

浊属阴邪。浊邪多易阻滞脉络，壅塞气机。毒属阳邪。毒邪性烈善变，损害气血营卫。浊、毒两者常相互胶结致病，故常浊毒并称。本病属本虚标实，脾气亏虚为本，浊毒为标，正虚邪实贯穿始终。正虚包括脏腑气血阴阳的虚损，以脾气亏虚为主。邪实则为浊毒内蕴。治疗上应标本兼治。

Turbidity belongs to Yin evil. It is easy to block the vein and abundantly obstruct the energy mechanism. Toxin belongs to Yang evil. Toxin evil is fierce and fickle, can damage qi and blood, damage the system of nourishment and defence. Turbidity and toxin often cause diseases by inter-cementing, so the combined word "turbid toxin" is invented. This disease belongs to syndrome of asthenia root and sthenia tip, deficiency of spleen qi is the root, and turbid toxin is the tip. Asthenia healthy qi and sthenia evil qi is manifested overthrough the whole process of the course. The deficiency of healthy qi includes the deficiency and damage of qi, blood, Yin and Yang, mainly the deficiency of spleen qi. Sthenia evil is actually the internal accumulation of turbid toxin. Dual attention should be paid to the tip and root treatment in clinical practice.

（一）调补脾胃以治本
3.1 To treat the root syndrome by regulating and tonifying the spleen and stomach

脾气亏虚是慢性肾衰竭的病因之一，随着病程进展，毒素蓄积，产生湿浊、溺毒，影响脾胃运化、水液代谢，导致脾胃功能失调，胃失和降，出现腹胀、纳呆、恶心、呕吐等症状。故在慢性肾衰竭治疗时以调补脾胃为本，多采用二陈汤、参苓白术散等方。

Spleen qi deficiency is one of the causes of chronic kidney failure. With the progress of the course of the disease, accumulation of toxin generates wet turbidity and urinary toxin, which affects the the transporting of spleen and stomach, metabolism of water and liquid, leads to dysfunction of the spleen and stomach, stomach looses harmonizing and descending, patients see abdominal distension, anorexia, nausea, vomiting and other symptoms. Therefore, treatment of chronic kidney failure should be based on regulating and tonifying the spleen and stomach. Prescriptions usually used are Erchen Decoction, Shenling Baizhu Powder and others.

（二）化浊解毒以治标

3.2 To treat the tip syndrome by turbidity resolving and toxin removing

1.浊毒在上焦

3.2.1 Turbid toxin is in upper energizer

（1）症状：胸闷咳喘，身热口渴，头晕，心烦失眠，面红目赤，甚则心悸怔忡，恶寒发热，身热不扬，午后热甚；甚或言语謇涩，神昏谵语；或胸痛，咳吐黄稠脓痰，心烦肢厥，舌暗红或紫暗，苔黄腻或厚腻，或薄黄，脉弦滑数。

3.2.1.1 Symptoms: chest distress, cough and asthma, hot in body and thirsty in mouth, dizziness, restless insomnia, red eyes and face, even palpitations, fever with adversion to cold, hidden fever, fever more severe in the afternoon; or difficult and astringent in speech, unconscious delirium; chest pain, coughing and vomiting yellow thick phlegm with pus, upset in mind and cold in limbs, dark or purple dark tongue, yellow greasy, or thick greasy or thin yellow moss, string slippery and rapid pulse.

（2）治法：清热解毒。

3.2.1.2 Treatment method: to clear heat and remove toxin.

（3）方药：黄连解毒汤加大黄、蒲公英、水牛角丝、土茯苓、栀子等药加减。

3.2.1.3 Prescription and medicines: decoction of Huanglian Jiedu (Coptis chinensis detoxification soup) with addition of da huang (Radix et Rhizoma Rhei), pu gong ying (Herba Taraxaci cum Radice), shui niu jiao si (Pieces of Cornu Bubali), tu fu ling (Rhizoma Smilacis Glabrae), zhi zi (Fructus Gardeniae) and other drugs.

2.浊毒在中焦

3.2.2 turbid toxin is in middle energizer

（1）症状：胃脘连及胁肋胀满疼痛，灼烧感、反酸，急躁易怒，嗳气频数，情志抑郁不舒，不思饮食，小便不利，大便溏滞不爽、色黄味臭或秘结不通，头晕目眩，胁有痞块，腹胀；或寒热往来，身目发黄；或面色晦暗，口干口苦，肢倦身重；或恶心干呕，舌质红或暗红，苔黄厚腻或薄黄，脉弦数或弦滑。

3.2.2.1 Symptoms: epigastric and flank distention and pain, sense of burning, acid reflux, irritability, frequent belching, depression, poor appetite, difficult urination, loose and stagnated stool, yellow, foul or constipation, dizziness, ruffian, abdominal distension; alterative cold and fever, yellow eyes and body; dark complexion, dry and bitter mouth, tired limbs and fatigue in body; or nausea, retching, red or dark red tongue, yellow thick and greasy moss, string rapid or string slippery pulse.

（2）治法：和胃降气，祛湿化浊。

3.2.2.2 Treatment method: to harmonize stomach and ascend qi, dispel dampness and resolve turbidity.

（3）方药：常用药物有藿香、薏苡仁、砂仁、紫豆蔻、陈皮、半夏、白术等；常用方剂为小半夏加茯苓汤、黄连温胆汤、三妙丸等加减。

3.2.2.3 Prescription and medicines: medicines generally used are huo xiang (Herba Agastaches seu Pogostemonis), yi yi ren (Semen Coisis), sha ren (Fructus Amomi), zi dou kou (Purple Cardamom Kernel), chen pi (Pericarpium Citri Reticulatae), ban xia (Rhizoma Pinelliae), bai zhu (Rhizoma Atractylodis Macrocephalae), etc.; prescriptions commonly used are Xiaobanxia Jia Fuling Decoction, Huanglian Wendan Decoction, Sanmiao Pill (Pill of three miraculous drugs) and so on.

3.浊毒在下焦

3.2.3 Turbid toxin is in lower energizer

（1）症状：小腹胀满，尿闭便坚；或尿频而急，尿痛，淋漓不畅，尿中带血，大便不畅；或下痢腹痛，便下脓血，里急后重，肛门灼热；妇女月经时来时断，带下秽浊，脘痞腹胀，身热呕恶，头晕头胀，神识昏蒙；或神识如狂，口干不欲饮，男女不育不孕，下肢浮肿，舌红苔黄腻，脉滑数。

3.2.3.1 Symptoms: small abdominal distension, urine closure and constipation; or frequent and abrupt urination, urinary pain, bleeding and difficult urine, difficult stool; or dysentery abdominal pain, stool with pus and blood, tenesmus, hot anus; female patients will have intermittent menstruation, foul secreted leukorrhagia, gastric ruffian and abdominal distention, dizziness and brain distention, mind unconsciousness; or mania, thirsty but with no want to drink, sterility and infertility, dropsy lower limbs, red tongue with yellow greasy moss, slippery rapid pulse.

（2）治法：淡渗利湿，排浊解毒；通腑泄浊解毒。

3.2.3.2 Treatment method: using bland herbs to eliminate dampness, resolve turbidity and remove toxin; to unblock fu-organs, purge turbidity and remove toxin.

（3）方药：①淡渗利湿，排浊解毒：常用药物有猪苓、茯苓、冬瓜皮、薏苡仁等；常用方剂为五苓散、五皮饮等加减。②通腑泄浊解毒：常用药物为大黄、厚朴、枳实等。还常选用解毒化浊、活血化瘀的中药（常用药物有大黄、蒲公英、生牡蛎、丹参、槐花、芒硝等）保留灌肠，使浊毒从大便而出。

3.2.3.3 Prescriptions and medicines: a. using bland herbs to eliminate dampness, resolve turbidity and remove toxin: medicines generally used are zhu ling (Polygorus Umbellatus), fu ling (Poria), dong gua pi (Benicasae Exocarpium), yi yi ren (Semen Coisis), etc.; prescriptions commonly used are Wuling Powder, Wupi Yin Decoction with addition and reduction. b. to unblock fu-organs, purge turbidity and remove toxin: medicines generally used are da huang (Radix et Rhizoma Rhei), hou po (Cortex Magnoliae Officinalis), zhi shi (Aurantii Fructus Immaturus), etc. Medicines for turbidity resolving and toxin removing, blood circulation promoting and blood stasis removing da huang (Radix et Rhizoma Rhei), pu gong ying (Herba Taraxaci cum Radice), sheng mu li (raw Ostreae Concha), dan shen (Salviae Miltiorrhizae), huai hua (Sophora Japonica), mang xiao (Natrii Sulfas), etc. are aslo used as enemata, so as to discharge turbid toxin through stool.

（三）兼顾活血化瘀通络

3.3 Giving dual consideration to promoting blood circulation, removing blood stasis and unblocking collateral

浊毒日久，深藏脏腑，可出现不同程度的血瘀症状和体征，所以在化浊解毒的同时需兼顾活血化瘀通络。

Turbid toxin deeply hidden in viscera for a long time, can generate different degrees of blood stasis symptoms and signs, so while resolving turbidity and removing toxin, dual attention should be paid to promoting blood circulation, resolving blood stasis and unblocking collateral.

1.症状　面色晦暗，手足麻木，腰痛有定处，唇甲紫暗，舌质淡紫或有瘀点、瘀斑，舌底脉络迂曲，脉细涩。

3.3.1 Symptoms　Dull complexion, numbness of hands and feet, fixed pain of lumbar, purple dark lips and nails, light purple tongue or with ecchymosis and petechia, circuitous vein at the bottom of tongue, thready astringent pulse.

2.治法　活血化瘀通络。

3.3.2 Treatment method　To promote blood circulation, resolving blood stasis and unblocking collateral.

3.方药　血府逐瘀汤、大黄䗪虫丸等加减。并选用僵蚕、水蛭、乌梢蛇、地龙等药物起到通络消散浊毒、攻毒散浊解毒的作用。

3.3.3 Prescriptions and medicines　Prescriptions as Decoction of Xuefu Zhuyu Decoction, Dahuang Zhechong Pill etc. And medicines of jiang cang (Bombyx Batryticatus), shui zhi (Hirudo), wu shao she (Zaocys), di long (Lumbricus) and other drugs are used to play the role of unblocking the collateral to disperse turbidity and remove toxin, attacking poison to disperse turbidity and remove toxin.

第二节　糖尿病肾病浊毒论
Section 2　On Turbid Toxin of Diabetic Nephropathy

一、糖尿病肾病的中医概述
1. Overview of traditional Chinese medicine of diabetic nephropathy

糖尿病肾病（DN）是糖尿病最主要的慢性并发症之一，是导致糖尿病患者死亡的主要原因。目前西医学对糖尿病肾病的治疗主要是控制血糖、降压、限制饮食等对症处理，晚期给予肾移植或血液透析。李佃贵教授经过多年的临床研究发现，中医药在治疗糖尿病肾病方面疗效显著，特别是其将"浊毒理论"用于糖尿病肾病的治疗，其认为浊毒是糖尿病肾病发病的关键所在。

Diabetic nephropathy (DN) is one of the most important chronic complications of diabetes, is the main cause of death of diabetes patients. At present, the western medical treatment of diabetic nephropathy is mainly controlling blood sugar, blood pressure and restricting diet due to specific symptoms, in late stage kidney transplantation or hemodialysis are provided. Professor Li Diangui found through many years of clinical research that using TCM especially turbid toxin theory in treatment of diabetic nephropathy is significantly effective. He thinks that turbid toxin is the key factor to generate diabetic nephropathy.

消渴之名首见于《黄帝内经》，中医古籍中并无"糖尿病肾脏病"这一病名，但依据其临床表现，可归属于中医学"消渴病""水肿""尿浊""关格""尿崩"等范畴。

The name of Xiao Ke (diabetes) is first seen in *Medical Classic of the Yellow Emperor*. There is no name of "diabetic kidney disease" in ancient traditional Chinese medicine works, but according to its clinical manifestations, it belongs to the categories of "Xiao Ke", "edema", "turbid urine", "frequent vomiting and dysuria" and "urine collapse" in traditional Chinese medicine.

二、糖尿病肾病浊毒证的病因病机
2. The etiology and pathogenesis of the turbid toxin syndrome of diabetic nephropathy

（一）病因
2.1 Etiology

本病是由糖尿病逐渐发展而来，主要为消渴日久，阴阳气血虚衰，痰湿瘀血蕴结，终致毒损肾络。其基本病理变化可能是"本虚、浊毒"。病变脏腑重在肺、脾、肾三脏，并涉及痰、瘀、水、湿、浊、毒等，现将本病病因归纳如下。

The disease is gradually developed from diabetes, mainly due to long course of diabetes, decline of Yin and Yang, qi and blood, accumulated stagnation of phlegmatic hygrosis and blood stasis, eventually cause toxic damage to kidney collateral. Its basic pathological change may be "asthenia root, turbid toxin". The pathological changes focus on three zang-organs including the lungs, spleen, and kidney, and involve phlegm, blood stasis, water, dampness, turbidity, toxin, etc. The etiology of this disease is summarized as follows.

1.先天不足　先天禀赋不足，肾气亏虚，气化失常或命门火衰，肾不制水，故见水肿或少尿。

2.1.1 Innate deficiency　Congenital endowment deficiency, deficiency of renal qi, gasification disorder or renal fire failure, kidney cannot control water, so edema or oliguria occur.

2.饮食不节，浊毒内生　饮食不节，过食肥甘，致脾胃运化失调，聚湿生痰，日久化热，热伏于下，肾体受伤，肾失气化，则水谷精微混杂趋下，则生消肾，湿热内蕴，日久化浊，聚而成毒，浊毒内生。因此糖尿病肾病的发病与浊毒密切相关。

2.1.2 Uncontrolled diet, and internal generation of turbid toxin　Uncontrolled diet, over-taking of fat and sweet food, causes irregular transportation of spleen and stomach, aggregation of dampness generating phlegm, transmitted into heat with time passes, the embedded heat burns and damages kidney organ, kidney lost the function of gasification, essence of water and grain moves downward, generates diabetic kidney, with time passes, internal accumulation of dampness and heat turns to be turbidity, aggregation of turbidity turns to be toxin, turbid toxin is endogenously generated. Therefore, the onset of diabetic nephropathy is closely related to turbidity toxicity.

3.情志不调，浊毒瘀结　情志不调，气机郁结，肝失疏泄，肝气乘脾，脾失健运，水液代谢失常，湿浊内生。肝气郁结，郁久化火，火热炽盛，上烁肺津，中灼胃液，下耗肾阴，火之甚为毒。

2.1.3 Abnormal state of mood, stagnated stasis of turbid toxin　Abnormal mood causes stagnation of energy mechanism, liver losses the function of dispersing, liver qi over-restricts spleen, spleen looses function of transporting, water and fluid metabolism is in disorder, wet turbidity generates endogenously. Depression of liver qi turns to be fire for long time, hot fire burns lung fluid in upper energizer, burning stomach liquid in middle energizer, consumes kidney Yin in lower energizer, severe fire turns to be toxin.

4.毒损肾络　糖尿病肾病之毒，既有内生之毒，又有外侵邪毒，其中主要是内生之毒。内毒指因脏腑功能和气血运行不利，使机体的生理或病理产物不能及时排出，出现气滞、痰凝、血瘀、湿浊中阻等的病理产物。糖尿病肾病之毒是由于消渴病日久，缠绵不愈而内生，毒邪循络而行，伤阴耗气，阴损及阳，致阴阳气血失调，脏腑亏损，病变波及三焦、脏腑经络，尤以毒损肾络为病因核心。

2.1.4 Toxin damages kidney collateral　The toxin of diabetic nephropathy has both endogenous toxin and external evil toxin, among which, endogenous toxin is dominate. Internal toxin refers that the abnormal operation of the viscera and abnormal circulation of qi and blood causes delayed discharging of physiological or pathological products from the body, generates pathological products as qi stagnation, phlegm coagulation, blood stasis, wet turbidity obstructed in middle energizer. The toxin of diabetic nephropathy is generated endogenously due to the prolonged lingering diabetes. The toxic evil moves along with the collateral, hurting Yin and consuming qi, bringing damages to Yang, leading to imbalance of Yin and Yang, irregular operation of qi and blood, viscera deficiency. The pathological changes affect triple energizers, viscera and meridians, among which especially the damage of kidney collateral by toxin is the core of the disease etiology.

（二）病机

2.2 Pathogenesis

李佃贵教授认为糖尿病肾病病机总属本虚标实，虚实夹杂。本虚是指正气亏虚，即五脏气血阴阳的虚损，标实即水湿潴留、浊毒内蕴、瘀血内停，所涉及的脏腑以肺、脾、肾为主。其中，湿浊瘀毒壅塞三焦为糖尿病肾病的主要病机。现主要概述如下。

Professor Li Diangui believes that the pathogenesis of diabetic nephropathy generally belongs to asthenia root and sthenia tip, with complication of asthenia and thenia. Asthenia root refers to the deficiency of healthy qi, that is, the deficiency of five zang-organs, and deficiency of qi, blood, Yin and Yang. Sthenia tip refers to the retention of water and dampness, internal accumulation of turbid toxin, and internal retaining of blood stasis. The viscera involved mainly include lungs, spleen and kidney. Among them, obstruction of wet turbidity and stasis toxin in triple energizers is the main pathogenesis of diabetic nephropathy. The overview is now illustrated as follows.

1.气阴两虚　李佃贵认为气阴两虚贯穿于DN的始终，其他均为气阴两虚之"变证"。病之初期以阴伤为主，迁延日久，阴伤及气，临床多表现为气阴两虚之证，且以肾脏气阴两虚最为突出。燥热为主要兼夹之邪，常贯穿于病理始终。随着病程进展，可逐渐转化为脾肾气虚、脾肾阳虚、肝肾阴虚、阴阳两虚。

2.2.1 Deficiency of both qi and Yin　Li Diangui believes that deficiency of qi and Yin runs through the whole process of DN, and the others are the "changed syndromes" of deficiency of qi and Yin. In the early stage of the disease, Yin injury is the main pathogenesis, prolonging for a long time, Yin damages qi, which is clinical manifested as deficiency of both qi and Yin, and the deficiency of kidney qi and Yin is most prominent. Dryness and heat is the main complex evil, often runs throughout the pathology. Along with the progress of the disease course, the pathogenesis can be gradually transformed into deficiency of spleen and kidney qi, deficiency of spleen and kidney Yang, deficiency of liver and kidney Yin, deficiency of both Yin and Yang.

2.湿浊　是糖尿病肾病的常见病机之一。湿浊指外来湿邪或体内津液化生障碍的病理产物，又是导致糖尿病肾病进展的致病因素。平素嗜食肥甘，或居处潮湿，涉水冒雨，损伤脾胃，脾失健运，水湿内生，湿困脾阳，甚或脾损及肾，脾肾阳虚，水湿浊邪不得运化，阻滞气机，变生诸证。

2.2.2 Wet turbidity　It is one of the common diseases of diabetic nephropathy. Wet turbidity refers to the pathological product of external dampness evil or generated internally from fluid metaplasia disorder, and it is also the pathogenic factor leading to the progress of diabetic nephropathy. Patients usually addicted to fat, sweet food, or living in damp houses, or having the experience of wading across a river or braving the storm, damage the spleen and stomach, causes the dysfunction of spleen transportation, endogenous, generation of water wet, which traps the spleen Yang, or even leading to damage of spleen, and kidney resulting in deficiency of spleen and kidney yang, water dampness and turbid evil which can not be transported, block the energy mechanism and generate various diseases.

3.瘀血　糖尿病肾病一般病程较长，久病必瘀，久病入络，故有瘀血阻滞之标实。瘀血是在脾肾气阴两虚的基础上发展而来的，阴虚和气虚是血瘀形成的基础，脾肾气阴两虚与瘀血内结使糖尿病肾病迁延不愈。

2.2.3 Blood stasis　DN (diabetic nephropathy) generally has a long course, long disease will generate blood stasis, long disease will develop into collateral, therefore causes sthenia tip of resistance of blood stasis. Blood stasis is developed on the basis of the deficiency of both spleen and kidney qi, deficiency of Yin and qi is the basis for generation of blood stasis, deficiency of both spleen and kidney qi and internal binding of blood stasis make DN linger and difficult to recover.

4.浊毒　李佃贵教授认为，消渴日久，气阴亏耗，脏腑功能失调，湿浊、水湿、瘀血等病理产物的代谢失常，而湿浊、水湿、瘀血均可视为"浊毒"，聚积体内从而诱发和（或）加重糖尿病肾病。因此，消渴的发生与浊毒密切相关。

2.2.4 Turbid toxin　Professor Li Diangui believes that prolonged diabetes causes over

-consumption of qi and Yin, irregular operation of viscera, metabolic disorder of pathological products as wet turbidity, water dampness and blood stasis, which can be regarded as "turbid toxin" aggregate and accumulate in the body to induce and (or) aggravate diabetic nephropathy. Therefore, the occurrence of diabetes is closely related to the turbid toxin.

李佃贵教授提出脾肾亏虚、水湿浊毒内停是糖尿病肾病发生的根源。其认为本病多因消渴病迁延日久或治不得法，加之先天禀赋不足，后天饮食不节等多种病因而致脾胃虚损。若病情持续发展，脾肾俱衰，久则阳衰浊毒瘀阻，内生之湿浊痰瘀滞于肾络。故糖尿病肾病为本虚标实之证，本虚责之脾肾，以肾为根本，标实为湿浊瘀血之毒。

Professor Li Diangui proposed that deficiency of spleen and kidney, retaining of water dampness turbid toxin is the root cause of diabetic nephropathy. It is believed that the disease is mostly due to a long delay or improper treatment of diabetes, coupled with congenital endowment deficiency, uncontrolled - diet and other causes resulting in deficiency of spleen and stomach. If the disease continues to develop, both the spleen and kidney will decline, over long time Yang decays and resistance of turbid toxin occurs, which generates endogenous dampness, turbidity, phlegm and stasis, stagnate in the kidney collateral. Therefore, diabetic nephropathy is the syndrome of the asthenia root and sthenia tip, root asthenia is caused by the spleen and kidney, and kidney is fundamental. Tip sthenia is the toxin of wet turbidity and blood stasis.

三、糖尿病肾病的浊毒证辨证论治
3. The differentiation treatment of diabetic nephropathy caused by turbid toxin syndrome

（一）辨证要点
3.1 Critical points of syndrome differentiation

蛋白尿为临床上诊断糖尿病肾病的最主要指标，临床上初期表现为气阴两虚或肝肾不足，水肿尚不明确，仅见气短懒言、腰酸耳鸣；后期脾肾两虚，可有畏寒怕冷、恶心呕吐、面色萎黄、神疲乏力等表现；晚期阴阳两虚，使水肿加重。若肾元衰竭，浊毒壅塞三焦，气化无力，肾关不开，则尿少而浮肿，甚至无尿，已发展到关格病的危重阶段。

Prominuria is the main index for clinical diagnosis of diabetic nephropathy. In early stage of the disease, the clinical performance is deficiency of both qi and Yin or insufficiency of liver and kidney, edema is not obvious, patients only have shortness of breath, lazy for speech, waist acid tinnitus. In the late stage of the disease, the clinical performance is deficiency of both spleen and kidney, fear of cold, nausea, vomiting, yellow complexion, fatigue in spirit and force. In the critical stage of the disease, the clinical performance is deficiency of both Yin and Yang, more severe edema. If the nephron declines, turbid toxin congest triple energizer, function of gasification is weak, kidney switch is not open, phenomenon of little urine, edema, or even no urine occur, the disease has developed to the critical stage of frequent vomiting and dysuria.

（二）治疗原则

3.2 Principles of treatment

李佃贵教授认为糖尿病肾病病机总属本虚标实、虚实夹杂。本虚是指正气亏虚，即气血阴阳虚损，标实即水湿、浊毒、瘀血等，所涉及的脏腑以肺、脾、肾为主。故李佃贵认为"健脾益肾、化浊解毒"应贯穿于糖尿病肾病的病程进展始终。

Professor Li Diangui believes that the pathogenesis of diabetic nephropathy generally belongs to asthenia root and sthenia tip, with complication of asthenia and thenia. Asthenia root refers to the deficiency of healthy qi, that is, the deficiency of five zang-organs, and deficiency of qi, blood, Yin and Yang. Sthenia tip refers to the retention of water and dampness, internal accumulation of turbid toxin, and internal retaining of blood stasis. The viscera involved are mainly lung, spleen and kidney. Therefore, Li Diangui believes that the principle of "reinforcing spleen and replenishing kidney, resolving turbidity and removing toxin" should be carried out through the whole progress of diabetic nephropathy treatment.

（三）辨证治疗

3.3 Syndrome differentiation treatment

1.气阴两虚型

3.3.1 Dual deficiency of qi and Yin

（1）症状：神疲乏力，面色无华，形体消瘦，自汗气短，口干欲饮，大便秘结或手足心热，舌红，少苔，脉弦细数。

3.3.1.1 Symptoms: fatigue in spirit and force, pale complexion, emancipated body, sweating and short of breath, dry mouth with want to drink, constipation or hot in hands and feet, red tongue, little moss, string thready rapid pulse.

（2）治法：益气养阴，佐化浊解毒。

3.3.1.2 Treatment method: replenishing qi and nourishing Yin, adjuvant with turbidity resolving and toxin moving.

（3）方药：参芪地黄汤加减。

3.3.1.3 Prescription: Shenqi Dihuang Decoction with addition or reduction.

（4）常用药物：人参、黄芪、茯苓、地黄、山药、山茱萸、牡丹皮、泽泻、茵陈、制大黄、黄连、黄芩、蒲公英、白花蛇舌草。

3.3.1.4 Medicines generally used: ren shen (Radix Ginseng), huang qi (Radix Astragali seu Hedysari), fu ling (Poria), di huang (Rehmannia), shan yao (Discoreae Rhizoma), shan zhu yu (Corni Fructus), mu dan pi (Cortex Moutan), ze xie (Rhizoma Alismatis), yin chen (Herba Artemisiae Scopariae), zhi da huang (prepared Radix et Rhizoma Rhei), huang lian (Rhizoma Coptidis), huang qin (Radix Scutellariae), pu gong ying (Herba Taraxaci cum Radice), bai hua she she cao (Herba Oldenlandiae Diffusae).

2.肝肾阴虚，瘀血内阻型

3.3.2 Deficiency of liver and kidney Yin, internal obstruction of blood stasis

（1）症状：两目干涩，五心烦热，头晕耳鸣，口干喜饮，口干咽燥，腰膝酸痛，梦遗，或月经不调，舌暗红少苔，脉弦涩或细数。

3.3.2.1 Symptoms: dry eyes, upset, dizziness and tinnitus, dry mouth with want to drink, dry mouth and throat, acid pain of waist and knee, nocturnal emission, or irregular menstruation, dark red tongue with little moss, string astringent or thready rapid pulse.

（2）治法：滋养肝肾，佐化瘀通络泄浊。

3.3.2.2 Treatment: nourishing the liver and kidney, assisted with resolving blood stasis, unblocking collateral and purging turbidity.

（3）方药：六味地黄丸和桃红四物汤加减。

3.3.2.3 Prescription: Liuwei Dihuang Pills and Taohong Siwu Decoction with addition or reduction.

（4）常用药物：生地黄、玄参、天花粉、丹参、枸杞子、山萸萸、太子参、茵陈、黄连、黄芩、蒲公英、白花蛇舌草、桃仁、红花、当归、赤芍。

3.3.2.4 Medicines generally used: sheng di huang (Radix Rehmanniae), xuan shen (Radix Scrophulariae), tian hua fen (Raidx Tricothanthis), dan shen (Salviae Miltiorrhizae), gou qi zi (Lycii Fructus), shan zhu yu (Corni Fructus), tai zi shen (Radix Pseudostellariae), yin chen (Herba Artemisiae Scopariae), huang lian (Rhizoma Coptidis), huang qin (Radix Scutellariae), pu gong ying (Herba Taraxaci cum Radice), bai hua she she cao (Herba Oldenlandiae Diffusae), tao ren (Semen Persicae), hong hua (Flos Carthami), dang gui (Radix Angelicae Sinensis), chi shao (Radix Paeoniae Rubra).

3.脾肾阳虚，湿浊瘀阻型

3.3.3 Deficiency of spleen and kidney Yang, congestion of wet turbidity

（1）症状：颜面及下肢浮肿，腰以下尤甚，畏寒肢冷，或胸闷气短，心悸，腹胀便溏，纳差恶心，或小便频数清长，或混浊如脂膏，或少尿无尿，或面色苍白，晦滞无华，舌质淡胖或暗淡，苔白腻，脉沉迟而无力。

3.3.3.1 Symptoms: facial and lower limb edema, more severe in the region below the waist, fear of cold and cold in limbs, or chest distress, short of breath, palpitations, abdominal distension, loose stool, anorexia and nausea, frequent, long and clean urination, or urination cloudy as fat ointment, or oliguria or no urination, or pale, dull complexion, pale or dull tongue, white and greasy moss, late sunk and weak pulse.

（2）治法：温补脾肾，利湿泄浊。

3.3.3.2 Treatment: to warm and tonify the spleen and kidney, disinhibit dampness and discharge turbidity.

（3）方药：真武汤和实脾饮加味。

3.3.3.3 Prescription: Zhenwu Decoction and Shipi Yin Decoction.

（4）常用药物：附子、桂枝、狗脊、杜仲、地龙、白茅根、白术、厚朴、泽泻、赤芍、茯苓、黄芪、牛膝、茵陈、制大黄、黄连、蒲公英、川芎。

3.3.3.4 Medicines generally used: fu zi (Radix Aconiti), gui zhi (Cmnamomi Mmulus), gou ji (Cibolti Rhizoma), du zhong (Cortex Eucommiae), di long (Lumbricus), bai mao gen (Rhizoma Imperatae), bai zhu (Rhizoma Atractylodis Macrocephalae), hou po (Cortex Magnoliae Officinalis), ze xie (Rhizoma Alismatis), chi shao (Radix Paeoniae Rubra), fu ling (Poria), huang qi (Radix Astragali seu Hedysari), niu xi (Radix Achyranthis Bidentatae), yin chen (Herba Artemisiae Scopariae), zhi da huang (prepared Radix et Rhizoma Rhei), huang lian (Rhizoma Coptidis), pu gong ying (Herba Taraxaci cum Radice), chuan xiong (Rhizoma Chuangxiong).

4.阴阳两虚，浊毒内蕴型

3.3.4 Dual deficiency of Yin and Yang, internal accumulation of turbid toxin

（1）症状：多饮多尿，混如脂膏，面色㿠白，畏寒肢冷，腰酸脚软痛，或烦热不得卧，口干欲饮，或有水肿，小便不利，大便稀溏，或阳痿早泄，舌淡胖，苔白而干，脉沉细无力。

3.3.4.1 Symptoms: more drink, more urine cloudy as fat ointment, white complexion, fear of cold, cold limbs, acid waist and soft pain in feet, or cannot lay down because of restless fever, dry mouth with want to drink, or with edema, adverse urine, loose stool, or impotence premature ejaculation, pale and fat tongue, white and dry moss, sunk thready and weak pulse.

（2）治法：阴阳双补，化浊解毒。

3.3.4.2 Treatment: tonifying both Yin and Yang, resolving turbidity and removing toxin.

（3）方药：肾气丸加减。

3.3.4.3 Prescription: Shenqi Pills (kidney qi reinforcing pills) with addition and reduction.

（4）常用药物：附子、肉桂、熟地黄、山茱萸、淫羊藿、巴戟天、黄芪、桃仁、当归、茵陈、大黄、黄连、黄芩、蒲公英、白花蛇舌草、翻白草、六月雪、莪术、赤芍。

3.3.4.4 Medicines generally used: fu zi (Radix Aconiti), rou gui (Cortex Cinnamomi), shu di huang (Radix Rehmanniae Praeparatum), shan yu rou (Corni Fructus), yin yang huo (Epimedii Folium), ba ji tian (Morindae Officinalis Radix), huang qi (Radix Astragali seu Hedysari), tao ren (Semen Persicae), dang gui (Radix Angelicae Sinensis), yin chen (Herba Artemisiae Scoperiae), da huang (Radix et Rhizoma Rhei), huang lian (Rhizoma Coptidis), huang qin (Radix Scutellariae), pu gong ying (Herba Taraxaci cum Radice), bai hua she she cao (Herba Oldenlandiae Diffusae), fan bai cao (Potentillae Discoloris Herba), liu yue xue (Herba Serissae),e zhu (Rhizoma Curcumae), chi shao (Radix Paeoniae Rubra).

第三节　高尿酸血症肾病浊毒论
Section 3 On Turbid Toxin of Hyperuricemia Nephropathy

一、高尿酸血症肾病的中医概述
1. Overview of TCM treatment of hyperuricemia nephropathy

"痛风"一词在我国最早出现在南北朝时期的医学典籍里，因其疼痛来得快如一阵风而得名，在中医学归属为"痹证""白虎历节"等范畴。《素问·痹论》曰："此亦其食饮居处，为其病本也。"《备急千金要方》认为："热毒气从脏腑出，攻于手足，手足则焮热、赤肿、疼痛也。"尤在泾在《金匮翼》中亦明确指出："历节风……亦有热毒流入四肢者，不可不知。"《太平圣惠方》云："夫白虎风病者，是风、寒、暑、湿之毒，因虚而起，将摄失理，受此风邪，经脉结滞，气血不行，蓄于滑节之间，或在四肢，肉色不变，其疾病昼静而夜发，夜彻骨髓疼，其痛如虎之噬，故名白虎风病也。"《格致余论》曰："痛风者，大率因血受热已自沸腾，其后或涉水或立湿地……寒凉外搏，热血得寒，汗浊凝滞，所以作痛，夜则痛甚。"痛风乃浊毒瘀滞使然，此浊毒之邪非受自于外，而主生于内。《丹溪心法》云："肥人肢节痛，多湿与痰饮流注经络而痛。"说明胖人多痰湿互结，阻滞经络。龚廷贤《万病回春》云："一切痛风肢体痛者，痛属火，肿属湿……所以膏粱之人，多食煎炒、炙酒肉，热物蒸脏腑，所以患痛风、恶疮、痛疽者最多。"

The word "gout" first appeared in the medical works of the Northern and Southern dynasties in China, because the pain occurs as fast as a gust of wind. In traditional Chinese medicine it belongs to the "arthromyodynia", "white tiger acute arthritis" and other categories. *Simple Conversation-Discussion* on arthromyodynia said: "This disease is also caused by improper diet and living environment." *Qianjin Prescription* believed that: "Hot toxic substance is generated from the viscera, when it attacks hands and feet, hands and feet will be hot, red, swelling and painful". You Zaijing also clearly pointed out in *Golden Chamber Wing* : "Acute arthritis wind... there is also hot toxin getting into the limbs, which should not be ignored". *Taiping Shenghui Prescription* said: "The white tiger acute arthritis, is the toxin of wind, cold, summer heat, dampness, is generated due to deficiency, will lead to irregular operation of energy mechanism, affected by the wind evil, meridian are stagnated, qi and blood are obstructed and stored between the slides, or in the limbs, meat color unchanged, the disease stops at day time and occurs at night, the pain stimulates the patients through bone marrow at night, it seems as being swallowed up by tiger, so it is named "white tiger wind pain". *Ge Zhi Yu Lun* says: "Gout, most probably because blood is self boiling due to heat attacking, then the patient experiences wading across river or staying in wetland... cold and cool attack from outside, boiling blood affected by coldness, sweat is coalgulational stagnated, so pain, especially night pain occurs." Gout is caused by congestion of turbid toxin, the evil of turbid toxin is not from the outside, but mainly born generated internally. *Danxi Xinfa (What I Have Learned From Clinical Treatment By Zhu Danxi)*: "Fat man feels painful in limbs, mostly because dampness and phlegmatic retention flow into meridians." It shows that fat people have more inter-binding of phlegm and dampness, which block the meridians. Gong Tingxian said in *Recovery of All Diseases*: "All gout patients feel painful in body, as pain is fire, swelling is dampness... so the rich people who eat more fried food, prepared wine and baked meat, as the hot substances steam the viscera, so most of them suffer from gout and superficial infection of evil ulcer."

二、高尿酸血症肾病浊毒证的病因病机
2. The etiology and pathogenesis of turbid toxin syndrome of hyperuricemia nephropathy

中医学认为其本质是机体代谢失常，气机壅滞，湿浊内瘀，酿生毒性，浊毒内蕴，相夹为患，阻滞气机，壅塞血脉，再伤脏腑气血。由浊致毒的变化与尿酸毒性的形成，两者均既为病理产物，亦为致病因素，对于机体都是一种渐进损害的病理过程。

Traditional Chinese Medicine believes that the essence of the said syndrome is that metabolism disorder of human body, qi stagnation, internal congestion of wet turbidity, brew toxin, turbidity and toxin accumulates internally, do evil together, which blocks the energy mechanism, obstructs blood vein, and then hurt the viscera, qi and blood. The pathological changes from turbidity to toxin and the formation of uricemia toxicity are both pathological products and pathogenic factors, which is a pathological process of gradual damage to the body.

李佃贵教授基于浊毒学说认为，过高的血尿酸作为病理产物，一旦成为致病因素影响人体的正常生理功能，即成为浊毒。本病病因为脾胃功能失调，复因饮食不节，酿生湿浊，流注关节，郁闭发热而为病，内生湿浊毒邪是痛风发病的关键。其发病主要因于以下几点：或禀赋不足，或调摄不慎，嗜欲无节，过食膏粱厚味，导致脾胃功能紊乱。

Professor Li Diangui believes according to the turbid toxin theory that once high blood uricemia as a pathological product becomes pathogenic factor affecting the normal physiological function of the human body, it has already become turbid toxin. This disease is because of the dysfunction of the spleen and stomach, un-controlled diet brew damp turbidity, which flows into joints, leading to depressed fever. Endogenous dampness and turbidity is the key factor to the incidence of gout. The onset of gout is mainly due to the following causes: insufficient endowment, or careless regulation, excessive sexual intercourse, over-taking of greasy diet, leading to function disorder of spleen and stomach.

（一）饮食不节，脾胃失和，浊毒内生
2.1 Irregular diet, discord of spleen and stomach, internal generation of turbid toxin

素日过食膏粱厚味、醇酒肥甘、辛辣腥腻之品，碍胃滞脾，则食物不归正化，反而酿生湿浊。湿浊停留中焦，影响气机升降，久蕴不消，则化生湿热浊毒。湿热浊毒随气血流行于周身，浸淫百脉，每于关节筋络之中纠结不行，损耗气血，经脉阻滞而出现红肿疼痛。此即浊毒伏于血脉，日久可随机体之阴阳偏盛而化，或从阳化热，或从阴化寒，但痛风以湿热浊毒多见。

Over-taking of greasy food, alcohol and fat and sweet, spicy and stinking products, hinder the stomach and block spleen, the food can not be normally digested, but leading to dampness and turbidity. Wet turbidity stays in middle energizer, affect the ascending and descending of the qi movement. If it accumulates for a long time without dispersing, it will be transmitted into damp heat and turbid toxin. The damp heat and turbid toxin circulates over through the whole body along with qi and blood, spreading over various veins, entangled in joints and tendon collateral, consuming qi and blood, obstructing meridians bringing phenomenon of red and swollen, ache and pain. This is so-called turbid toxin embedded in the blood veins, will make changes according to the excess of Yin and Yang with time passes, either be transformed to heat along with Yang, or transformed into coldness along with Yin, but most of the gout disease see damp heat turbid toxin.

（二）浊毒内伏，外因触动，毒攻关节

2.2 Turbid toxin inside, or external toxin attacking the joints

毒伏血中，若无触动，仅暗耗气血。若遇外因触动，如局部关节损伤、饱餐饮酒、过度劳累、感受风寒湿邪等，则浊毒阻滞脉络，气血不畅。营气欲推动血行，反而加重阻滞，所以疼痛突发而严重。外感六淫可诱发本病，但并非唯一的诱因，且本病既作，则有自身的演变规律，而不遵六经或卫气营血传变。

When toxin is in hidden in blood, if not touched, it consumes qi and blood silently. In case of external touching, such as local joint injury, full drinking, overwork, feeling cold dampness, etc. the toxin block the veins, qi and blood are not smooth. Nutrient qi desire to promote blood flow, but aggravate the block, so the pain is sudden and severe. External six sex can induce this disease, but not the only inducement, and this disease is done, it has its own evolution law, and do not follow the six meridians or Wei-defence, qi, ying nutrients and blood transmission.

李佃贵教授认为本病的病机不外湿热、浊毒、痰瘀、虚损，本病多以脾肾亏虚为本，湿热、浊毒、痰瘀闭阻为标，形成本虚标实之证。初起实邪为主要矛盾，风寒湿热之邪侵袭经络，气血运行不畅，郁而化热，湿热互结，滋生痰瘀，久稽致病，痹阻关节，不通则痛。或素体阳盛之人，脾肾功能失调，复因饮食不节，嗜酒肥甘，或劳倦过度，情志过极，脾失健运，肝失疏泄，聚湿生痰，血滞为瘀，久蕴不解，酿生浊毒。本病属湿热浊毒之邪，其性重浊，湿热下注，故多见于下肢关节，久则浊毒胶固以致僵肿畸形。日久内损脏腑，脾运失健，痰浊内生，脾肾亏虚，湿毒内聚，复感风寒湿热之邪，如遇劳倦、酗酒、贪食膏粱厚味，则致湿热内生，湿浊瘀血流注关节，可致关节肿大畸形、僵硬，关节结节，甚则内损脏腑，引起"关格"。

Professor Li Dianui believes that the pathogenesis of this disease is not dampness and heat, turbidity, phlegm stasis, deficiency, this disease is mostly due to spleen and kidney deficiency, dampness and heat, turbidity, phlegm stasis as the standard, forming the evidence of this deficiency standard. Early real evil is the main contradiction, cold and dampness of evil attack meridians, qi and blood operation is not smooth, depression and heat, dampness and heat each knot, breeding phlegm stasis, long history disease, bi joint, not common pain. Or people, spleen and kidney dysfunction, due to diet, alcohol, fat and sweet, or excessive fatigue, emotional ambition, spleen loss, liver loss, wet phlegm, blood stagnation for blood stasis, long accumulation, lead to turbidity poison. This disease is the evil of damp heat and turbidity poison, its heavy turbidity, dampness and heat injection, so it is more seen in the lower limb joints, for a long time, the turbidity poison glue fixed rigidity and swelling deformity. Days damage the viscera, spleen loss, phlegm endogenous, spleen and kidney deficiency, wet poison cohesion, feeling the evil of wind and heat, such as fatigue, drinking, greedy cream, endogenous, heat and heat, wet stasis blood flow into the joint, can cause joint enlargement, stiffness, joint nodules, even internal damage to the viscera, cause "frequent vomiting and dysuria".

（三）脾肾亏虚，酿生浊毒

2.3 Deficiency of spleen and kidney brew turbid toxin

机体超量、异常的代谢产物，若对机体产生急剧、严重的损害，可谓之毒。正常情况下，通过脏腑的协调作用，机体代谢产物可以及时排出体外，不致蓄积为害。若素体阴阳失衡，或外邪侵袭，或七情内伤，致使脏腑功能失调，不能及时将代谢产物排出体外，则蕴结成毒，留而为害。脾肾两虚，脾失运化，肾失气化，水液和代谢产物留存体内。如《素问·逆调论》曰："肾者水脏，主津液。"若肾气本弱，或浊毒内蕴，耗伤气血，肾之气化不利，开阖无权，则浊毒留而不去，深伏血脉。同时因脾失健运，水湿不化，痰湿内生，与浊毒相合，为害日甚。

Excessive and abnormal metabolites, which can make abrupt and severe damages to the body, can be called toxin. In normal circumstances, the metabolites can be discharged from the body in time through the coordinated action of the viscera without harmful accumulation. However, the imbalance of Yin and Yang of the body, the invasion of external evil, or internal injury of seven emotions, may cause dysfunction of the viscera, abnormal or delayed discharging of the metabolites, which will accumulate into toxin retaining inside to make damages. Dual deficiency of spleen and kidney, spleen fails to transport, kidney fails to gasify, water liquid and metabolites retained in the body. For example, *Simple Conversation-Discussion on Disharmony* said: "Kidney is the organ of water, controlling fluid and liquid". If the kidney qi is originally weak, or affected by internal accumulation of turbid toxin, over consumption of qi and blood, the abnormal gasification of the kidney, failure to control urination and defecation, then turbid toxin will stay in body without leaving, hidden deep blood veins. At the same time, as spleen fails to transport, water wet can not be dissipated, phlegmatic hygrosis is generated endogenously, and aggregate with turbid toxin to make damages.

（四）热毒煎熬，酿生痰瘀

2.4 Torments of heat toxin brew phlegm stasis

热痹不已，必伤阴耗气，气虚者不足以推血运行，则血因之而瘀。阴虚者，津液亏耗，不能载血运行，亦可致瘀血。更有热毒蒸灼气血津液，血受熏灼则易凝结瘀塞，瘀阻于脉中，又可郁而化热，加重热毒。如《灵枢·痈疽》言："营血稽留于经脉之中，则血泣而不行，不行则卫气从之而不通，壅遏不得行，故热。"湿邪为热熏灼，凝滞为痰，痰湿循行经脉，无处不到。痰瘀互结，深入骨骺、经隧之中，因而痼疾根深，病情缠绵难愈。因痰瘀阻滞的部位不同，而有不同的表现。血脉瘀阻，肌肤失养，则皮肤紫暗。痰瘀结于骨节、筋脉，则见关节周围结节、关节肿大畸形、屈伸不利等证。痰瘀结于肾，可形成石淋、癃闭等证。总之，痛风初起病在血脉，继则浊毒流注骨节、经络、肌肤，损伤脾肾。其病初为邪盛的实热证，继则出现气血亏虚和痰湿瘀血阻滞。由于本病为内生毒邪，外因触动所致，与其他外感风寒湿热之邪痹阻经络，由浅入深的痹病截然不同。

Consisting pyretic arthralgia will hurt Yin and consumes qi. Deficient qi is not powerful to push blood circulation, thus blood stasis occurs. Deficiency of Yin, which over-consumes body fluid and liquid, can not carry blood to run, can also cause blood stasis. Moreover, heat toxin steams and burns qi and blood, fluid and liquid. Blood is easy to be coagulated and stagnated in veins when being fumigated, and can be depressed into heat, aggravating heat toxin. For example, *Pivot-Discussion on Carbuncle* said: "When nutrient blood is left in the meridians, it will be coagulated without flowing in case of cold attacking. If the blood fails to flow, the defensive qi following blood will be abundantly blocked, therefore fever occurs." Wet evil fumigated by heat, coagulates into phlegm, phlegmatic hygrosis moves along with meridians, spreading over everywhere of the body. Phlegm and stasis agglutinate, deep into the articulation of bone and meridian tunnel, so the chronic disease with deep root, lingers long and is difficult to heal. Because the phlegm stasis is resisted in different areas, thus different manifestations are presented. When resistance is in Blood veins, skin nourishment is absent, then the skin is purple and dark. When phlegm stasis is resisted in the bone joints and tendon veins, joint peripheral nodule, enlargement and deformity of joints, function difficulty in flexion and extension and other symptom occur. When phlegm stasis is resisted in the kidney, it will cause stone stranguria, uroscheesis and other symptoms. In short, gout disease is initially generated in the blood veins, then turbid toxin of gout enters and retains in bone joints, meridians, skin, make damages to the spleen and kidney. The disease is the sthenia heat of excessive evil at the very beginning, then followed by deficiency of qi and blood and obstruction of phlegmatic hygrosis and blood stasis. As the disease is generated from endogenous toxic evil which is attacked by external cause, it is absolutely different from the arthromyodynia which is generated because the external wind, coldness, dampness and heat evil, arthralgialy block meridians from shallow to deep.

三、高尿酸血症肾病的浊毒证辨证论治
3. The differential treatment of turbid toxin syndrome of hyperuricemia nephropathy

（一）急性发作期
3.1 Stage of abrupt occurrences

1.症状　多为起病急骤，关节红肿发热，痛如刀割或剧烈咬噬样，口干口渴，面红目赤，大便干，小便黄赤，舌质红，脉数。

3.1.1 Symptoms　Generally the disease occurs suddenly and fiercely, with edema and heat in joints, with intolerable pain as knife-cutting or severe biting of animals, dry and thirsty in mouth, red eyes and face, dry stool, yellow red urine, red tongue, rapid pulse.

2.治法　清热解毒，利湿通络。

3.1.2 Treatment method　Clearing heat and removing toxin, dissipating dampness and unblocking collateral.

3.方药　五味消毒饮合四妙散加减。常用药物有金银花、蒲公英、紫花地丁、苍术、薏苡仁、牛膝、黄柏、虎杖、大黄、茯苓、山慈菇、苦参、猪苓、泽泻、车前草、滑石、竹叶等。

3.1.3 Prescription and medicines　Wuwei Xiaodu Yin Decoction combined with Simiao Powder with addition and reduction. Medicines generally used are: jin yin hua (Lonicerae Japonicae Flos), pu gong ying (Herba Taraxaci cum Radice), zi hua di ding (Herba Violae), cang zhu (Rhizoma Atractylodis), yi yi ren (Semen Coisis), niu xi (Radix Achyranthis Bidentatae), huang bo (Cortex Phellodendri), hu zhang (Rhizoma Polygoni Cuspidati),da huang (Radix et Rhizoma Rhei), fu ling (Poria), shan ci gu (Pseudobulbus Cremastrae Variabilis), ku shen (Sophorae Flavescentis Radix), zhu ling (Polygorus Umbellatus), ze xie (Rhizoma Alismatis), che qian cao (Plantaginis Herba), hua shi (Talcum), zhu ye (Folium Phillostachydis Nigrae) and so on.

（二）慢性缓解期

3.2 Stage of chronic remission

1.症状　关节红肿热痛症状明显缓解，但某些关节仍肿痛不适，舌质略红，苔薄黄，脉弦细。

3.2.1 Symptoms　The symptoms of joint redness, heat and pain are significantly relieved, but some joints are still swollen painful and uncomfortable, with slightly red tongue, thin yellow moss and string thin pulse.

2.治法　清热利湿。

3.2.2 Treatment method　Clearing heat and disinhibiting dampness.

3.方药　萆薢分清饮加减。常用药物有萆薢、石菖蒲、黄柏、白术、茯苓、车前子、莲子心、丹参、薏苡仁、土茯苓等。

3.2.3 Prescription and medicines　Beixie Fenqing Yin Decoction with addition and reduction. Medicines generally used are: bi xie (Rhizoma Dioscoreae), shi chang pu (Rhizoma Acori Graminei), huang bo (Cortex Phellodendri), bai zhu (Rhizoma Atractylodis Macrocephalae), fu ling (Poria), che qian zi (Semen Plantaginis), lian zi xin (Plumula Nelumbinis), dan shen (Salviae Miltiorrhizae), yi yi ren (Semen Coisis), tu fu ling (Rhizoma Smilacis Glabrae) and so on.

（三）间歇期

3.3 Stage of intermission

1.症状　患者关节基本不痛，症状消失。

3.3.1 Symptoms　The patient's joints are basically painless, and the symptoms disappear.

2.治法　健脾除湿，通腑泄浊，补益肝肾。

3.3.2 Treatment method　Reinforcing spleen and removing dampness, unblocking the fu-organ and discharging turbidity, invigorating the liver and replenishing kidney.

3.常用药物　党参、白术、薏苡仁、土茯苓、制大黄、萆薢、猪苓、泽泻、车前草、滑石、牛膝、地龙、苍术等。

3.3.3 medicins generally used　Dang shen (Radix Codonopsitis Pilosulae), bai zhu (Rhizoma Atractylodis Macrocephalae), yi yi ren (Semen Coisis), tu fu ling (Rhizoma Smilacis Glabrae), zhi da huang (prepared Radix et Rhizoma Rhei), bi xie (Rhizoma Dioscreae), zhu ling (Polygorus Umbellatus), ze xie (Rhizoma Alismatis), che qian cao (Herba Plantaginis), hua shi (Talcum), niu xi (Radix Achyranthis Bidentatae), di long (Lumbricus), cang zhu (Rhizoma Atractylodis), etc.

第四节　膜性肾病浊毒论
Section 4 On Turbid Toxin of Membranous Nephropathy

一、膜性肾病的中医概述
1. Overview of traditional Chinese medicine of membranous nephropathy

膜性肾病属中医学"水肿""尿浊"等范畴。《素问·水热穴论》指出："勇而劳甚，则肾汗出，肾汗出逢于风，内不得入于脏腑，外不得越于皮肤，客于玄府，行于皮里，传为胕肿。"故其本在肾，其末在肺。《素问·至真要大论》又指出："诸湿肿满，皆属于脾。"明代李梴《医学入门·水肿》提出疮毒致水肿的病因学说。《景岳全书·肿胀》云："凡外感毒风，邪留肌肤，则亦能忽然浮肿。"《景岳全书·水肿》云："大人小儿素无脾虚泄泻等证，而忽尔通身浮肿，或小便不利者，多以饮食失节，或湿热所致。"

Membranous nephropathy belongs to the category of "edema", "turbid urine" and so on in traditional Chinese medicine. *Simple Conversation-Discussion on Water and Heat Disease* points out: "If a person parades his strength and overstrains himself, it induces sweating from the kidney. Invasion of wind during sweating cannot deepen into the viscera, or get out of the skin, but maintains in the Xuan-Fu (sweat pores), moves in the skin, eventually leading to swollen instep." So the root is in the kidney, the end is in the lung. *Simple Conversation-Major Discussion on the Most Important and Abstruse Theory* also points out: "All dampness diseases characterized by swelling and fullness, are associated with The spleen." Ming dynasty Li Ting in his book *Medical Introduction-Edema* put forward the etiology theory that ulcer toxin generates edema. *Jingyue Quanshu-Swelling* said: "Attacked by external toxic wind, evil retains in the skin, can also generates abrupt swelling." *Jingyue Quanshu -Edema* said: "Adults and children without spleen deficiency, diarrhea and other symptoms, suddenly has edema in overall body, or difficult urine, mostly due to improper diet, or invasion of dampness and heat."

综上所述，我国古代医家已经认识到水肿发病的基本病机为肺失通调，脾失健运，肾失开阖，三焦气化失司。肺主一身之气，主通调水道；脾主运化，可将水谷精微布散周身；肾主水，水液的输化有赖于肾阳的蒸化及其开阖功能。肺虚则气不化精而化为水，脾虚则土不制水，肾虚则水无所主而妄行；气虚则固摄无力，精微外泄，自小便而出，则见蛋白尿、血尿。

Summarizing the above, ancient Chinese doctors have realized that the basic pathogenesis of edema are pulmonary maltuning of the lungs, dysfunction of spleen transportation, dysfunction of kidney control of urination and defecation, and dysfunction of triple energizer control gasification. The lungs control qi circulation of the whole body, are responsible for dredging and regulation of water channel; the spleen controls transportation, spreading the essence of water and grain over through the whole body; the kidney controls water, the vaporizing of water and grain essence depends on the steaming function of kidney Yang, and the discharging of water liquid depends on the urination controlling function of kidney Yang. If the lung is deficient, the qi cannot be turned into essence but into water. If the spleen is deficient, the soil cannot control water; if the kidney is deficient, water will flow rashly without restriction; if qi is deficient, it will be unable to astringe the essence, the essence might be discharged with urine, therefore proteinuria, hematuria occur.

二、膜性肾病浊毒证的病因病机
2. The etiology of turbid toxin syndrome of membranous nephropathy

本病的发生主要由于先天禀赋不足，或后天失养，加之外邪侵袭，损伤脾肾，致脾失健运，肾失气化，水湿内停，泛溢肌肤，脾肾失于固摄则精微下注而见小便浑浊。脾气虚则无以运化和敷布水谷精微，水湿津液代谢发生障碍；肾气虚则全身各脏腑组织得不到充分的温煦与濡养，无力推动血行，"血不利则为水"，并进一步转化为致病的代谢产物——湿浊，且久病入络，湿浊瘀血互结，加之激素热化和外感热毒之邪，导致痤疮满布或感染等症，均为热毒，湿热毒邪互结日久伤肾，故湿、瘀、虚、浊、毒互结是本病致病的关键。浊毒既是疾病的病理产物，又是脏腑功能失调的病因。李佃贵认为膜性肾病基本病机是本虚标实，脾肾气虚为本，湿热、血瘀、浊毒为标，并重点指出肾络瘀阻，浊毒内蕴是本病发病与产生各种并发症的根本病机，并贯穿于疾病的整个发病过程中。对于本病的病因病机，主要从以下几方面进行论述。

The occurrence of this disease is mainly due to the deficiency of innate endowment, or insufficient acquired recuperation, assisted by the invasion of external evil, which damage the spleen and kidney, causing the dysfunction of spleen transportation, and the dysfunction of kidney gasification. Water wet retains internally, overflow the skin. Spleen and kidney loose the astringing function, so essence is discharged with urine resulting in turbid urine. Deficient spleen qi fails to transport and spread water and grain essence over through the whole body, so metabolism disorder of water, dampness, fluid and liquid takes place; if kidney qi is deficient, viscera tissue of the whole body cannot be sufficiently warmed and nourished, uncapable to promote blood circulation, "if the blood cannot flow smoothly, it will generate water", and further it will be transformed into pathogenic metabolites -- damp turbidity. Disease of long course will surely get into collateral. Agglutinateing of damp turbidity and blood stasis, plus hormone pyretic generation and attacking of external heat toxin, lead to generation or infection of acne in whole body, they are all heat toxin. Agglutinating of dampness, heat, toxin and evil for long time will damage kidney. The agglutinating of dampness, stasis, deficiency, turbidity and toxin is the key factor of this disease. Turbid toxin is the pathological product of the disease, as well as the etiology of the viscera dysfunction. Li Diangui believes that the basic pathogenesis of membranous nephropathy is asthenia root and sthenia tip. Deficiency of spleen, kidney and qi is the root, damp and heat, blood stasis, turbid toxin is the tip. It is importantly pointed out that congestion of renal collateral, the internal accumulation of turbid toxin is the fundamental pathogenesis of the disease and runs throughout the whole process of the disease. The etiology and pathogenesis of this disease is mainly discussed from the following aspects.

（一）脾肾气虚

2.1 Deficiency of spleen and kidney qi

脾肾气虚是膜性肾病发病的基本病机。脾为制水之脏，脾虚则水无所制而泛滥，肾为主水之脏，肾虚则水失所主而妄行，终致水湿外淫肌肤、内渍脏腑，从而出现面部四肢水肿、胸水、腹水。脾主升清，若脾虚则精微失升而下陷，肾司封藏，肾虚则精微失藏而外泄，则又可导致蛋白尿。而脾肾阳虚是病变中后期病情久延，气伤及阳的病理转变。

Spleen and kidney qi deficiency is the basic pathogenesis of membranous nephropathy. The spleen is the zang - organ to restrict water, if the spleen is deficient, water will overflow is without restriction. The kidney is the zang-organ to control water, if kidney is deficient, water will flow rashly without control, water wet overflows externally in the skin, and internally in viscera, eventually leading to facial edema, limbs edema, hydrothorax, ascites. The spleen controls lucidity ascending, if spleen is deficient, the cereal essence does not ascend but sinks down. Kidney is responsible for sealing and storing, if kidney is deficient, the cereal essence will not be stored but leaks out with urination, leading to albuminuria. The spleen and kidney Yang deficiency is the pathological change in the middle and late stage of the disease when the disease lingers long and qi damages Yang.

（二）脉络瘀滞、湿热内蕴

2.2 Congestion in vessels, internal accumulation of dampness and heat

脉络瘀滞、湿热内蕴是膜性肾病反复发作、缠绵难愈的病理基础。本病病程中常因气虚无以推血，则血行瘀滞，瘀血形成之后又可作为新的致病因素而阻滞经络，阻碍气化，从而形成瘀、水互结。脾肾气虚，水湿内生，湿有内湿和外湿两种，内湿是脾失运水湿所致，三焦气化功能失常，水溢肌肤；外湿指感受六淫之湿，雾露之气伤于皮腠所致，水湿之邪既可由外侵入人体，是肾脏病的重要病理产物。水湿致病与肺、脾、肾密切相关，肺失通调水道，脾失转输津液，肾失蒸腾水液，膀胱气化不利，三焦决渎失职，以致水湿聚积，加之脾肾气虚故易于招引外邪，以致湿热之客邪再至。湿热是膜性肾病病情加重的重要病理因素。正如徐灵胎所云："有湿必有热，虽未必尽然，但湿邪每易化热。"虚实错杂，交互为害，终成湿热蕴滞，胶着不化；水瘀积久，氤氲化热，又造成湿、热、瘀相互攀援，纠集结聚，交相济恶之势，常可导致水肿、蛋白尿加重，病情反复发作、缠绵难愈。湿热互结，蕴结不解，久而由实致虚，由虚致瘀，随着阴阳气血的不断消耗，湿瘀浊毒在体内潴留，不断耗伤正气，终至肾气衰微。

Congestion in vessels and internal accumulation of dampness and heat are the pathological basis of lingering, repeated attacks and difficult recovering of membranous nephropathy. In the course of this disease, blood is often difficult to be pushed forward, then congested due to qi deficiency. The formation of blood stasis will reversely become new pathogenic factor to block the meridians, hindering gasification, resulting in the agglutinating of stasis and water retention. Deficiency of spleen and kidney qi, water dampness will generate endogenously. Dampness can be divided into internal dampness and external dampness. Internal dampness is caused by dysfunction of spleen transportation of water dampness. The gasification of the triple energizer does not work normally, thus water overflows in the muscle and skin; external dampness refers to the invasion of the dampness of the six excessive evil, substance of fog and dew injury the skin striae. The evil of water dampness can invade the human body from outside, simultaneously, it is also an important pathological product of kidney disease. Diseases caused by water dampness are closely related to lung, spleen, kidney. The lung fails to unblock water channel, the spleen fails to transport fluid and liquid, the kidney fails to transpire water liquid, the bladder fails in gasification, the triple energizer fails to dredge water channel, so water dampness aggregates and accumulates, in addition, the spleen and kidney qi is deficient, thus it is easy to be invaded by external evil, which brings the guest evil of dampness and heat to come again. Dampness and heat is an important pathological factor to aggravate the membranous kidney disease. As Xu Lingtai said: "Although it is not one hundred percent right that where there is wet there must be heat, but dampness evil can easily be transformed into heat." Mixture of asthenia ansd sthenia makes interactive damages, eventually causes accumulation and stagnation of dampness and heat, which is densely cemented and cannot be dispelled for long time; long-time of condensed accumulation of water and stasis will be transformed into heat. Dampness, heat and stasis inter-twine and aggregate to do evil together, lead to aggravation and repeated attacks of lingering edema and proteinuria which is difficult to heal. Agglutinating of dampness and heat, accumulate and knot over a long time, from sthenia to asthenia, from deficiency to stasis, continuously consume Yin and Yang, qi and blood. Dampness, stasis, turbidity and toxin retain in the body, constantly wear out the healthy qi and finally lead to to failure of kidney qi.

（三）浊毒内蕴

2.3 Internal accumulation of turbid toxin

浊毒内蕴是本病发病与产生各种并发症的根本病机。李佃贵教授认为浊与湿同源，浊之源乃湿，浊乃湿之甚，浊为湿之重。湿与浊常兼夹为害，并可以互相转化。毒与火热同类，热乃毒之渐，毒乃热之极。热与毒常兼夹为害，并可以互相转化。

Internal accumulation of turbid toxin is the fundamental pathogenesis of the occurrence of this disease and generation of various complications. Professor Li Diangui believes that turbidity and dampness share the same source, the source of turbidity is dampness, turbidity is the extreme of dampness, turbidity is seriously damp. Dampness and turbidity often make damages together, and can be transformed into each other. Toxin has similarity with fire and heat, heat is the gradual progress of toxin, toxin is the extreme of heat. Heat and poison often make damages together, and can be transformed into each other.

浊毒既是膜肾的病理产物，又是致病因素。浊毒作为其主要的病理机制而贯穿于疾病的整个过程。浊毒致病，常兼夹为患，易夹湿夹痰夹瘀，气血失和，诸症百出；浊毒致病广泛，胶滞难解，易阻遏气机，可侵犯上中下三焦，但以中焦脾胃最为常见；浊毒蕴于中焦，既可加重气滞湿阻，又能入血入络伤阴耗气；浊毒致病缠绵难愈，病情重，治疗难，疗程长。由于浊毒致病的以上特点，所以浊毒内蕴是本病发病与产生各种并发症的根本病机。

Turbid toxin is both the pathological product and pathogenic factor of membrane kidney. As the main pathogenesis, turbid toxin runs throughout the whole process of the disease. Turbid toxin disease, often mixed with other pathogenic factors, easy to be mixed with dampness, phlegm, and stasis, in case of discord of qi and blood, various kinds of diseases occur. Turbid toxin can generate disease in wide area, which is cemented and difficult to resolve. It can easily resist the energy mechanism, invade the upper, middle and lower energizers, but most probably, the spleen and stomach of middle energizer. Turbid toxin accumulates in middle energizer, can aggravate the stagnation of qi and obstruction of dampness, as well as getting into blood and collateral damaging Yin and consuming qi. Turbid toxin syndrome is lingering, and difficult to heal, the disease condition is severe, the disease course is long, and the treatment is more complicated. Due to the above characteristics of turbid toxin, internal accumulation of turbid toxin is the fundamental pathogenesis of the occurrence of this disease and generation of various complications.

三、膜性肾病的浊毒证辨证论治
3. The differentiation treatment of turbid toxin syndrome of membrane nephropathy

膜性肾病治疗时要给浊毒以出路，化浊解毒要贯穿始终。《素问·汤液醪醴论》曰："开鬼门，洁净府。"对浊毒的治疗也要遵循此法则，使浊毒尽快排出，以减少对机体的损害。根据浊毒的部位、轻重，可采用通腑泄浊的方法，使浊毒从大便排出；也可渗湿利浊解毒，使浊毒从小便排出；或达表透浊解毒，使浊毒从汗液排出。

Treatment of membranous nephropathy should leave a way out for turbid toxin, and carry out the principle of resolving turbidity and removing toxin through the whole process. *Simple Conversation-Discussion on Decoction and Wine* says: "Open the Guimen (sweat pores), clean the bladder (to eliminate the retention of fluid)." The treatment of turbid toxin should also follow this principle, so that turbid toxin can be discharged as soon as possible while reducing the damages to the body. According to the location and severity of turbid toxin, the method of unblocking fu-organs and purging turbidity can be used to discharge the turbid toxin through defecation; method of draining dampness, resolving turbidity and removing toxin can be used to discharge turbid toxin through urination; method of outthrushing turbidity to surface of body and removing toxin to discharge turbid toxin through sweating.

（一）治则特点
3.1 The characteristics of Treatment principle

1.强调通络泄浊解毒　浊毒内蕴贯穿于膜性肾病的整个发病过程中，病程长、迁延难愈。病久入络，加之本病病位在肾络，浊毒深入肾络，难以排出。常选用可以通经入络的虫类药和藤类药以通络化浊解毒。藤类植物多绕木攀援，屈曲而生，善走经络，取其祛风湿、解筋之效。正如《本草便读》所云："凡藤蔓之属，皆可通经入络。盖藤者缠绕蔓延，犹如网络，纵横交错，无所不至，其形如络脉。"常加用青风藤、海风藤。两药具有祛风湿、通经络、利小便的功效，既有行散之性又能利水消肿。常用血肉有情之品的虫类药物，取其搜剔之性，以通络消散浊毒。常用药有僵蚕、水蛭、乌梢蛇、地龙等。

3.1.1 Emphasizing unblocking collateral, purging turbidity and removing toxin　Internal accumulation of turbid toxin runs through the whole process of membranous nephropathy, and the disease is lingering, long in course and difficult to heal. Long -time of disease will develop into

collateral, as the said disease is located in collateral of kidney, turbid toxin get deep into the kidney collateral, and is difficult to be discharged. Medicines of insects and liana plants are used to unblock the collateral, resolve turbidity and remove toxin. Most of the liana plants climb up twining the wood, growing flexibly. Being used as medicine they are good at running along with meridians, with effect of dispelling wind damp, unblocking the meridians. As *Bencao Biandu (Materia)* says: "Medicines of liana plants can pass through the meridians and collateral, as the vine twines and creeps like network, crisscrossing everywhere, and the shape is similar to collateral vessels." Generally qing feng teng (Caulis Senomomentii seu Sabiae), hai feng teng (Caulis Piperis Kadsurae) are used. The two drugs have the effect of removing wind and dampness, unblocking meridians and improving urination, with nature of dispersing and ability to improve ruination and reduce swelling. Medicines of insects with flesh, blood and emotions are used to unblock the meridians and disperse turbid toxin taking the advantage of their exorcising function. Medicines generally used are jiang can (Bombyx Batryticatus), shui zhi (Hirudo), wu shao she (Zaocys), di long (Lumbricus), etc.

2.注重调理脾胃，恢复脾之升清、胃之和降之职　脾胃为后天之本，为气机升降枢纽，脾主运化水谷精微、水湿，胃主受纳腐熟。若脾失运化，胃失和降，则出现纳呆、腹胀等症状。调理脾胃有利于运化水湿，而渗湿利水又可使脾土不被湿困，恢复其健运功能。升降相因，纳食好转，精微物质化生正常，并得以统摄，濡养敷布全身，减少蛋白尿。

3.1.2 Emphasizing on spleen and stomach regulating to recover the function of lifting and ascending　As acquired root of life, the spleen and stomach is the lifting and ascending hub of the qi movement. The spleen controls transporting of cereal essence and water dampness. The stomach controls acceptance and digesting. If the spleen fails to transport, stomach fails to harmonize and descend, anorexia, abdominal distension and other symptoms will occur. Conditioning the spleen and stomach is conducive to transport water wet, and draining dampness and dissipating water can release the spleen soil from dampness trapping, and restore its transportation function. Operation of ascending and descending become normal, appetite is improved, transformation and generation of cereal essence restores, and sufficient to control, cover and nourish the whole body, reducing proteinuria.

（二）治疗大法

3.2 General Method of Treatment

1.气虚瘀水交阻型

3.2.1 Qi deficiency and cross-resistance of blood stasis and water

（1）症状：全身浮肿，面色黧黑萎黄，腰痛固定，口中黏腻，腰酸乏力，小便短少，大便不畅，舌质暗紫或有瘀点瘀斑，苔白腻，脉沉滑或弦滑。

3.2.1.1 Symptoms: edema in whole body, dark and yellow complexion, sticky mouth, fixed pain of loin, acid waist and fatigue, short and little urine, difficult stool, dark purple tongue or with ecchymosis or petechia, white and greasy moss, sunk slippery or string slippery pulse.

（2）治法：益气化瘀利水。

3.2.1.2 Treatment method: replenishing qi, resolving blood stasis and disinhibiting water.

（3）方药：桂枝茯苓丸加减。党参、桂枝、茯苓、桃仁、牡丹皮、赤芍、益母草、炙甘草。

3.2.1.3 Prescription and medicines: Guizhi Fuling Pill with addition or reduction. Medicines: dang shen (Radix Codonopsitis Pilosulae), gui zhi (Cmnamomi Mmulus), fu ling (Poria), tao ren (Semen Persicae), mu dan pi (Cortex Moutan), chi shao (Radix Paeoniae Rubra), yi mu cao (Herba Leonuri), zhi gan cao (fried Radix Glycyrrhizae).

2.气虚湿热互结型

3.2.2 Agglutination of qi deficiency, dampness and heat

（1）症状：下肢浮肿，口干咽燥，纳差，口苦乏力，小便短赤，大便干结，或见面部痤疮，或见皮肤湿疹，舌质红，苔薄黄，脉濡或濡数。

3.2.2.1 Symptoms: edema in lower limbs, dry mouth and throat, poor appetite, bitter mouth, fatigue, short and red urine, dry stool, acne in face, or skin eczema, red tongue, thin yellow moss, weak or weak rapid pulse.

（2）治法：清利湿热，益气活血。

3.2.2.2 Treatment method: clear heat and disinhibit dampness, replenish qi and promote blood circulation.

（3）常用药物：党参、白术、丹参、白花蛇舌草、黄芩、石韦、车前草、猪苓、当归、益母草等。

3.2.2.3 Medicines generally used: dang shen (Radix Codonopsitis Pilosulae), bai zhu (Rhizoma Atractylodis Macrocephalae), dan shen (Salviae Miltiorrhizae), bai hua she she cao (Herba Oldenlandiae Diffusae), huang qin (Radix Scutellariae), shi wei (Pyrrosia Folium), che qian cao (Herba Plantaginis), zhu ling (Polygorus Umbellatus), dang gui (Radix Angelicae Sinensis), yi mu cao (Herba Leonuri), etc.

3.阳虚湿浊内聚型

3.2.3 Yang deficiency, internal aggregation of dampness and turbidity

（1）症状：下肢浮肿，腰酸乏力，畏寒怕冷，面色晦暗，易感外邪，小便清长或短少，恶心呕吐，纳差腹胀，大便溏薄，舌淡，苔白腻或秽浊，或边有齿痕，脉沉细无力。

3.2.3.1 Symptoms: edema in lower limbs, acid waist and fatigue, fear of cold, dark complexion, prone to external evil, long lucid or short urine, nausea and vomiting, anorexia, abdominal distension, thin and loose stool, light tongue, white and greasy or dirty moss, or with teeth marks, sunk thready weak pulse.

（2）治法：温阳活血，化湿降浊。

3.2.3.2 Treatment method: to warm Yang and promote blood circulation, dispel dampness and resolve turbidity.

（3）常用药物：党参、黄芪、白术、肉苁蓉、淫羊藿、丹参、益母草、山药、薏苡仁、苍术、制大黄等。

3.2.3.3 Medicines generally used: dang shen (Radix Codonopsitis Pilosulae), huang qi (Radix Astragali seu Hedysari), bai zhu (Rhizoma Atractylodis Macrocephalae), rou cong rong (Cistanches Herba), yin yang huo (Epimedii Folium), dan shen (Salviae Miltiorrhizae), yi mu cao (Herba Leonuri), shan yao (Discoreae Rhizoma), yi yi ren (Semen Coisis), cang zhu (Rhizoma Atractylodis),zhi da huang (prepared Radix et Rhizoma Rhei), etc.

4.浊毒内蕴型

3.2.4 Internal accumulation of turbid toxin

（1）症状：全身浮肿，腰以下肿甚，尿中有泡沫，面色晦暗，头晕头痛，腰膝酸软，恶心呕吐，纳差腹胀，舌红，苔黄腻或秽浊，脉细弱。

3.2.4.1 Symptoms: edema of the whole body, more severe below the waist, foam in urine, dark complexion, dizziness and headache, lassitude loin and knees, nausea and vomiting, poor appetite, abdominal distension, red tongue, yellow and greasy moss or filth, weak thready pulse.

（2）治法：化浊解毒。

3.2.4.2 Treatment method: to resolve turbidity and remove toxin.

（3）常用药物：翻白草、积雪草、金雀根、六月雪、白花蛇舌草、蒲公英、茵陈、黄连、川朴、大黄、茯苓、泽泻、车前子、青风藤、海风藤、僵蚕、水蛭、乌梢蛇、地龙等。

3.2.4.3 Medicines generally used: fan bai cao (Potentillae Discoloris Herba), ji xue cao (Centellae Herba), jin que gen (Radix Caraganae Sinicae), liu yue xue (Herba Serissae), bai hua she she cao (Herba Oldenlandiae Diffusae), pu gong ying (Herba Taraxaci cum Radice), yin chen (Herba Artemisiae Scopariae), huang lian (Rhizoma Coptidis), hou po (Cortex Magnoliae Officinalis), da huang (Radix et Rhizoma Rhei), fu ling (Poria), ze xie (Rhizoma Alismatis), che qian zi (Semen Plantaginis), qing feng teng (Caulis Senomomentii Et Sabiae), hai feng teng (Caulis Piperis Kadsarae), jiang cang (Bombyx Batryticatus), shui zhi (Hirudo), wu shao she (Zaocys), di long (Lumbricus), etc.

第五节　狼疮性肾炎浊毒论
Section 5　On Turbid Toxin of Lupus Nephritis

一、狼疮性肾炎的中医学概述
1. The traditional Chinese medicine overview of lupus nephritis

古代中医学中并无"狼疮性肾炎"这一病名的记载，但根据其临床表现可归属于中医学"丹疹""红蝴蝶疮病""阴阳毒""温毒发斑""虚劳""水肿""腰痛"等范畴。

There is no record of "lupus nephritis" in ancient Chinese medicine, but according to its clinical manifestations, it belongs to the categories of "red rash""red butterfly disease", "Yin Yang Toxin", "warm toxin muculae", "consumptive disease", "edema", "low back pain" and so on.

近代睢书魁等认为红斑狼疮累及肾脏，出现水肿、蛋白尿且有关节疼痛等临床表现，应属"肾痹"。尽管这些病名在一定程度上反映了红斑狼疮的部分特征性表现，但目前仍无法用一个统一的病名来概括其多系统受累的表现。

Sui Shukui in Modern times believes that lupus erythematosus involves the kidney, with clinicalmanifestations as edema, proteinuria and joint pain and others, should belongs to "kidney bi". Although these disease names partly reflect the characteristic manifestations of lupus erythematosus, up to now, there is not yet a uniform disease name to generalize the manifestations of multisystem involvement.

二、狼疮性肾炎浊毒证的病因病机
2. The etiology and pathogenesis of turbid toxin of lupus nephritis

李佃贵教授认为狼疮性肾炎的发病是内外因共同作用的结果，两者相互影响，使疾病反复发作，缠绵不愈。

Professor Li Diangui thinks that the onset of lupus nephritis is the result of combined reaction of internal and external causes, the two influence each other, make the disease repeatedly occur, lingering and difficult to heal.

（一）禀赋不足，肾精亏虚为本
2.1 Insufficient endowment, kidney essence deficiency is the root

"肾为先天之本，脾为后天之本"，先天滋养后天。若先天禀赋不足，则五脏六腑失养；若后天脾主运化失常，则气血生化乏源，肾精失于充养，终致脾肾两虚。狼疮性肾炎的患者先天禀赋不足，后天失于调养，机体正气虚弱，防御功能降低，易感受外邪，百病由生。故禀赋不足、肾精亏虚是狼疮性肾炎发生的重要内因。

"Kidney is the root of congenital endowment, the spleen is the acquired root." Congenital root nurtures the acquired root. If the congenital endowment is insufficient, the viscera cannot be sufficiently nourished; if the acquired spleen is abnormal to transport, the source to generate and transform qi and blood is insufficient, kidney essence cannot be sufficiently nourished, eventually lead to dual deficiency of spleen and kidney. Patients of lupus nephritis are deficient in congenital endowment, lack of acquired recuperation, weak in healthy qi and defense function, easy to be attacked by external evil, therefore various diseases occur. Therefore, insufficient endowment and deficiency of kidney essence are the important internal causes of lupus nephritis.

（二）感受外来疫疠之邪
2.2 Attacked by external epidemic evil

外感邪毒既包括烈日暴晒皮肤、农药污染、有毒食品添加剂、染发剂等，又包括外感风、寒、湿等，其侵袭人体，郁而化毒，形成狼疮性肾炎发病的外在条件。

External evil includes not only burning sun exposure, pesticide pollution, toxic food additives, hair dye, etc. but also external wind, cold, dampness, which attack human body, transformed from depression to toxin, forming the external conditions of the onset of lupus nephritis.

（三）风湿、湿热、瘀血、浊毒贯穿疾病始终

2.3 Wind and dampness, dampness and heat, blood stasis, turbid toxin run through the whole process of disease

首先狼疮性肾炎患者先天之本亏虚，日久脾肾虚损，水湿内蕴，湿浊壅塞三焦，阻滞气机，水湿郁久生热，热则生毒，形成浊毒内壅之势。浊毒互结，壅塞经络，致气机不畅，津液不得输布，血液不得运行，水湿停留，化生痰浊瘀血，反复日久，造成络脉受阻，浊毒瘀滞。又因虚致瘀，血水同源，血运受阻而致瘀，三焦气化不利，久则酿为浊毒，蒙蔽清窍，损伤五脏六腑。

First, lupus nephritis patients is deficient in congenital endowment, deficient in spleen and kidney with time being, with internal accumulated water dampness, and congestion of damp turbidity in triple energizer, obstruct the operation of qi movement, prolonged depression of water dampness will be transformed into heat, heat generates toxin, forming the potential of internal accumulation of turbid toxin. Agglutination of turbidity and toxin, obstruct meridians, causes abnormal operation of qi movement, body fluid can not be transported and spread, blood can not circulate, water dampness retains, then transforms and generates phlegm, turbidity and blood stasis. The above process repeat for a long time, results in blocking of collateral, congestion of turbid toxin. Besides, deficiency causes blood stasis, blood and water shares the same source, resistance of blood circulation may generate stasis, sustainable abnormal gasification of triple energizer will brew turbid toxin, blind clear orifices, damage viscera.

其次感受外界六淫疫疠之邪，湿热内盛，浊毒内生，气机不畅，气滞血瘀，壅结日久不化，浸渐及肾，开阖不利，小便点滴，四肢肿胀，而发为狼疮性肾炎。

Second, attacked by the epidemic evil of six exopathogens, internal abundance of dampness and heat will generate internal turbid toxin, cause abnormal operation of qi movement, qi stagnation and blood stasis. Congestion for a long time will gradually immerse kidney, affect the control of bladder, lead to drip urine, limbs swelling, and finally lupus nephritis.

综上所述，狼疮性肾炎的病因包括禀赋不足、感受六淫疫疠之邪等。其病机主要有以下几个方面：肾精亏虚，风湿、湿热、浊毒、瘀血互结，导致脾、肾两脏俱损，体内代谢失衡而发病。故病位主要在脾肾两脏，临床上以虚实夹杂证，本虚标实证居多。

In conclusion, the causes of lupus nephritis include insufficient endowment and attacking of the epidemic evil of six exopathogens. Its pathogenesis mainly includes the following aspects: kidney essence deficiency, agglutination of wind and dampness, dampness and heat, turbidity and toxin, and blood stasis, which bring damages to both spleen and kidney, metabolic imbalance in the body and finally the occurrence of the disease. Therefore, the disease is mainly located in the spleen and kidney, clinically see the syndrome of mixture of asthenia and sthenia, asthenia in root and sthenia in tip.

三、狼疮性肾炎的浊毒证辨证论治
3. The differentiation treatment of turbid toxin syndrome of lupus nephritis

李佃贵教授认为狼疮性肾炎病机复杂，临床变化多端，主张分期辨证论治。目前，临床上主要应用糖皮质激素，而糖皮质激素相当于中医理论中的"纯阳"之品，日久耗竭阴液，出现阴虚火旺的证候。故李佃贵强调中西医结合治疗狼疮性肾炎。

Professor Li Diangui believes that the pathogenesis of lupus nephritis is complicated and has many clinical changes, and advocates syndrome differentiation according to different stages. At present, glucocorticoids are mainly used in clinical practice of western medicine. But glucocorticoids are equivalent to the "pure Yang" products in traditional Chinese medicine theory, which exhaust Yin fluid over time, see the syndrome of Yin deficiency and fire flourishing. Therefore, Li Diangui emphasizes the combination of Chinese and western medicine in treatment of lupus nephritis.

狼疮性肾炎的治疗分为急性期、缓解期、维持期。急性期治疗主要是为了尽快控制狼疮活动，减少蛋白尿，改善肾功能；缓解期治疗主要为了稳定病情，进一步减少蛋白尿；维持期治疗则主要是为了防止狼疮复发，保护肾功能，减少并发症的发生，并尽量减少药物的不良反应。是在狼疮性肾炎的各期，糖皮质激素都是基础药物之一。急性期患者的病情凶险，单纯使用中药效果欠佳，因此中药常作为辅助用药。李佃贵教授经过多年临床研究发现，急性期主要证型为热毒炽盛兼有血瘀证，缓解期为阴虚内热证，而维持期患者，因为长期使用激素，证型以阴阳两虚证为主。

The treatment of lupus nephritis is divided into acute stage, remission and maintenance stage. Treatment in the acute stage is mainly to control lupus activity as soon as possible, reduce proteinuria and improve renal function; treatment in the remission stage is mainly to stabilize the condition and further reduce proteinuria; treatment in the maintenance stage is mainly to prevent lupus from recurring, protect renal function, reduce the occurrence of complications, and minimize the adverse reactions of drugs. In any stage of lupus nephritis treatment, glucocorticoid is one of the basic drugs. The disease condition of patients in acute stage is more dangerous, only using Chinese medicine is not obviously effective, so Chinese medicines are usually used as auxiliary medicine. Professor Li Diangui found through years of clinical research that the main syndrome in acute stage of the disease is excessive abundance of heat and toxin accompanied by blood stasis, the main syndrome in remission stage of the disease is Yin deficiency and internal heat. The main syndrome of the patients in maintenance stage of the disease is dual deficiency of Yin and Yang due to long-term use of hormones.

（一）热毒炽盛型
3.1 Burning exuberance of heat and toxin

1.症状　高热，烦躁易怒，面色潮红，面部环形或蝶形红斑，口腔溃疡，血尿，口渴，大便秘结，舌红脉数，甚则神昏谵语等。

3.1.1 Symptoms　High fever, irritability, flushing, hectic red complexion, ring or butterfly erythema in face, oral ulcer, hematuria, thirsty in mouth, constipation, red tongue, rapid pulse, or even confused in mind and delirium, etc.

2.治法　清热解毒，清营凉血消斑。

3.1.2 Treatment method　Clear heat and remove toxin, clear nourishing qi, cool blood and eliminate spots.

3.方药　犀角地黄汤加减。

3.1.3 Prescription　Xijiao Dihuang Decoction with addition or reduction.

4.方义　本方以犀角清心凉血解毒为主，配生地黄可以凉血止血及养阴清热，芍药、牡丹皮既能凉血，又能散瘀。本方特点是凉血与活血散瘀并用，以共收清热解毒、凉血散瘀之功。药味加减方面，可酌用大蓟、小蓟、侧柏叶等以凉血止血，蒲公英、紫花地丁等以加强清热解毒的效果。

3.1.4 Explanation of the prescription　The prescription uses rhinoceros horn as the main medicine to clear heart, cool blood and remove toxin; auxiliarily using sheng di huang (Radix Rehmanniae) to cool blood and stop bleeding and nourish Yin and clear heat. Using bai shao (Radix Paeoniae Alba) and mu dan pi (Cortex Moutan) to cool blood and disperse blood stasis. This prescription is characterized by cooling blood while promoting blood circulation and resolving stasis, in order to realize the effect of clearing heat and removing toxin, cooling blood and dispersing stasis. Referring addition and reduction to the prescription, da ji (Herba Cirsii Japonici), xiao ji (Herba seu Radix Cephalanoploris), ce bai ye (Platycladi Cacumen) can be used to cool blood, stop bleeding, pu gong ying (Herba Taraxaci cum Radice), zi hua di ding (Herba Violae) can strengthen the effect of clearing heat and removing toxin.

（二）瘀血型

3.2 Blood stasis

1.症状　面部出现环形或蝶形红斑，关节疼痛，腰部疼痛，固定不移，入夜尤甚，舌暗红，舌边有瘀斑，脉涩或弦紧。

3.2.1 Symptoms　Annular or butterfly erythema on the face, joint pain, waist pain, fixed, especially severe at night, dark red tongue, ecchymosis on the side of the tongue, astringent or tight string pulse.

2.治法　活血祛瘀，行气止痛。

3.2.2 Treatment method　Promote blood circulation and remove blood stasis, exercise qi and relieve pain.

3.方药　身痛逐瘀汤加减。

3.2.3 Prescription　Shentong Zhuyu Decoction with addition or reduction.

4.方义　因瘀血痹阻于经络关节，故见关节、腰部疼痛等。方中以川芎、当归、桃仁、红花为基础，有活血祛瘀止痛的作用，配有通络宣痹之秦艽、羌活、地龙等，多用于瘀血痹阻于经络而致的关节疼痛或肢体痹痛等症，可随症加用延胡索、郁金、蒲黄以收活血止痛之功。

3.2.4 Explanation of the prescription　As blood stasis is obstructed in meridian and joints, so the pain of joint and waist occur. Based on chuan xiong (Rhizoma Chuanxiong), dang gui (Radix Angelicae

Sinensis), tao ren (Semen Persicae) and hong hua (Flos Carthami), the prescription has the effect of promoting blood circulation, removing blood stasis and relieving pain. The auxilary medicines like qin jiao (Radix Gentianae Macrophyllae), qiang huo (Notopterygii Rhizoma), di long (Lumbricus), etc. which are mostly used to treat joint pain or limb pain caused by obstruction of blood stasis in meridians, are selected to unblock the collateral and diffuse the numbness. According to the condition of diseasecan, yan hu suo (Rhizoma Corydalis), yu jin (Radix Curcumae) and pu huang (Pollen Typhae) can be added to promote blood circulation and relieve pain.

（三）阴虚内热型
3.3 Yin Deficiency and Intrinsic Heat

1.症状　蛋白尿，血尿，兼见口干心烦，自汗盗汗，潮热，眼睛干涩，舌红少津，脉细数。

3.3.1 Symptoms　Proteinuria, hematuria, and dry mouth, upset, sweat and night sweat, hectic fever, dry eyes, red tongue little fluid, thready rapid pulse.

2.治法　滋阴清热，益气养阴。

3.3.2 Treatment method　Enriching Yin and clearing heat, replenishing qi and nourishing Yin.

3.方药　二至丸合杞菊地黄汤或知柏地黄汤加减。

3.3.3 Prescription　Erzhi Pill, Qiju Dihuang Decoction or Zhibai Dihuang Decoction with addition or reduction.

4.方义　患者长期使用激素，易出现阴虚内热证的表现，二至丸取女贞子甘苦凉，滋肾养肝，配墨旱莲甘酸寒，养阴益精凉血止血，全方药味少而性平和，为补阴之平剂。杞菊地黄汤系将六味地黄丸加枸杞子、菊花而成。六味地黄丸为滋补肾阴的主方，加枸杞子、菊花兼有滋水明目的作用。另外，可考虑加白薇、地骨皮以退虚热。

3.3.4 Explanation of the prescription　Patients who have been using hormones for long-term, are prone to syndrome of Yin deficiency and internal heat. Erzhi Pill uses nv zhen zi (Fructus Ligustri) which is sweet and cold, to enrich kidney, nourish liver, assisted by mo han lian (Herba Ecliptae) which is sweet, acid and cold to nourish Yin, replenish essence, cool blood and stop bleeding. The whole prescription is few in number of medicines and peaceful in nature and taste, is the peaceful agent to tonify Yin. Qiju Dihuang Decoction (Qi ju rehmannia soup) is formed by Liuwei Dihuang Pill (six rehmannia pills) with addition of gou qi zi (Lycii Fructus), ju hua (Chrysanthemi Flos). Liuwei Dihuang Pill is the main prescription for nourishing kidney Yin, adding gou qi zi (Lycii Fructus), ju hua (Chrysanthemi Flos) which also have function of enriching water and brightening eyes. Besides, bai wei (Cynanchi Atrati Radix Et Rhizoma), di gu pi (Lycii Cortex) are suggested to retreat asthenia heat.

（四）阴阳两虚型
3.4 Dual deficiency of Yin and Yang

1.症状　面部红斑不明显，颜面、双下肢浮肿，大量蛋白尿，且兼见神疲乏力，面色无华，畏寒肢冷，胃纳差，大便溏烂，舌淡苔白，脉沉细弱。

3.4.1 Symptoms Facial erythema is not obvious, edema in face and lower limbs, large amount of proteinuria, spiritual overexertion and fatigue, dull complexion, fear of cold, cold in limbs, poor appetite, loose and mashed stool, light tongue, white moss, sunk thready and weak pulse.

2.治法　补益阴阳，健脾温肾。

3.4.2 Treatment method Tonifying Yin and Yang, invigorate spleen and warm kidney.

3.方药　真武汤或右归丸加减。

3.4.3 Prescriptions Zhenwu Decoction or Yougui Pill with addition or reduction.

4.方义　真武汤中附子为君药，用其大辛大热之性以温肾暖土，以助阳气。臣药以茯苓健脾渗湿，以利水邪，生姜既助附子之温阳祛寒，又伍茯苓以温散水气；佐以白术健脾燥湿，配合白芍以利小便。右归丸是在《金匮要略》肾气丸的基础上，减去茯苓、泽泻和牡丹皮，加鹿角胶、菟丝子、杜仲、枸杞子而成。方中附子、肉桂、鹿角胶均属温补肾阳之药，熟地黄、山茱萸、山药、菟丝子、枸杞子、杜仲俱为滋阴益肾健脾之品，更加当归补血，可加用猪苓、泽泻以加强利尿退肿的疗效。

3.4.4 Explanation of prescription In Zhenwu Decoction, fu zi (Radix Aconiti) is used as the principal medicine, with nature of extremely spicy extremely hot to warm kidney, warm soil and assist Yang qi. Fu ling (Poria) is used as subordinate (minister) medicine to reinforce spleen and drain dampness, to disinhibit water evil. Sheng jiang (Rhizoma Zingiberis Recens) is used as guiding medicine, not only helping the fu zi (Radix Aconiti) to warm Yang and dispel coldness, but also combining with fu ling (Poria) to warm and disperse water retention. Bai zhu (Rhizoma Atractylodis Macrocephalae) is used as adjuvent medicine to reinforce spleen and dry dampness, cooperating with bai shao (Radix Paeoniae Alba) to improve urination. Yougui Pill is formed on the basis of Shenqi Pill prescription of "Synopsis of Golden Chamber", minus fu ling (Poria), ze xie (Rhizoma Alismatis) and mu dan pi (Cortex Moutan), plus lu jiao jiao (antler glue), tu si zi (Cuscutae Semen), du zhong (Cortex Eucommiae), gou qi zi (Lycii Fructus). In the prescription, fu zi (Radix Aconiti), rou gui (Cortex Cinnamomi) and lu jiao jiao (Colla Cornus Cervi) are the medicines to warm kidney and tonify Yang, shu di huang (Radix Rehmanniae Praeparatum), shan zhu yu (Corni Fructus), shan yao (Discoreae Rhizoma), tu si zi (Cuscutae Semen), gou qi zi (Lycii Fructus), du zhong (Cortex Eucommiae) are medicines for enriching Yin, replenishing kidney and reinforcing spleen. Dang gui (Radix Angelicae Sinensis) is used to tonify blood. Besides, zhu ling (Polygorus Umbellatus), Ze xie (Rhizoma Alismatis) can be added to strengthen the effect of improve urination and retreat swelling.

此外，李佃贵教授还根据激素的使用情况，针对各个阶段所表现的症状进行辨证分析。但毒邪最易伤阴，故临证治疗时应在清热解毒的基础上加用滋阴降火之中药，如知母、黄柏、生地黄、玄参等；在激素减量过程中应酌情加用太子参、麦冬、党参、沙参、黄芪等益气养阴之品；在激素维持阶段宜选用桑寄生、熟地黄、山茱萸等平补阴阳之品。

In addition, professor Li Diangui also differentially analyzed the symptoms in each stage of the disease according to the condition of hormones using. Toxic evil is the most likely to hurt Yin, so in clinical treatment, zhi mu (Rhizoma Anemarrhennae), huang bo (Cortex Phellodendri), sheng di huang (Radix Rehmanniae), xuan shen (Radix Scrophulariae) and other products should be used to enrich Yin and counterbear fire. Tai zi shen (Radix Pseudostellariae), mai dong (Radix Ophiopogonis), dang shen (Radix Codonopsitis Pilosulae), sha shen (Glehniae Radix),huang qi (Radix Astragali seu Hedysari) and other medicines for replenishing qi and nourishing Yin should be used in the process of reducing the amount of hormone. Sang ji sheng (Talxilli Herba), shu di huang (Radix Rehmanniae Praeparatum), shan zhu yu (Corni Fructus) and other products should be used to tonify Yin and Yang in the process of maintaining the use of hormone.

总之，对于狼疮性肾炎的治疗，急性期在西医免疫抑制药治疗的基础上加用中药可以增加疗效、减少西药的不良反应，缓解期使用中药则有利于西药的撤减，并在防止复发方面具有一定优势，而对于疾病后期则应中西并重，各自扬长避短，以西药纠正可逆因素，用中药保护肾功能，微调体内阴阳气血在低水平状态下达到相对平衡，着眼于改善临床症状，提高患者的生存质量。

In short, for the treatment of lupus nephritis, in acute stage to add Chinese materia medica on the basis of immunosuppressive drugs in western medicine can increase the curative effect, reduce the adverse reactions of western medicine. In the alleviate stage using Chinese medicine is beneficial for reduction of western medicine, and has certain advantages in preventing recurrence. In late stage of the disease, both Chinese and western medicine should be used cooperatively and foster strengths and circumvent weaknesses of each other. While using western medicine to correct reversible factors, use Chinese medicine to protect kidney function, mildly adjust the low state of Yin and Yang, qi and blood in body to relative balance, in order to improve clinical symptoms, improve the life quality of patients.

第六节　乙肝相关性肾小球肾炎浊毒论
Section 6 On Turbid Toxin of Hepatitis B-related Glomerulonephritis

一、乙肝相关性肾小球肾炎的中医学概述
1. TCM overview of hepatitis B-related glomerulonephritis

乙肝相关性肾小球肾炎中医学虽无本病的病名记载，可将本病归属"尿血""水肿""虚劳""郁证"等范畴。本病多由于禀赋薄弱，正气不足，复因饮食不洁，或劳累过度，或情志内伤，湿热毒邪乘虚而入，内蕴肝脏；肝肾同源，肝肾互传，一脏有病，累及他脏。具体可概述为以下三方面：①外感湿热毒邪，内蕴脏腑；②饮食不节，湿热邪毒内伤；③先天禀赋不足或素体虚弱，劳累过度，情志内伤，以及其他疾病损伤元气，湿热毒邪乘虚而入。李佃贵教授认为乙肝病毒感染乃湿热之邪稽留。湿为有形之邪，阻碍气机运行。肝失疏泄，三焦、脾肾升降失常，脾不升清而精微下注，肾不固摄而精微外泄，故见尿中蛋白漏出。肝气郁结，气滞血瘀，故见舌边有瘀斑。长期蛋白尿漏出，必损精血，肝血既亏，其疏泄通达之事又何以济？于是，子病及母，肾气不能固摄，终成顽固性蛋白尿。

Although there is no record of this disease in the name hepatitis B-related glomerulonephritis, this disease can be attributed to "urine blood", "edema""consumptive disease", "depression" and other categories. This disease is mostly due to weak endowment, lack of healthy qi, unclean diet, or overwork, or internal emotional injury, attacked by dampness and heat toxic evil, accumulated internally in liver; liver and kidney shares the same source, liver and kidney inter - transform to each other, one zang - organ has disease, will involve the other. Specifically it can be summarized in the following three aspects: a. exogenous dampness and heat toxic evil, accumulate internally in viscera; b. irregular diet, evil of dampness, heat and toxin make internal injury; c. congenital deficiency or physical weakness, overwork, emotional injury, and other diseases damage vitality, invasion of damp and heat toxic evil. Professor Li Diangui thinks that hepatitis B virus infection is the retaining of dampness and heat evil. Dampness is a tangible evil hindering the operation of the qi movement. When liver looses the function of dispersing, the ascending descending of triple energizer, of spleen and kidney turns to be abnormal. If spleen does not ascend lucidity and cereal essence will move downwards. If kidney can not seal and store, the cereal essence will leak outside, so protein is leaked in urine. Depression of liver qi, qi stagnation and blood stasis occur, so stasis spots can be seen on the tongue side. Long-term proteinuria leakage, will surely damage essence and blood. Since both liver and blood are deficient, how to maintain the normal operation of dispersing and and dredging? Therefore, the disease of son involves mother, kidney qi can not be sealed and stored, eventually stubborn proteinuria is generated.

由此可见，乙肝相关性肾小球肾炎初期以湿热邪毒瘀阻三焦气机之标实证为主，而在疾病发生变化的过程中，气滞血瘀又是必然的结果。邪毒日久不去，耗气伤阴，则终致肝脾肾的虚损。由此可知本病实邪与正虚并存，虚实夹杂，病位主要在肝、肾、脾，湿热瘀毒蕴结肝肾是本病的基本病机。治疗上多采用祛邪扶正的方法，祛邪扶正，虚实兼顾；祛邪以清热解毒、祛湿化瘀为主，以消灭体内病毒，改善机体微循环，促使组织的修复；扶正以益气健脾、滋补肝肾为主，以改善机体的免疫功能，促使病情的恢复；前期以重在祛邪佐以扶正；后期以重在扶正兼顾祛邪。

It can be seen that in the initial stage, hepatitis B-related glomerulonephritis is mainly syndrome of sthenia tip characterized by dampness and heat toxic evil blood stasis congesting the qi mechanism of triple energizer. In the process of disease change, qi stagnation and blood stasis is an inevitable result. Evil toxin does not leave over time, wears out qi and injures Yin, finally lead to deficiency of the liver, spleen and kidney. It can be seen that excess of evil and deficiency of healthy qi coexist in this disease, sthenia and asthenia are mixed together. The location of disease is mainly in the liver, kidney, spleen. The accumulation and binding of dampness, heat, stasis, and toxin in liver and kidney is the basic pathogenesis of the disease. In the treatment, the method of dispelling evilness, and reinforcing healthy qi is generally use to dually care asthenia and sthenia. To dispel evilness, we should mainly clear heat and remove toxin, dispel dampness and resolve blood stasis, in order to eliminate viruses in human body, improve the micro - circulation, and promote the recovery of tissues. To reinforce the healthy qi, we should mainly enrich qi and reinforce the spleen, diffuse the liver and tonify the kidney, so as to improve the immune function of the body and promote the recovery of the disease. In the former stage, stresses should be layed on evil dispelling, giving proper consideration to healthy qi reinforcement; in the latter stage, stresses should be layed on healthy qi reinforcing, giving proper consideration to evil dispelling.

二、乙肝相关性肾小球肾炎浊毒证的病因病机

2. Etiology and pathogenesis of turbid toxin syndrome of hepatitis B-related glomerulonephritis

　　李佃贵教授认为本病的根本病机是肝肾阴虚，湿热瘀毒蕴结。肝肾同源，肝肾互传，一脏有病，累及他脏，或多脏同病，致肝失疏泄，气机不利，气滞湿阻，脉络瘀滞，而见胁胀胁痛，脘腹痞满，或腹胀如鼓，尿色黄赤；肝病及脾，或湿毒伤脾，脾失健运，运化失司，升降失常，湿热壅滞三焦，而见乏力，纳差，口苦口黏，大便不爽，浮肿难消；病程迁延日久，湿热毒邪久羁伤肾，肾络损伤，气化封藏失职，精微下注，而见腰膝酸软，头晕目眩，尿浊尿赤等。热毒伤阴，湿毒伤气，肝肾同源，脾肾相生互化，以致肝肾阴虚，脾肾阳虚，久病入络，瘀血内停，终致瘀毒互结，深伏久滞，肾络大伤，正气大败。反之，因虚可以致实，脾肾阳虚则虚寒内生，温煦失常，运化无权，肾虚水无所主而水湿内生；肝肾阴虚化火，热灼脉络，迫血妄行，血不循经而外溢，积于体内，则瘀血内生。由此可见，因实致虚，因虚致实，相互转化，循环往复。故肝肾俱虚、湿热瘀毒互结，虚实夹杂为病机关键。早期以邪实为主，渐至虚实夹杂；后期以正虚为主，邪实与正虚并存为其病机特点。本病的病机主要有以下几方面。

Professor Li Diangui believes that the root pathogenesis of this disease is deficiency of liver and kidney Yin, accumulation and binding of dampness, heat, stasis and toxin. Liver and kidney shares the same source, liver and kidney inter-transform to each other, one zang-organ has disease, will involve the other or multi zang - organs. Liver looses function of dispersing, operation of air mechanism become abnormal, qi is stagnated, veins are congested, symptoms of hypochrondrium swelling and pain, abdominal distension and fullness, abdominal swelling, yellow red urine occur; liver disease affect the spleen, or dampness and toxin hurt spleen, spleen looses the function of transportation, ascending and descending is abnormal. Dampness and heat are abundantly stagnated in triple energizer, patients have fatigue, anorexia, dry and bitter mouth, difficult stool, and swelling which is difficult to be dispersed. As the disease lingers long, retaining of dampness,heat, toxin and evil injures kidney. When kidney collateral are damaged, function of vaporization, sealing and storing fail to work, cereal essence moves downward, patients have lassitude in loin and knees, dizziness, turbid and red urine. Heat toxin injures Yin, wet toxin injures qi, liver and kidney share the same source, spleen and kidney inter- promote and can be transformed to each other, causing Yin deficiency of liver and kidney, Yang deficiency of spleen and kidney. Long disease will enter collateral, blood stasis retains inside, eventually lead to agglutinateing of stasis and toxin, deeply hidden and long-time stagnation, kidney collateral seriously injured, vital qi severely declined. On the contrary, because deficiency can transform into excess, spleen and kidney Yang deficiency causes deficiency and coldness generates endogenously, warming is irregular, transportation does not work. Kidney is deficient, water is out of control, water dampness generates endogenously. Deficiency of liver and kidney Yin is transformed into fire, burning veins, force blood to flow rashly, blood does not follow the meridian and overflows, if accumulated in the body, blood stasis generates internally. Thus it can be seen that sthenia may lead to asthenia, asthenia can also lead to sthenia. Asthenia and sthenia can be inter-transformed to each other, the process may repeat in endless cycles. Therefore, dual deficiency of the liver and kidney, agglutinating of dampness, heat, stasis, and toxin, mixture of asthenia and sthenia is the key of pathogenesis.In the early stage, the syndrome is mainly evil excess, and then mixture of asthenia and sthenia; in the later stage, the syndrome is mainly deficiency of healthy qi, evil excess coexists with deficiency of healthy qi. The pathogenesis of this disease mainly has the following aspects:

（一）禀赋不足

2.1 Deficient endowment

先天不足，脾胃易伤，出现腹胀、纳呆、乏力等症。

Congenitally deficient, easy to be injured in spleen and stomach, patients see abdominal distension, anorexia, fatigue and other diseases.

（二）情志不遂

2.2 Discomfort in emotions

情志不遂，肝失疏泄，气机不利，致使肝郁脾虚出现两胁胀满，腹胀午后为甚，腰酸，食欲不振，大便稀溏等症。

Emotional dissatisfied, liver looses the function of dispersing, abnormal operation of qi mechanism, resulting in liver depression and spleen deficiency, hypochondrium distension and fullness, abdominal distension especially in the afternoon, lassitude loin, poor appetite, loose stool and other symptoms.

（三）湿热蕴结

2.3 Accumulation and binding of dampness and heat

湿热毒邪内蕴，累及于肝，肝失疏泄，气机不利，见口干口苦，厌食油腻，上腹胀满，大便干燥或黏滞不爽，或双下肢浮肿，形体倦怠，舌质红苔黄，脉弦滑。

Internal accumulation of dampness, heat, toxin and evil affects the liver, liver looses the function of dispersing, abnormal operation of qi mechanism occurs. Patients have dry and bitter mouth, anorexia of greasy food, abdominal distension and fullness, dry or sticky stool, or edema in lower limbs, body burnout, red tongue and yellow moss, string slippery pulse.

（四）肝肾阴虚

2.4 Deficiency of liver and kidney Yin

素体肝肾阴虚，肾阴亏虚，不能气化水津，阴虚生内热，肾络迫血妄行。临床见头晕耳鸣，五心烦热，咽干口燥，下肢浮肿，尿黄或尿血，舌红少苔，脉弦细或细数。

Liver and kidney Yin is usually deficient, deficient kidney Yin can not gasify fluid. Yin deficiency generates internal heat, kidney collateral force blood to flow rashly. Clinically patients have dizziness tinnitus, upset in five feverish centers, dry throat and mouth, edema in lower limbs, yellow urine or blood urine, red tongue little moss, string thready or thready rapid pulse.

（五）脾肾阳虚

2.5 Deficiency of spleen and kidney Yang

素体脾胃虚弱，脾为制水之脏，肾主水，脾阳虚损及肾阳，以致脾肾阳虚。故临床可见面色㿠白，畏寒肢冷，腰酸痛，神疲，便溏，尿少，浮肿，舌质淡嫩，脉沉细无力。

Spleen and stomach are usually weak. Spleen is the the zang - organ to restrict water, kidney controls water generation. Deficiency of spleen Yang affects kidney Yang, leads to deficiency of spleen and kidney Yang. Therefore, patients have white pale face, cold limbs and fear of coldness, waist acid and painful, spiritual fatigue, loose stool, little urine, edema, tender tongue, sunk thready and weak pulse.

三、乙肝相关性肾小球肾炎的浊毒证辨证论治
3. Differential Treatment of Turbid Toxin Syndrome of hepatitis B - related glomerulonephritis

（一）湿热疫毒，热毒浸淫型
3.1 Heat, dampness and epidemic toxin, immersion of heat toxin

1.症状　心中懊侬，口干口苦，厌食油腻，不思饮食，上腹胀满，大便干燥或黏滞不爽，尿黄，或双下肢浮肿，形体倦怠，舌红苔黄腻，脉弦数。

3.1.1 Symptoms　Upset in the heart, dry and bitter mouth, anorexia of greasy food, do not think about diet, epigastric distension and fullness, dry stool or sticky uncomfortable, yellow urine, or edema in lower limbs, physically fatigue, red tongue, yellow greasy moss, string rapid pulse.

2.治法　清热利湿解毒。

3.1.2 Treatment method　Clearing heat, disinhibiting dampness and removing toxin.

3.常用药物　茵陈、青蒿、制大黄、炒栀子、土鳖虫、水蛭、地龙、羚羊角粉、白芍、桃仁、柴胡、黄芩、牡丹皮、薏苡仁、白茅根等。

3.1.3 Medicines generally used　Yin chen (Herba Aretemisiae Scorpariae), qing hao (Artemisiae Annuae Herba), zhi da huang (prepared Radix et Rhizoma Rhei), chao zhi zi (fried Fructus Gardeniae), tu bie chong (Eupolyphaga Steleophaga), shui zhi (Hirudo), di long (Lumbricus), ling yang jiao fen (powder of Saigae Tataricae Cornu), bai shao (Radix Paeoniae Alba), tao ren (Semen Persicae), chai hu (Radix Bulpleuri), huang qin (Radix Scutellariae), mu dan pi (Cortex Moutan), yi yi ren (Semen Coisis), bai mao gen (Rhizoma Imperatae), etc.

（二）瘀毒闭阻肾络型
3.2 Stasis toxin obstructs renal collateral

1.症状　面色晦暗，两胁胀满，腹胀，腰酸，腰痛固定，肢困乏力，食欲不振，大便干燥，全身或下肢浮肿，尿赤有泡沫，舌质暗，有瘀点瘀斑，脉细涩。

3.2.1 Symptoms　Dark complexion, hypochondrium distention and fullness, abdominal distension, waist acid, fixed pain in loin, fatigue in limbs, poor appetite, dry stool, edema in whole body or lower limbs, red urine with foam, dark tongue, with petechia or ecchymosis, thready and astringent pulse.

2.治法 活血化瘀，佐以化湿解毒。

3.2.2 Treatment method Promoting blood circulation and resolving blood stasis, assisted by dispelling dampness and removing toxin.

3.常用药物 桃仁、红花、丹参、当归、川芎、虎杖、郁金、益母草、地龙、僵蚕、猪苓、泽泻、白术、茯苓等。若伴气滞者，可加香附、柴胡；若血热者，可加生地黄、赤芍、牡丹皮以凉血；若寒凝者，可加桂枝、当归、淫羊藿。

3.2.3 Medicines generally used Tao ren (Semen Persicae), hong hua (Flos Carthami), dan shen (Salviae Miltiorrhizae), dang gui (Radix Angelicae Sinensis), chuan xiong (Rhizoma Chuanxiong), hu zhang (Rhizoma Polygoni Cuspidati), yu jin (Radix Curcumae), yi mu cao (Herba Leonuri), di long (Lumbricus), jiang can (Bombyx Batryticatus), zhu ling (Polygorus Umbellatus), ze xie (Rhizoma Alismatis), bai zhu (Rhizoma Atractylodis Macrocephalae), fu ling (Poria), etc. If accompanied by qi stagnation, add xiang fu (Rhizoma Cyperi) , chai hu (Radix Bulpleuri). In case of blood fever, add sheng di huang (Radix Rehmanniae), chi shao (Radix Paeoniae Rubra), mu dan pi (Moutan Cortax) to cool blood. In case of cold coagulation, add gui zhi (Cmnamomi Mmulus), dang gui (Radix Angelicae Sinensis), yin yang huo (Epimedii Folium).

（三）肝肾阴虚型

3.3 Deficiency of liver and kidney Yin

1.症状 腰膝酸软，头晕目眩，耳鸣健忘，两目干涩，失眠多梦，胁肋隐痛，五心烦热，口咽干燥，小便短赤夹有泡沫，大便秘结，舌红少苔，脉细数。

3.3.1 Symptoms Lassitude in loin and knees, dizziness, tinnitus, amnesia, dry eyes, insomnia with more dreams, hypochondrium vague pain, upset in five feverish centres, dry oropharynx, short red urine with foam, constipation, red tongue little moss, thready rapid pulse.

2.治法 养阴清热，补益肝肾，佐以祛湿化瘀。

3.3.2 Treatment method Nourishing Yin and clearing heat, tonifying the liver and replenishing kidney, and assisted by removing dampness and resolving blood stasis.

3.常用药物 生地黄、山药、山茱萸、牡丹皮、女贞子、墨旱莲、知母、龟甲、黄柏等。若湿热内蕴，可加车前子、泽泻、白茅根、土茯苓、白花蛇舌草等以清利湿热；若头晕目眩，可加菊花、夏枯草、炙鳖甲等以滋阴潜阳；活血化瘀可选用水蛭、泽兰、川牛膝、莪术等。

3.3.3 Medicines generally used Sheng di huang (Radix Rehmanniae), shan yao (Discoreae Rhizoma), shan zhu yu (Corni Fructus), mu dan pi (Cortex Moutan), nv zhen zi (Fructus Ligustri Lucidi), mo han lian (Herba Ecliptae), zhi mu (Rhizoma Anemarrhennae), gui jia (Plastrum Testudinis), huang bo (Cortex Phellodendri), etc. In case of internal accumulation of dampness and heat, add che qian zi (Semen Plantaginis), ze xie (Rhizoma Alismatis), bai mao gen (Rhizoma Imperatae), tu fu ling (Rhizoma Smilacis Glabrae), bai hua she she cao (Herba Oldenlandiae Diffusae) to clear dampness and heat; if dizziness, add ju hua (chrysanthemi Flos), xia ku cao (Spica Prunellae), zhi bie jia (prepared Trionycis Corapax) to enrich Yin and subdue Yang; to promote blood circulation and resolve blood stasis, add shui zhi (Hirudo), ze lan (Herba Lycopi), chuan niu xi (Radix Achyranthis Bidentatae), e zhu (Rhizoma Curcumae), etc.

（四）脾肾阳虚型

3.4 Deficiency of spleen and kidney Yang

1.症状　腰膝酸软，面浮肢肿，按之凹陷，神疲乏力，畏寒肢冷，脘腹胀满，纳少便溏，面色苍白，小便短少或清长，舌质淡胖，苔白，脉沉细无力。

3.4.1 Symptoms　Lassitude in loin and knees, edema in face and limbs, sunken when being pressed, spiritually and physically fatigue, fear of coldness and cold limbs, epigastric distension and fullness, poor appetite, loose stool, pale complexion, short little or long lucid urine, light fat tongue, white moss, sunk thready and weak pulse.

2.治法　温补脾肾，化湿解毒，佐以化瘀。

3.4.2 Treatment method　Warm and tonify the spleen and kidney, resolve dampness and remove toxin, assisted with resolving blood stasis.

3.常用药物　干姜、附子、草果、桂枝、白术、茯苓、炙甘草、生姜、大枣、泽泻、车前子、木瓜、木香、厚朴、大腹皮等。若气虚甚者，可加人参、黄芪以健脾益气；若伴呕吐者，可加吴茱萸以止呕；若伴五更泄泻者，可加补骨脂、肉豆蔻以补肾止泻；若脘腹冷痛，可加肉桂以温经通脉，散寒止痛。

3.4.3 Medicines generally used　Gan jiang (Zingiberis Rhizoma), fu zi (Radix Aconiti), cao guo (Fructus Tsaoko), gui zhi (Cmnamomi Mmulus), bai zhu (Rhizoma Atractylodis Macrocephalae), fu ling (Poria), zhi gan cao (fried Radix Glycyrrhizae), sheng jiang (Rhizoma Zingiberis Recens), da zao (Jujubae Fructus), fu ling (Poria), ze xie (Rhizoma Alismatis), che qian zi (Semen Plantaginis), mu gua (Chaenomelis Fructus), mu xiang (Radix Aucklandiae), hou po (Cortex Magnoliae Officinalis), da fu pi (Arecae Pericarpium), etc. In case of qi deficiency, add ren shen (Radix Ginseng) and huang qi (Radix Astragali seu Hedysari) to inforce spleen and replenish qi; if accompanied by vomiting, add wu zhu yu (Euodiae Fructus) to stop vomiting; in case of morning diarrhea, add bu gu zhi (Psoraleae Fructus), rou dou kou (Semen Myristicae) to tonify kidney and stop diarrhea; in case of epigastric cold pain, rou gui (Cortex Cinnamomi) can be added to warm meridians and unblock vessles, dissipate coldness and relieve pain.

第七节　肥胖相关性肾病浊毒论
Section 7　On Turbid Toxin of Obesity-related Nephropathy

一、肥胖相关性肾病的中医学概述
1. Overview of TCM for obesity-related nephropathy

肥胖相关性肾病属于中医"肥胖""尿浊""水肿""溺毒"等范畴。

Obesity-related nephropathy belongs to the category of "obesity", "urine turbidity", "edema" and "toxic urine" in traditional Chinese medicine.

中医学认为肾为先天之本，"肾者，主蛰，封藏之本，精之所处"。肾气充沛，则精气封藏固密；肾虚则不能藏精，水谷精微物质随尿液排出而形成尿浊。脾为后天之本，与先天之本相互滋养，为气血生化之源。饮食不节，过食肥甘厚腻，可致水谷精微在体内堆积成为膏脂，形成肥胖；也可损伤脾胃，导致水谷精微布散无力，水湿内停形成痰湿，日久则成肥胖，精微外泄。

Traditional Chinese medicine believes that the kidney is the congenital root, "the kidney controls hibernating, to seal and store essence". If kidney qi is abundant, essence qi is densely sealed and stored; if kidney is deficient, it can not store essence, cereal essence is discharged with urine and form turbid urine. The spleen is the acquired root, it inter-nourish with kidney, is the generation and transforming source of qi and blood. Irregular diet, over-taking of fat, sweet, thick and greasy food, can cause water valley accumulated into greasy fat in the body, forming obesity; it can also damages the spleen and stomach, lead to weak spreading of cereal essence, water dampness stop internally and turns to be phlegmatic hygrosis, with time passes, it becomes fat, cereal essence is leaked out.

二、肥胖相关性肾病浊毒证的病因病机
2. The etiology and pathogenesis of turbid toxin syndrome of obesity-related nephropathy

《素问·至真要大论》曰："审察病机，无失气宜……谨守病机，各司其属。"唐代王冰阐释道："得其机要，则动小而功大，用浅而功深。"刘完素进一步发挥说："察病机之要理，施品味之性用，然后明病之本焉，故治病不求其本，无以去深藏之大患。"从本病的发病机制来看，先天禀赋失常，脾胃虚弱，运化脂质能力受限；或中年以后，肾气渐衰，以致冲任不足，天癸衰减，肾脏气化失司，不能化气消脂，以及七情不畅，肝气郁滞，不能疏理脾运，通达三焦，以致痰湿脂浊停滞是疾病发生和发展之关键，是病之本；而痰湿脂浊内停，浸淫于肌肤脉络，浊毒内蕴于脏腑是病之标。

Simple Conversation - Major Discussion on the Important and Abstuse Theory said: "Carefully check the pathogenesis of disease, do not make mistake in following the suitability of qi, the pathogenesis should be carefully examined according to the nature." Tang dynasty Wang Bing explained:

"when the pathogenesis is accurately grasped, small action in treatment will make big effect, shallow effort will make deep achievement." Liu Wansu further explained: "Doctors should check the key factor of pathogenesis, use the nature and function of the medicines, and acknowledge the essence of the disease, so treating disease without seeking its root, it's no difference than hiding the greater disaster deeply." Observing from the pathogenesis of the disease, the root and key factor to decide the occurrence and development of the disease is that short of congenital endowment, weak spleen and stomach limit lipid substances transporting capacity; or after middle age, kidney qi declines causes deficiency of thoroughfare and conception vessles, decline of Tiangui (substance promoting sexual maturity) insufficient, dysfunction of kidney gasification, unable to gasify and dissipate lipid, disorder of seven emotions, liver qi depression, failing to disperse spleen transportation, drain triple energizer, leading to retaining of phlegmatic hygrosis and lipid turbidity. The internal retaining of phlegmatic hygrosis and lipid turbidity spreading over muscles, skin, and veins, and internal accumulation of turbid toxin is the tip of the disease.

肥胖之人体内痰湿瘀脂蓄积，阻塞脉道，痰瘀互结，故清阳不升，浊阴不降，毒邪内生，滞于肾络，使肾开阖启闭失常，而致肾脏损害，肾虚封藏失职，固摄无权，则精微物质流失于外而致蛋白尿。肾失封藏致脾胃运化失司，使脾气虚弱，则脂浊聚于体内。先天不足，肾精不充，或年老肾亏，或久病伤肾，导致肾精亏耗，不能生髓，上下俱虚，致血压升高，出现头痛、眩晕。

Internal aggregation of phlegmatic hygrosis blocks the meridians obesity people, phlegm and stasis agglutinates, so lucidity does not ascend, turbid yin does not descend, toxic evil generates endogenously, stagnated in kidney collateral, causes abnormal controlling of urination and defecation, damage kidney, lead to dysfunction and powerless of sealing and storing because of kidney deficiency, cereal essence leaks outside resulting in proteinuria. Renal dysfunction of sealing and storing causes dysfunction of spleen and stomach transportation and weak spleen qi, fat turbidity aggregate in the body. Innate deficiency, kidney essence insufficiency, or kidney decline due to ages, or kidney injured by long disease, result in deficient kidney essence unable to generate pulp. Up and down all deficient causes elevated blood pressure, headache and vertigo.

总之，本病的特点为本虚标实，致病因素为痰、虚、浊毒，病位在脾肾，治疗时应以补虚泻实、补气化湿、化浊解毒为重点，补肾健脾、化痰利湿为治疗原则。《金匮要略》曰"病痰饮者，当以温药和之"，是治疗痰湿所致疾病的治疗大法。古人云："治痰不理脾胃，非其治也。"故治疗本病应健脾益气、补肾固涩以补虚，祛湿化痰、化浊解毒、祛脂活血以泻实。本病病程较长，古人云"久病必瘀，久病入络"，痰与瘀血有相关性，因此如果患者有血瘀的症状，则应兼顾活血化瘀。本病的临床症状多，治疗时应谨守病机，辨证施治。若气虚则应补气健脾，若阳虚为主应温补脾肾之阳，随证加减，充分利用中医的优势以提高本病的治疗效果。

In short, the characteristics of the disease is asthenia root and sthenia tip. Pathogenic factors are phlegm, deficiency and turbid toxin. The location of the disease is in spleen and kidney. The focal point of the treatment is to tonify the asthenia, purge the sthenia, tonify qi and resolve dampness, resolving turbidity and removing toxin. The principle of the treatment should be to tonify the kidney and reinforce the spleen, resolve phlegm and dissipate the dampness. *The Synopsis of Gold Chamber* says: "To treat the disease of phlegmatic retention, use warm medicine to harmonize". This is the treatment principle to deal with diseases caused by phlegmatic retention. The ancient people said: "Treat phlegm disease without regulating the spleen and stomach, is not the right way." So the treatment of the disease should reinforce the spleen and replenish qi, tonify kidney and strengthen the astringent in order to tonify deficiency, dispelling dampness and resolving phlegm, resolving turbidity and remove toxin, removing lipid and promoting blood circulation in order to purge sthenia. The disease course is longer, the ancients said: "long disease will surely generate stasis, long disease will surely get into collateral". Phlegm is relative to blood, stasis, so if patients of phlegmatic retention have blood stasis symptoms, promoting blood circulation and resolving blood stasis should be simultaneously considered. As there may be many clinical symptoms of the disease, doctors should keep pathogenesis, treat according to syndrome differentiation. If qi is deficient, tonify qi and reinforce the spleen. If Yang is deficient, doctors should warm and tonify spleen and kidney Yang, selecting proper prescriptions with addition and reduction due to difference of syndromes, making full use of the advantages of traditional Chinese medicine to improve the treatment effect of the disease.

三、肥胖相关性肾病的浊毒证辨证论治
3. The differential treatment of turbid toxin syndrome of obesity-related nephropathy

中医学将肥胖病患者称为"脂人""膏人""肉人"。《素问·经脉别论》云："饮入于胃，游溢精气，上输于脾，脾气散精，上归于肺，通调水道，下输膀胱，水精四布，五经并行。"因此，脾胃健运则气血生化有源，且水谷精微输布、转化井然有序。反之，若脾失健运，则气血生化无源，水谷精微不能正常输布全身，留而为痰，积聚体内，膏脂内蓄而发为肥胖。正如《脾胃论》所言："脾胃俱旺，则能食而肥。脾胃俱虚，则不能食而瘦，或少食而肥，虽肥而四肢不举。"而脾气虚损，则精微失于统摄，下渗于膀胱导致精微外泄。然脾气亏虚，则肾精得不到滋养，则肾的封藏功能失于正常，则导致精微物质外泄，损伤肾络，久之则导致关格等病证的发生。因此，脾肾亏虚为本，邪实侵袭肾脏，而痰浊、气滞、水湿、瘀血阻滞肾络贯穿始终。《太平圣惠方》载："饮水随饮便下，小便味甘而白浊，腰腿消瘦者，肾消也。"《圣济总录》亦载："消渴病久，肾气受伤，肾主水，肾气虚衰，气化失常，开阖不利，能为水肿。"《张氏医通·杂门》曰："肾消之病，古曰强中，又名内消。"以上文献中记载的水肿、蛋白尿与肥胖相关性肾病的症状相一致。可以看出，肥胖相关性肾病患者多有痰、湿、瘀等病理产物，而浊毒理论认为，痰、瘀、湿等病理产物不断堆积凝聚胶结而成浊毒，属瘀毒、湿毒、痰毒、燥毒等多方面。其形成的主要机制为气虚无力运血，血行不畅而瘀滞，瘀久化湿成浊毒；湿热灼伤津血，津血凝滞瘀结，久而化为浊毒；此外寒邪可入里化热，内热灼伤津血而瘀，久瘀亦可化为浊毒，此为外邪之毒。所以浊和毒是肥胖相关性肾病的重要病机。禀赋不足、过食肥膏厚味、情志所伤、劳欲过度等耗气伤阴，气阴两虚，气虚则血行不畅，滞而成瘀，阴虚则生内热，耗血成瘀结痰，瘀阻肾络，久而滋生邪毒，而成肥胖相关性肾病。

Traditional Chinese medicine call obese patients as "fat people", "paste people", "meat people". *Simple Conversation-Special Discussion on Channels and Vessels* says: "When water is taken into the stomach, Jingqi (essence qi) is distributed around and is transported up to the spleen. The spleen distributes jing (essence) and transports it upward to the lung. The lung regulates water passage and transports (water) to the bladder. In this way, the jing (essence) of water is distributed all through the body and into the five channels in conformity with the changes of the four seasons (and the changes of Yin and Yang of the five -zang organs). These are normal changes of the Channels." When the spleen and stomach operates normally, there is the source for generating and transforming of the qi and blood. The transporting, distributing and transforming of cereal essence is in order. On the contrary, if the spleen can not work normally, there is no source for generating and transforming of the qi and blood, the cereal essence cannot be normally transported and spread over the whole body, it stays and turns to be phlegm, accumulated in the body, retention of greasy lipid is aggregated into obesity. As *Discussion on Spleen and Stomach* says: "When spleen and stomach are flourishing, people can eat grow fat. If the spleen and stomach are dual deficient, people can not eat and grow thin, or eat little but grow fat, although they look fat, but are unable to raise limbs." When the spleen qi is deficient and injured, the cereal essence cannot be thoroughly ingested, it will be infiltrated into the bladder leading to cereal essence leakage. But as the spleen qi is deficient, the kidney essence can not be enriched, the sealing and storing function of the kidney is abnormal, causes the leakage of cereal essence, damages the kidney collateral, with time passes leads to the occurrence of frequent vomiting and dysuria and other diseases. Therefore, the spleen and kidney deficiency is the root, evil sthenia invades the kidney, and phlegm turbidity, qi stagnation, water dampness, and blood stasis obstructing kidney collateral throughout the whole process of the disease. It is written in *Taiping Shenghui Prescriptions* that "Water is discharged soon after drinking, urine tastes sweet with white turbidity, thin waist and legs, that is the syndrome of renal diabetes." *Shengji General Record* also writes: "Diabetes for a long time will injure kidney qi, kidney controls water, when kidney qi is deficient, gasification is in disorder, the controlling of opening and closing is abnormal, water aggregates in the body and generates edema." *Zhang's Medical Works-Division of Miscellaneous Diseases* says: "Renal diabetes in ancient times is called Super Strong in Yang, also called as internal diabetes." The edema and proteinuria documented in the above literature coincide with the symptoms of obesity-related nephropathy. It can be seen that most patients with obesity-related nephropathy have pathological products such as sputum, dampness and blood stasis. Turbid toxin theory holds that turbid toxin is generated from constant accumulation, coagulation and glue binding of pathological products such as sputum, blood stasis and dampness, which belong to blood stasis toxin, wet toxin, phlegm toxin, dry toxin and other aspects. The main pathological mechanism is deficient qi unable to transport blood, blood stagnation and stasis occurs because of blocking. Long time of blood stasis turns to be dampness, then transformed into turbid toxin. Dampness and heat burns and damages fluid and blood, fluid and blood coagulates and congested, transformed into turbid toxin with time passes; besides, cold evil invades human body and is transformed into heat, internal heat burn fluid and blood generating stasis, long stasis can also become turbid toxin, which is the toxin of external evil. Therefore, turbidity and toxin are the important pathogenesis of obesity-related kidney disease. Insufficient endowment, excessive taking of fat sweet thick and tasty food, emotional injury, excessive labour and sexual intercourse consumes qi and injures Yin, causing dual deficiency of qi and Yin. Qi deficiency obstruct the blood circulation, stagnation generates blood stasis. Yin deficiency generates internal heat, consumes blood, generates stasis and binding phlegm. Blood stasis resists in kidney collateral long time, generates evil toxin and obesity-related kidney disease.

肾为"先天之本"，脾为"后天之本"，两者在功能上相辅相成，互相促进。脾主运化、统血，输布水谷精微，为气血生化之源。肾藏精，主水，纳气。脾阳健运，气能津布，脾虚日久，则水谷不能化生精微，脏腑功能亏虚，肾精不足，脾肾同虚，开阖失司，清浊不分，精微不循常道而外泄。因此，肥胖相关性肾病的发病基础是脾虚，最终病位在肾，属于脾肾同病。

The kidney is the "congenital root", the spleen is the "acquired root", the two complement each other in function and promote each other. Spleen controls transporting and distributing of blood, spreading cereal essence, is the source to generate and transform qi and blood. Kidney stores essence, controls water, qi in-taking. When spleen yang works normally, qi can spread and distribute fluid. When spleen is deficient over time, the water valley can not brew essence, viscera function becomes deficient, kidney essence is deficient, spleen and kidney are both deficient, open and closing function does not work, lucidity and turbidity cannot be separated, cereal essence does not follow the usual way and leaks out. Therefore, the pathological basis of obesity-related nephropathy is spleen deficiency, the final location is in the kidney, belongs to dual disease of spleen and kidney.

因此，治疗肥胖相关性肾病应固护脾肾、化浊解毒并举。健脾补肾的同时，针对结滞经络、阻碍气血津液运行输布的无形之浊毒邪气，用茯苓、猪苓、泽泻、白术等淡渗利湿之品，健脾助运；用砂仁、茵陈、紫豆蔻、藿香、佩兰、木香、陈皮等芳香温化之品，醒脾健运。根据证机的不同，结合随证施治，助脾运化，则湿去浊化，毒无所依。用连翘、地榆、牡丹皮、玄参、栀子、黄芩、板蓝根等清热凉血之品，清除体内毒邪。并根据体内浊、毒邪气的偏胜不同，而侧重有所不同。浊重毒轻则化浊为主，解毒为辅；毒重浊轻则解毒为主，化浊为辅；浊邪与毒邪并重，则解毒化浊并重。然而诸药配合，重在化浊，使毒随浊去，以达解毒化浊之功效。

Therefore, the treatment of obesity - related nephropathy should strengthen the spleen and kidney, resolve turbidity and remove toxin simultaneously. While invigorating the spleen and tonifying kidney, regarding the invisible turbid toxin evil which stagnate in meridians and resist the operation and spreading of qi, blood, fluid and liquid, use medicines of dampness draining and disinhibiting as fu ling (Poria) zhu ling (Polygorus Umbellatus), ze xie (Rhizoma Alismatis), bai zhu (Rhizoma Atractylodis Macrocephalae) to reinforce spleen and assist transportation; use sha ren (Fructus Amomi), yin chen (Herba Artemisiae Scopariae), zi dou kou (Purple Cardamom Kernel), huo xiang (Herba Agastaches seu Pogostemonis), pei lan (Herba Eupatorii), mu xiang (Radix Aucklandiae) and chen pi (Pericarpium Citri Reticulatae), to invigorate the spleen and normalize the transportation. Use differential treament according to the different pathogenesis to help spleen to transport, dampness will be removed, turbidity will be resolved, toxin fails to survive. Use lian qiao (Forsythiae Fructus), di yu (Radix et Rhizoma Sanguisorbae), mu dan pi (Cortex Moutan), xuan shen (Radix Scrophulariae), zhi zi (Fructus Gardeniae), huang qin (Radix Scutellariae), ban lan gen (Radix Isatidis) and other products of clearing heat and cooling blood, to remove toxin evil in the body. Medication is made according to difference of priority and focusing of turbidity, toxin and evilness in the body. When turbidity is severe, toxin is light, lay stress on turbidity resolving, assisted by toxin removing; when toxin is severe, turbidity is light, lay stress on toxin removing, assisted by turbidity resolving; when turbidity is as severe as toxin, pay dual consideration to turbidity resolving and toxin removing. Generally speaking, the purpose of combination of different drugs is to lay stress on turbidity resolving, let the toxin be removed along with turbidity, so as to realize the effect of removing toxin and resolving turbidity.

第十章 代谢性疾病浊毒论
Chapter 10 On Turbid Toxin of Metabolic Diseases

第一节 高脂血症浊毒论
Section 1 On Turbid Toxin of Hyperlipidemia

一、病因
1. The etiology

（一）主要病因
1.1 Main causes

1.外因

1.1.1 External causes

（1）饮食不节，过食肥甘厚味：饮食不节，可损伤脾胃，导致脾胃的腐熟、运化功能失常。饮食不节主要表现为嗜食肥甘厚味和长期饱食等。

1.1.1.1 Diet is not regular, over-taking of fat, sweet, thick and tasty food: irregular diet can damage the spleen and stomach, resulting in the abnormal function of digesting and transporting of the spleen and stomach. Irregular diet is mainly manifested as in favor of fat, sweet, thick and tasty food and long-time of satiety.

（2）过度安逸，少有劳作：过逸少劳致使气血运行不畅，同样可致脾气虚弱，人体气血壅滞，水谷精微化生乏力，清浊混淆而发为高脂血症。

1.1.1.2 Excessive comfort, little work: excessive comfort and little work causes abnormal operation of qi and blood, can also cause weak spleen qi, stagnation of qi and blood in human body, inability to generate and transform water and grain essence, confusion of lucidity and turbidity, and results in hyperlipidemia.

（3）情志不遂，多思易怒：忧思伤脾，郁怒伤肝，情志过极可影响精、气、血、津液的正常化生和运行，致营养物质代谢障碍，痰饮、瘀血等病理产物生成。

1.1.1.3 Dissatisfied in emotion, more thinking and irritability: worried thinking hurts the spleen, depression anger hurts liver, extreme emotion can affect the normal generation, transformation and operation of essence, qi, blood, fluid liquid, causes obstruction of nutrient metabolism, generate phlegmatic retention, blood stasis and other pathological products.

2.内因

1.1.2 Internal causes

（1）脾失健运：是高脂血症最关键的病理基础。脾主运化，为后天之本、气血生化之源，膏脂的生成与转化皆有赖于脾的健运。若脾胃虚弱，脾失健运，则水谷精微失于输布，易致膏脂输化障碍而成高脂血症。

1.1.2.1 Abnormal transportation of the spleen: it is the most critical pathological basis of hyperlipidemia. The spleen controls transporting and transformation, is the acquired foundation of life, the source to generate and transform qi and blood, and the generation and transformation of paste lipid all depends on the normal transporting of the spleen. If the spleen and stomach are weak and the spleen transporting is abnormal, the water and grain essence cannot be transported and distributed, which causes transporting and transforming obstacle of ointment fat, finally generate hyperlipidemia.

（2）肾精亏虚，肾阳衰微：肾为先天之本，肾精亏虚，肾阳不足，则不能蒸化津液，于是脂凝液积而体肥胖。部分高血脂患者体常发胖，即阳虚气化功能衰退之象。

1.1.2.2 Deficiency of kidney essence, decline of kidney Yang: kidney is the congenital foundation of life, deficiency of kidney essence, kidney Yang deficiency, can not steam body fluid, so coagulation of lipid, accumulation of liquid are transformed into body obesity. Some patients with hyperlipidemia often get fat, that is the phenomenon of the gasification function decline due to Yang deficiency.

（3）肝失疏泄：肝失疏泄，气机失常，脏腑功能受累，气、血、津液运行失常，气机不利，气滞则血瘀、水停，津血运行失常，日久为痰为瘀，化生浊毒。

1.1.2.3 Dysfunction of liver dispersing: dysfunction of liver dispersing, abnormal operation of energy mechanism, increases load to the viscera function, qi, blood, fluid and liquid can not operation normally, causes qi stagnation, blood stasis, water retaining, which will be turned into phlegm and stasis, then transformed into turbid toxin.

（4）心阳痹阻：是指气血津液痹阻胞络的病理改变。心阳虚衰，不能温运血脉，即可以引起心脉不通，瘀血阻滞。七情所伤导致气机郁结，气滞血瘀，或因痰浊内阻脉络，皆可化生浊毒，造成心脉痹阻。

1.1.2.4 Heart Yang obstruction: refers to the pathological changes due to resistance of qi, blood, fluid, and liquid in pericardium collateral. As deficient heart Yang can not warm blood vessel, vessel blocking and obstruction of blood stasis might occur. Depression of qi mechanism, qi stagnation and blood stasis caused by injuries of seven emotions, or internal obstruction of phlegm turbidity in vessels, can be converted to turbid toxin resulting in pulse obstruction.

3.浊毒相干为致病的关键　内外因相合导致体内的"浊毒化"，形成浊毒内壅之势。浊性黏滞，易结滞脉络，阻塞气机，缠绵耗气；毒邪性烈善变，易化热耗伤阴精，壅腐气血。浊毒互结，胶着难愈，邪壅经络，气机不畅，邪不得散，血不得行，津不得布，津液停留，化生痰浊瘀血，日久痰浊、瘀浊相互搏结，反复日久，造成浊毒蕴壅，积滞络阻，脾不升清，胃失和降，阴血耗伤，气虚血郁的证机变化，而浊毒相干为致病的关键。

1.1.3 The involving of turbid toxin is the key pathogenic factor　The combination of internal and external causes leads to the "turbid toxin changes" in the body, forms the potential of internal accumulation of turbid toxin. The nature of turbidity is sticky, easy to be stagnated in veins, blocks qi mechanism, lingering and consuming qi; the nature of toxin is fierce and changeable, easy to be transformed into heat and wear out Yin essence, corrupts qi and blood. Agglutinating of turbidity and toxin, cemented and difficult to heal. Evil obstructs meridian, causes abnormal operation of qi mechanism. Evil cannot be dissipated, blood cannot move, fluid cannot be spread. Retaining of fluid liquid is transformed into turbid phlegm. Turbid phlegm and turbid stasis fights against and agglutinates with each other repeatedly, with time being, cause the syndrome changes of abundant accumulation of turbid toxin stagnates and resists collateral, the spleen cannot ascend lucidity, stomach fails to harmonize and descend, Yin blood is consumed and injured, with qi deficiency and blood depression, but involving of turbid toxin is the key factor to generate the disease.

（二）其他病因

1.2 Other causes

1.遗传及体质因素　原发性高脂血症多数是因遗传或先天体质影响，受之于先天，属先天之肾的范畴。由于先天真阴真阳不足，后天之本失却温煦推动，营血化生必受影响，轻则可致血脂代谢异常，重则可因严重的脂质代谢紊乱而夭亡。

1.2.1 Genetic and physical factors　Primary hyperlipidemia is mostly affected by genetic or congenital constitution, suffered from congenital, which belongs to the category of congenital kidney. Because of congenital deficiency of naive Yin and true Yang, the acquired foundation looses warm promotion, blood generation and transformation will be affected, as light result, it can cause abnormal metabolism of blood lipid, as severe result, patient might die of serious lipid metabolism disorder.

2.生活方式影响　不良饮食习惯、体力活动不足、肥胖、抽烟、酗酒等都是血脂升高的因素。

1.2.2 Influence of lifestyle　Bad diet habits, insufficient physical activity, obesity, smoking and alcohol abuse are all factors of elevated blood lipids.

3.年龄效应　随着年龄的增加，体重也会增加。老年人的低密度脂蛋白受体活性减退和低密度脂蛋白分解代谢率降低。绝经后妇女雌激素缺乏，血胆固醇会逐渐高于男性，已知在人类和哺乳动物中，雌激素能增加低密度脂蛋白受体的活性。

1.2.3 Age effect　Weight increases with ages. LDL receptor activity and LDL catabolism of old people will be reduced. Postmenopausal women have estrogen deficiency, blood cholesterol will be gradually higher than men. Estrogen is known to increase LDL receptor activity of human and mammals.

4.某些疾病导致继发性高脂血症　糖尿病、肾病综合征、肝脏疾病、甲状腺功能减退、多囊卵巢综合征等。

1.2.4 Certain diseases lead to secondary hyperlipidemia　such as diabetes mellitus, nephrotic syndrome, liver disease, hypothyroidism, polycystic ovary syndrome, etc.

5.长期应用某些药物可能引起高脂血症　糖皮质激素、噻嗪类利尿剂、β-受体阻滞剂、部分抗肿瘤药物等。

1.2.5 Long-term application of some drugs　May cause hyperlipidemia such as glucocorticoids, thiazide diuretics, beta-blockers, some anti-tumor drugs, etc.

二、病机
2. Pathogenesis

（一）脾胃虚弱，运化失常
2.1 Weak spleen and stomach, abnormal transporting

水谷精微的输布有赖于脾之运化，脾虚胃弱，气血生化不足，元气不能充，为浊毒的产生提供了可能。虽然浊、毒的产生皆有不同的途径，但均与脾失运化，脾不升清，胃失和降密切相关。另外浊毒结滞经络，阻碍气血津液运行输布，脾胃受困而不能运化，元气不能充足，气机不能通畅；浊毒积滞体内，脾胃升降受限，气机无法升降沉浮。如此邪不得散，津血停滞，日久进一步使浊毒加重。如此循环反复，使病情不断加重。

Spreading of water and grain essence depend on the transporting of the spleen. Deficient spleen and weak stomach cause insufficient generation and transformation of qi and blood, insufficient renal qi, provide the possibility to generate turbid toxin. Although turbid toxin is generated from different ways, but they are all closely related with dysfunction of spleen transportation, dysfunction of lucidity ascending of the spleen, and dysfunction of harmonious descending of the stomach. Besides, turbid toxin congests in meridians, obstructs the operation and spreading of qi, blood, fluid, and liquid, traps the spleen and stomach to loose function of transportation and digestion, the renal qi can not be sufficient, the operation of qi mechanism cannot be normal; when turbid toxin is accumulated in human body, the ascending and descending of spleen and stomach is restricted, the ascending and descending, rising and sinking of qi movement is abnormal. Therefore, evil cannot be dissipated, fluid and blood stays and stagnates, further aggravate turbid toxin. The process repeat in constant cycle aggravate the disease condition.

（二）肝失疏泄，痰湿内阻
2.2 Dysfunction of liver dispersing, internal resistance of phlegmatic hygrosis

肝主疏泄是保持脾胃正常消化吸收的重要条件，若肝失疏泄，犯脾克胃，必致脾胃升降失常，即可出现胃气不降、脾气不升等肝脾不调的症状，必致气机不调，影响气血的运行。气机阻滞，则气滞而血瘀。同时肝失疏泄，三焦气机阻滞，气滞则水停，从而导致水、湿、痰、饮内停。气血、津液、水饮、痰湿内阻，阻碍经脉气血运行，停滞于中，易于阻遏气机，壅塞脉道，致血运不畅，脉络瘀涩，痰瘀互结日久化热，变生浊毒，使脏腑气机升降失常。

Liver controlling dispersing is an important condition to maintain the normal digestion and absorption of the spleen and stomach. If the liver looses the function of dispersing, affects spleen and restrict the stomach, it will cause the abnormal ascending and descending of the spleen and stomach, cause symptoms of discord of liver and spleen which manifest as the stomach qi does not ascend, the spleen qi does not descend, it will cause abnormal operation of qi mechanism, affect the operation of qi and blood. When qi mechanism is resisted, qi stagnation and blood stasis occur. At the same time, liver looses the function of dispersing, qi mechanism is resisted in triple energizer, qi stagnation causes water staying, results in retaining of water, wet, phlegm, and drinking. The internal resistance of qi and blood, body fluid and liquid, water drink, phlegmatic hygrosis hinder the operation of qi and blood in meridians, easy to restrain the qi movement, obstruct the artery, affect the blood circulation, generate stasis and astringent in veins, agglutinating of phlegm and stasis for a long time transforms into heat, generates turbid toxin, leading to abnormal ascending and descending of the viscera qi mechanism.

（三）浊毒内蕴，脏腑失调，气血不和
2.3 Internal accumulation of turbid toxin, viscera disorder, discord of qi and blood

"浊"性黏滞、重浊，易结滞脉络、伤气浊血、阻塞气机，导致疾病缠绵难愈；"毒"性暴戾、顽固、多发、内损、染易，易耗气伤阴，损伤脏腑功能，致脏腑失调，其致病表现为凶险怪异、繁杂难治。浊与毒因性质相近，同气相求，而极易相生互助为虐，合为一体，如油入面，故以"浊毒"并称。

The nature of turbidity is sticky, easy to be stagnated in veins, affects qi and turbid the blood, blocks qi mechanism, making the diseases lingering and difficult to recover; the nature of toxin is fierce and stubborn, frequently encountered, internal injuring, easy to be infected, and consuming qi and injuring Yin, damaging viscera function, causing disorder of viscera, the pathogenic manifestation of toxin is fierce and monstrous, complicated and difficult to treat. The nature of turbidity and toxin is similar, like attracts like, easy to combine with and promote each other to do evil as a unity, just like mixing flour with oil, so the combined unity is called "turbid toxin".

浊毒之病理特性兼"浊""毒"两者之长，侵犯机体后具有暴戾性、迁延性、难治性、顽固性、传染性、正损性、增生性、广泛性等致病特性。浊毒致病具有"易耗气伤血，入血入络；易阻碍气机，胶滞难解；易积成形，败坏脏腑"的特点。浊毒既是疾病过程中的病理产物，也是疾病发生中重要的致病因素。

The pathological characteristics of turbid toxin has the advantages of both "turbidity" and "toxin", have the pathogenic characteristics of violence, delay, refractory, stubborn, infectious, destructive to healthy qi, proliferative and extensive after invading the body. The turbid toxin syndrome has the characteristics of "easy to consume qi and hurt blood, enter blood and collateral; hindering qi mechanism, glue-stagnated and difficult to be resolved; easy to accumulate and corrupt viscera". Turbid toxin is not only a pathological product in the disease process, but also an important pathogenic factor in disease generation.

三、治疗原则
3. Principles of treatment

（一）病证结合
3.1 Combination of disease and syndrome

高脂血症是一种病因病机较复杂的疾病，在分析病情时，首先要运用中医的辨证来认

识疾病，还要辨明高脂血症病理发展的阶段。这样将辨证与辨病很好地结合起来，才能整体把握疾病的程度及发展变化趋势，以便更好地指导治疗。

Hyperlipidemia is a disease with more complex etiology and pathogenesis. In the analysis of the disease condition, we should first use TCM syndrome differentiation to understand the disease, and also identify the stage of the pathological development of hyperlipidemia. In this way, the syndrome differentiation and disease differentiation can be well combined to grasp the overall degree and the development trend of the disease, so as to better guide the treatment.

在辨病与辨证相结合的过程中，还应充分考虑季节、地区、人的体质、年龄等不同而采用相应的治疗方法，即所谓因时、因地、因人制宜。

In the process of combining disease differentiation and syndrome differentiation, we should choose proper treatment method on the basis of fully considering the different season, region, human constitution, age of the patient, so-called "making treatment according to specific time, place and person".

（二）标本缓急，注重治本

3.2 To make treatment according to root, tip, gradual and urgent, laying stress on root treatment

高脂血症的治疗，应按照"急则治其标，缓则治其本"的原则。就其发病而言，脾胃虚弱、肝失疏泄、肾阳不足而化生湿浊、痰浊、血瘀，痰瘀在体内瘀积日久，瘀久化热，热毒侵袭，变成浊毒之证，治宜标本兼顾，在化浊解毒、祛瘀除湿的同时根据不同病因病机辨证分析，益气健脾、疏肝理气、温阳益肾以从根本祛除浊毒化生之源，而达到治病防变的效果。

The treatment of hyperlipidemia should be made according to the principle of "for urgent disease, treat the tip first; for gradual disease, first treat the root." Regarding the onset of hyperlipidemia, spleen and stomach weakness, dysfunction of liver dispersing, kidney Yang deficiency, generate damp turbidity, turbid phlegm, blood stasis, phlegmatic stasis, which are congested in the body, for long time, then transformed into heat, invaded by heat toxin, the disease become turbid toxin syndrome. To treat it, we should care both the root and the tip, while resolving the turbidity and removing the toxin, dispelling and removing the dampness, make syndrome differential analysis according to different etiology and pathogenesis, replenish qi and reinforce spleen, disperse liver and regulate qi, warm Yang and replenish kidney in order to fundamentally remove the source of turbid toxin generation and transformation, and achieve the effect of curing and preventing the disease.

（三）扶正祛邪，权衡轻重

3.3 Strengthening the healthy qi and dispelling evil, weighing the heavier and the lighter

扶正和祛邪是相互联系的两个方面。扶正是通过增强正气的方法，驱邪外出，从而恢复健康，即所谓"正盛邪自祛"。祛邪是消除致病因素的损害而达到保护正气，恢复健康的目的，即所谓"邪去正自安"。应以"扶正不致留邪，祛邪不致伤正"为度。具体如下。

Strengthening the healthy qi and dispelling evil are two interrelated aspects. Strengthening the healthy qi is to ward away evil by enhancing healthy qi, so as to restore health, so-called "Evil has to leave when healthy qi is sufficient". Eliminating evil is to eliminate the damage of pathogenic factors and achieve the purpose of protecting healthy qi and restoring health, so-called: "Healthy qi is safe when evil is eliminated". The specific degree and principle should be followed that "Strengthening healthy qi without leaving evil, dispelling evil without damaging healthy qi".

1.扶正　扶正适用于以正虚为主，而邪不盛实的虚证。

3.3.1 Strengthening healthy qi　Strengthening healthy qi is properly applicable to the asthenia syndrome manifested as asthenia in healthy qi but evil is not abundantly sthenia.

2.祛邪　适用于以邪实为主，而正未虚衰的实证。

3.3.2 Eliminating evil　It's adaptable to the syndrome of sthenia evil, but healthy qi is not declined yet.

3.先攻后补　即先祛邪后扶正。其适用于虽然邪盛、正虚，但正气尚可耐攻，以邪气盛为主要矛盾，若兼顾扶正反会助邪的病证。

3.3.3 First attacking then tonifying　First dispel evil then strengthening the healthy qi. It is applicable to the syndrome of sthenia evil, deficient healthy qi, but the healthy qi can still bear attacking. Sthenia evil is the main contradiction, taking into account the healthy qi will help evil.

4.先补后攻　即先扶正后祛邪。其适用于正虚邪实的虚实错杂证而正气虚衰不耐攻的情况。

3.3.4 First tonifying then attacking　First strengthen the healthy qi, then dispel the evil. It is applicable to the syndrome of mixture of asthenia and sthenia, with asthenia healthy qi and sthenia evil, but the healthy qi is too deficient to bear attacking.

5.攻补兼施　即扶正与祛邪并用。其适用于正虚邪实，但两者均不甚重的病证。具体运用时必须区别正虚邪实的主次关系，灵活运用。

3.3.5 Simultaneous attacking and tonifying　That is, to strengthen the healthy qi and dispel evil at the same time. It is adaptable to the syndrome of asthenia healthy qi and sthenia evil, but both are not very severe. In specific clinical practice, we must distinguish the priority relationship of asthenia healthy qi and sthenia evil, to use the method flexibly.

高脂血症的主要病因病机为浊毒内蕴、弥散入血，脾胃虚弱、运化失常，肝失疏泄、痰浊内阻，脏腑失调、气血不和，进而产生湿浊、痰瘀而化生浊毒，浊毒内蕴有进一步阻碍人体气血运行，影响脏腑功能，故在临床辨证治疗时，要分清疾病的病理阶段，辨明寒热虚实，对证施治，方可奏效。

The main etiology and pathogenesis of hyperlipidemia is internal accumulation of turbid toxin diffused into the blood, spleen and stomach weakness, dysfunction of transporting and transforming, liver looses the function of dispersing, phlegm turbidity resisted internally, viscera disorder, discord of qi and blood, and then produce wet turbidity, phlegm stasis which are transformed into turbid toxin. Internal accumulation of turbid toxin further hinder the operation of qi and blood, affect the viscera function. So in clinical syndrome differentiation treatment, doctors should make clear the pathological stage of the disease, distinguish cold, heat, asthenia and sthenia, suit the remedy to the disease, so as to make effect.

四、常用治疗方法
4. Common treatment methods

（一）化浊解毒法
4.1 Method of turbidity resolving and toxin removing

该法是高脂血症论治的关键，中医治疗过程的"化浊解毒"，就是要把浊毒化的病理产物，通过解毒化浊，使其重新回归到生理状态，参与到人体的代谢之中去。因此，在高脂血症的治疗方面，应注意适时应用芳香化浊、清热解毒法，并随症变通，从浊毒论治，以改善患者证候，逆转病势，此乃治疗高脂血症的关键环节。总结起来，化浊解毒药可分为淡渗利湿之品、苦寒燥湿之品、芳香化浊之品、化瘀解毒之品、疏肝理气之品等。即使对于以正虚为主者，辨治时在扶正方中酌加芳香化浊之品，亦有增效作用。从"治未病"角度而言，无论高脂血症患者辨证是浊毒盛为主还是正气虚为主，久病都可酿毒。尽早使用芳香化浊、清热解毒法可扭转病势。

This method is the key of the treatment of hyperlipidemia. "Resolving turbidity and removing toxin" in the process of TCM treatment is to return the pathological products of turbid toxin to the physiological state and participate in the metabolism of human body. Therefore, in the treatment of hyperlipidemia, attention should be paid to timely use the method of resolving turbidity with aroma, clearing heat and removing toxin, and make proper adjustment flexibly according to the syndrome. Treat from the turbid toxin to improve the syndrome of the patients and reverse the disease tendency, this is the key point in the treatment of hyperlipidemia. To sum up, the medicines of turbidity resolving and toxin removing can be divided into dampness draining and dissipating medicines, bitter, cold and dampness easing medicines, aroma and turbidity resolving medicines, blood stasis resolving toxin removing medicines, liver dispersing and qi regulating medicines etc. Even those who are mainly asthenia in healthy qi, the effect will be improved if we properly add some aroma and turbidity resolving medicines in differential treatment. From the perspective of "curing the future disease" no matter the syndrome differentiation of the hyperlipidemia patients is mainly excess in turbid toxin or deficient in healthy qi, long disease can brew toxin. Using aroma and turbidity resolving medicines and heat clearing and toxin removing medicines as early as possible can reverse the disease trend.

（二）祛湿化浊法
4.2 Method of dampness dispelling and turbidity resolving

调理脾胃、祛湿化浊是治疗血脂异常的常用方法。该方法针对引起血脂异常的"湿浊""痰饮""血瘀"或"痰瘀互阻"这一主要的病理机制，多从"痰浊""血瘀"入手，或祛痰化浊，或活血化瘀，或痰瘀同治，或祛邪扶正，总以恢复人体脏腑功能为宗旨。

To regulate the spleen and stomach, dissipate dampness and resolve turbidity is a common treatment method of dyslipidemia. This method aims at the main pathological mechanism of "wet turbidity", "phlegmatic retention", "blood stasis" or "phlegm stasis", which cause the abnormal lipid, to treat from "phlegm turbidity" and "blood stasis", dispel phlegm and resolve turbidity, promote blood circulation and resolve blood stasis, or to treat phlegm and stasis simultaneously, or dispel evil and strengthen the healthy qi, the final purpose is to restore the function of human viscera.

　　湿浊是脂代谢紊乱出现痰、瘀的根本，湿可生痰，渐次致瘀。津从浊化为膏，凝则为脂，一旦膏脂在体内的转输、排泄等发生异常，则化为病理性的脂浊痰湿，注入血脉，继而引发脂代谢紊乱。若脾失健运，升清降浊失调，运化水谷精微失司，水湿内停，聚湿生痰，滞留脉中，久则形成浊脂；病湿者又多有脾虚存在，导致水湿内停，阻滞气机，引起脏腑功能失调，水津停滞成饮，精化为浊，痰浊内聚，浊脂沉积形成脂代谢紊乱。若痰浊过重或日久，则必然妨碍气血运行，以瘀血相继。故而脾失健运生湿，进而生成痰浊瘀血，湿浊是疾病发生时最早出现的病理产物，健脾化浊祛湿是从源头治疗血脂异常的有效方法。

Wet turbidity is the basis to generate phlegm and stasis due to lipid metabolism disorder, wet can produce phlegm and gradually cause stasis. Fluid transforms from turbidity to ointment, when coagulated, it becomes lipid, once the transporting and discharging of paste and lipid in the body does not work normally, it becomes pathological lipid, turbidity, phlegm, and dampness, when they enter the blood veins, will cause lipid metabolism disorder. When the spleen looses normal transportation, disorder of lucidity ascending and turbidity descending, dysfunction of cereal essence transporting and transforming occur, water dampness stops internally, dampness aggregates to produce phlegm, all the above substances stay in the veins for a long time, will generate turbid lipid; most of the patients of dampness disease are deficient in the spleen, which causes water wet stopping internally, blocking the qi mechanism, lead to irregular function of viscera, water fluid stagnated into retention, essence transformed into turbidity, phlegm and turbidity aggregate inside, turbidity and lipid are deposited and generate lipid metabolism disorder. If the phlegm is too serious or stays long, it will inevitably hinder the operation of qi and blood, followed by stasis blood. Therefore, the spleen looses normal transportation and generates dampness, and then produces phlegm, turbidity and blood stasis. Wet turbidity is the earliest pathological product when the disease occurs, and reinforcing spleen, resolving turbidity and dispelling dampness is the effective method to treat dyslipidemia from the source.

（三）调理脾胃法
4.3 Method of regulating spleen and stomach

　　脾失健运是高脂血症形成的一个非常重要的病机，脾虚湿滞先于"痰浊""血瘀"产生，故健脾助运化浊祛湿法先用药，截断病势，能从源头治理血脂异常。即运用辛平芳香、健脾运化之品，祛除体内的陈腐浊毒之气，使脾运恢复，水谷精微得以吸收布散，脏腑得以受气血及津液濡养。同时根据临床辨证，分清虚实，并辅以益气养阴、清热解郁、化痰除湿、活血化瘀等法，做到辨病与辨证相结合，以求标本同治。当然我们在治疗时要注重整体观念，强调脾在高脂血症发展过程中的核心地位，但并不意味着因此而忽视肝、肾等脏腑。从上述病因病理看，治疗应以调理脾胃、消食导滞、化痰泄浊为主，佐以疏肝利胆、活血化瘀。

Dysfunction of spleen transportation is a very important pathogenesis for the generation of hyperlipidemia. Spleen deficiency and dampness stagnation occur before "phlegm turbidity" and "blood stasis". The method of reinforcing spleen, assisting transportation, resolving turbidity and dispelling the dampness first uses medicines to cut off the disease potential, can cure dyslipidemia from the source. That is, to use the medicines of acrid-peace and fragrance, medicines to reinforce the spleen and promote transporting, remove the stale and poisonous substance in the body, so as to restore the spleen transportation, ensure the absorption and spreading of cereal essence, nourish the viscera with qi, blood and body fluid and liquid. At the same time, according to the clinical syndrome differentiation, distinguish the asthenia and sthenia, supplemented by replenishing qi and nourishing Yin, clearing heat and relieving depression, resolving phlegm and dissipating dampness, promoting blood circulation and resolving blood stasis, combining disease differentiation with syndrome differentiation in order to treat both the root and the tip. Of course, we should pay attention to the wholistic concept in the treatment, emphasizing the core position of the spleen in the development process of hyperlipidemia does not mean that the liver, kidney and other viscera should be ignored. Observing the above etiology and pathology, the treatment should be mainly regulating the spleen and stomach, digesting food and conducting stagnation, resolving phlegm and purging turbidity, assisted with soothing the liver and dissipating the gallbladder, promoting blood circulation and removing blood stasis.

五、高脂血症浊毒证的分期、分层治疗
5. Stage and stratified treatment of hyperlipidemia syndrome

浊毒既可以是高脂血症发病的始动机制，也是病程进展中多种因素相互作用的结果，并主导着病机的变化，贯穿疾病的全程。

Turbid toxin is not only be the initiation generation mechanism of hyperlipidemia, but also the result of the interaction of various factors in the course of the disease, and dominate the changes of the pathogenesis throughout the whole course of the disease.

病变早期，"浊毒"初生，以浊为主，此阶段往往临床症状隐匿不显，患者化验检查时发现血脂升高。病变中期，浊毒渐盛，胶结不去而变生百病，临床症状开始显现或明显。若浊毒之邪害清，壅塞清窍，常表现为头昏沉、眩晕，浊毒之邪困脾则乏力、纳差、困倦等。此阶段往往邪气盛实而正气不虚。病变后期，浊毒壅滞，以毒为主，并深入脉络，正气渐亏，最终因毒损脏腑之不同而表现出心、脑、肾等受损症状，病情复杂而缠绵难愈。故在临床治疗中也应分期论治，根据浊毒化生的不同阶段，辨证施治。

In the early stage of the pathological process, "turbid toxin" is initially generated, mainly turbidity, clinical symptoms in this stage are usually vague, patients find lipid elevated in chemical examination. In the middle stage of the pathological process, turbid toxin is gradually abundant, cemented and generate various diseases. Clinical manifestation becomes obvious and significant, if the turbid toxin evil affects the lucidity, obstructed in the clean orifices, patients see dizziness, vertigo and fatigue, poor appetite, drowsiness due to evil of turbid toxin trapping the spleen, in this stage, the evil is excess, but the healthy qi is not deficient. In the late stage of the pathological process, turbid toxin is abundantly stagnated, toxin dominates, which enter the vessels, the healthy qi gradually becomes deficient, finally manifesting symptoms of damages in the heart, brain, and kidney due to different degree of injuries made by toxin to the viscera. The disease condition is complicated lingering and difficult to recover. Therefore, in the clinical practices doctors should treat by stages, make syndrome differentiation treatment according to the different stages of turbid toxin generation and transformation.

浊毒致病具有难治性、顽固性的特点，因此分离浊毒，孤立邪势，是治疗的关键。浊邪秽浊不清，故治以芳香化浊、渗湿化浊、健脾化浊、通腑泄浊、行气降浊等。毒由热生，变由毒起，毒不除，变必生，故治以清热解毒、通络解毒等。浊毒病邪有轻、中、重的相对划分，治疗上也要根据浊毒病邪之轻重分而治之。治疗浊毒应根据邪之浅深、病之新久、在气、在血以及是否入络成积等情况分层选药。芳香化浊常选用藿香、佩兰、砂仁等芳香之品运脾化浊；渗湿化浊取猪苓、泽泻之淡渗之品；健脾化浊用茯苓、白术、山药等。治毒按照毒之浅深量邪用药：毒轻者常用板蓝根、连翘、金银花、黄连、黄芩等；毒重者可选用全蝎、蜈蚣之属；毒邪介于轻与重之间者用半边莲、半枝莲、白花蛇舌草、败酱草、冬凌草等。

Turbid toxin syndrome has the characteristics of refractory and stubbornness, so separating turbidity and toxin, isolation of evil tendency is the key to treatment. As turbidity evil is foul, so it should be treated with method of resolving turbidity with aroma, resolving turbidity by draining dampness, resolving turbidity by reinforcing the spleen, purging turbidity by unblocking fu-organs, reducing turbidity by moving qi, etc. Toxin is generated from heat, changes are made from toxin, if toxin is not removed, pathological changes will surely take place, so the treatment should use the method of removing toxin by clearing heat and removing toxin by unblocking collateral. There is a relative division of light, medium and heavy degree of turbid toxin evil. It should also be treated according to the severity of turbid toxin disease evil. In the treatment of turbid toxin, drugs should be selected according to the shallow and depth of evil, recent occurrence or long history of disease, in qi, in blood, and whether has entered the collateral and formed accumulation. Medicines to resolve turbidity with aroma: huo xiang (Herba Agastaches seu Pogostemonis), pei lan (Herba Euopatori), sha ren (Fructus Amomi) and are often used to transport the spleen and resolve turbidity. Medicines for draining and resolving turbidity: zhu ling (Polygorus Umbellatus) and ze xie (Rhizoma Alismatis). Medicines for reinforcing the spleen and resolving turbidity: fu ling (Poria), bai zhu (Rhizoma Atractylodis Macrocephalae) and shan yao (Discoreae Rhizoma). Dosage of drugs is used according to the shallow and depth of the toxin: ban lan gen (Radix Isatidis), lian qiao (Forsythiae Fructus), jin yin hua (Lonicerae Japonicae Flos), huang lian (Rhizoma Coptidis), huang qin (Radix Scutellariae) are generally used for patients with lighter toxin; quan xie (Scorpio) and wu gong (Scolopendra) are used for patients with severe toxin; ban bian lian (Herba Lobelcae Radicantis), ban zhi lian (Scutellariae Barbatae Herba), bai hua she she cao (Herba Oldenlandiae Diffusae), bai jiang cao (Herba Patriniae), and dong ling cao (Rabdosiae Rubescentis Herba) are used for patients with toxin between lightness and severity.

六、常见辨证论治
6. Syndrome differentiation treatment generally used

近代医家根据自己及前人的经验，在中医药辨证治疗高脂血症上有着各种尝试，收效显著。综合各位医家的临床治疗经验，可大致总结为以下几种证型：痰湿阻遏型、痰浊内阻型、湿热壅滞型、气血瘀滞型、痰瘀阻滞型、脾肾阳虚型、气阴两虚型、肝肾阴虚型、气虚血瘀型。高脂血症临床辨证分型虽多，但根据其病因病机，首要应从浊毒内蕴分析，以化浊解毒为治疗宗旨。

Modern doctors have made various kinds of efforts on the TCM syndrome differentiation treatment of hyperlipidemia according to the experiences of the predecessors, have made significant effect. Summarizing the clinical treatment experience of modern doctors, patterns of syndromes include the following aspects: resistance of phlegmatic hygrosis, internal resistance of phlegmatic retention, abundant stagnation of dampness and heat, congestion of qi and blood, obstruction of phlegm and stasis, deficiency of spleen kidney Yang, dual deficiency of qi and Yin, deficiency of liver, kidney and Yin, qi deficiency and blood stasis. Although there are many clinical syndrome differentiation of hyperlipidemia, but according to its etiology and pathogenesis, the most important analysis should be made from internal accumulation of turbid toxin, the principal aim of the treatment is resolving turbidity abd removing toxin.

现代研究认为，血中总胆固醇、三酰甘油和低密度脂蛋白升高是高脂血症痰浊的主要特征和生化物质基础。浊毒症状为诊断高脂血症的外在特征，表现为面色浮肿，口唇紫红，舌质紫暗，脉象弦滑。基础方药如下：三棱、莪术、郁金、丹参、茵陈、黄连、砂仁、香附、苏梗、何首乌、桑葚。本方中三棱、莪术、郁金为一组药。三棱、莪术疏肝气，畅心血，解郁滞，伍以凉血活血、解郁除烦之郁金，共名为三郁，统治一切郁证以心烦、抑郁胀闷为主要表现者。其用于治疗高脂血症，效果良好，确有畅郁降脂祛浊的治疗作用。丹参养血活血，通达血脉。茵陈、黄连用于化浊解毒，两药合用具有清解肠胃浊毒的作用，为防其苦寒败胃，加入砂仁以佐制。香附、紫苏梗疏肝理气，和胃降逆；何首乌、桑葚补益肝肾，扶正降脂。全方标本兼治，可以久服，具有良好的近期和远期疗效。

Modern studies believe that elevated total cholesterol, triacylglycererol and low-density lipoprotein in blood are the main characteristics and biochemical material basis of hyperlipidemia. The symptoms of turbid toxin are the external features of the diagnosis of hyperlipidemia: swollen complexion, purple lips, purple dark tongue, and string sippery pulse. The basic prescription is as follows: san leng (Rhizoma Sparganii), e zhu (Rhizoma Curcumae), yu jin (Radix Curcumae), dan shen (Salviae Miltiorrhizae), yin chen (Herba Artemisiae Scopariae), huang lian (Rhizoma Coptidis), sha ren (Fructus Amomi), xiang fu (Rhizoma Cyperi), su geng (Caulis Perillae), he shou wu (Radix Polygoni Multiflori), sang shen (Mori Fructus). San leng (Rhizoma Sparganii), e zhu (Rhizoma Curcumae), yu jin (Radix Curcumae) is one medicine group. San leng (Rhizoma Sparganii), e zhu (Rhizoma Curcumae) which sooth the liver and regulate the qi, unblock the circulation of blood, can remove depression and stagnation, cooperated with yu jin (Radix Curcumae) with function of cooling and promoting the blood circulation, removing depression and eliminating restless rage. This group of three medicines is called San Yu (three medicines specially for depression releasing), can cure all kinds of depression syndromes which is manifested as restlessness in mind, depressing and distention bored, and make significant effect in treatment of blood, stagnation. To cool blood circulation, remove depression, depression gold, a total name of Three Yu, rule all depression to upset, depression as the main manifestations. It is used in the treatment of hyperlipidemia. Dan shen (Salviae Miltiorrhizae) promotes and nourishes blood circulation, dredges blood veins. Yin chen (Herba Artemisiae Scopariae) and huang lian (Rhizoma Coptidis) are used to resolve turbidity and remove toxin. The combination of the two drugs has the effect to clear the and remove gastrointestinal turbid toxin. In order to prevent the bitter cold medicine from spoiling the appetite, sha ren (Fructus Amomi) is added to restict it. Xiang fu (Rhizoma Cyperi) , zi su geng (Caulis Perillae), soothe liver and regulate qi, and harmonize the stomach to downbear the counterflow; he shou wu (Polygoni Multiflori Radix), sang shen (Mori Fructus) tonify and replenish liver and kidney, strengthen the healthy qi and reduce lipid. The whole prescription pays dual attention to treatment of the root and the tip, can be taken for a long time with present and future efficacy.

第二节　糖尿病浊毒论
Section 2 On Turbid Toxin of Diabetes

一、糖尿病的病因病机
1. The etiology and pathogenesis of diabetes

糖尿病是一种常见的内分泌代谢疾病，属于中医学"消渴病"的范畴。本文总结李佃贵教授多年临床经验，从"热毒"论治消渴并对其病因病机、辨证论治进行深入探讨。

Diabetes is a common endocrine and metabolic disease, belonging to the category of "xiaoke disease" of TCM. This paper summarizes professor Li Diangui's years of clinical experience of treating the diabetes from "heat toxin" and discusses the syndrome differentiation treatment according to the etiology and pathogenesis of the disease.

（一）饮食因素
1.1 Diet factors

随着现在人们生活水平的提高，饮食结构发生改变，长期嗜食肥甘、醇酒厚味、腥腻辛辣之物，以致脾失运化，湿热蕴生，积久为毒，热毒互结，消谷耗津，而发为消渴。

With the improvement of people's living standards, the diet structure has changed, long-term appetite for fat and sweet, alcohol, greasy and spicy things, cause the dysfunction of spleen transportation, accumulate and generate dampness and heat, which transforms into toxin with time being. Agglutinating of heat and toxin consumes grains and fluid and results in diabetes.

（二）情志因素
1.2 Emotional factor

当今社会生活方式加快，社会竞争激烈、人际关系紧张，这种长期过度的精神刺激致使肝气郁结，气机不疏，气滞则血瘀，血液壅滞不行，则郁久化火成毒，灼伤脾胃阴津而发为消渴。

Today's social life style change is accelerated, social competition is fierce, interpersonal relation becomes tension, this long-term excessive mental stimulation causes liver depression and qi stagnation, abnormal operation of qi mechanism. Qi stagnation generates blood stasis, abundant stagnation of blood will be transformed into fire and toxin in a long time, which burns the spleen and stomach, damages the Yin fluid, results in diabetes.

（三）体质因素
1.3 Factor of physical constitution

早在春秋战国时代，即已认识到先天禀赋不足是引起消渴病的重要内在因素。《灵枢·五变》谓："五脏皆柔弱者，善病消瘅。"尤其以阴虚体质最易罹患。阴虚体质之人体内津液精血等阴液亏虚，阴不制阳，阳热之气相对偏旺而生内热，引发消渴。

Early in the Spring and Autumn and the Warring States times, it had been realized that insufficient congenital endowment is an important internal factor to generate diabetes. *Spiritual Pivot-Five Changes* says: "When five viscera are all weak, Xiaodan (diabetes) disease occurs." Especially people with constitution of Yin deficiency is most probably to suffer from. People with constitution of Yin deficiency are usually deficient in Yin fluid including body fluid, liquid, essence and blood, Yin can not restrict Yang, the qi of Yang heat is relatively prosperous to generate internal heat, causing diabetes.

（四）劳欲过度
1.4 Excessive desire and exercises, excessive sexual intercourse

房事不节，劳欲过度，肾精亏损，虚火内生，则火因水竭益烈，水因火烈而益干，终致肾虚、肺燥、胃热俱现，发为消渴。如《外台秘要·消渴消中》说："房室过度，致令肾气虚耗，下焦生热，热则肾燥，肾燥则渴。"

Excessive desire and exercises, wears out the kidney essence loss, generates internal deficient fire, fire will be more fierce due to water exhaustion, water will be worn out due to fierce fire, eventually causes kidney deficiency, lung dryness, heat in stomach, resulting in diabetes. Such as *Collection of Secret Prescriptions Outside Palace-Xiaoke, Xiaozhong* says: "excessive sexual intercourse wears out kidney qi, heat is generated in lower energizer, heat makes kidney dry, dry kidney leads to diabetes."

（五）热毒
1.5 Heat poison

热毒是消渴的基本病机，并贯穿于消渴病程的始终。根据《黄帝内经》中的有关论述，并且按照消渴自身的发生发展及病变规律，消渴可分为脾瘅期、消渴期、消瘅期。

Heat poison is the basic disease machine of thirst elimination, and throughout the course of thirst elimination. According to the relevant discussion in *The Medical Classic of The Yellow Emperor*, and according to the occurrence and development of thirst itself and the law of lesions, thirst can be divided into spleen hate period, thirst period and depression period.

（六）其他因素
1.6 Other factors

1.遗传因素　目前尚不清楚，但现在清楚的是糖尿病遗传不是糖尿病本身，而是容易得糖尿病的体质，是容易得糖尿病的基因类型，有望逐步揭开并运用基因疗法彻底防治。

1.6.1 Genetic factors　It is not clear whether there is any genetic factor for diabetes generation, but it is clear that the inheritance of diabetes is not diabetes itself, but the constitution which is prone to diabetes, and the gene type which is easy to get diabetes. It is expected to gradually reveal and completely cure the diabetes with gene therapy.

2.环境因素　主要有感染、肥胖、饮食、体力活动、妊娠等，另外随着年龄的增长，糖尿病的患病率也显著上升。

1.6.2 Environmental factors　Mainly includes infection, obesity, diet, physical activity, pregnancy, etc. In addition, with the increase of age, the prevalence of diabetes will increase significantly.

二、治疗原则
2. Principles of treatment

（一）预防为主

2.1 Prevention as the priority

糖尿病慢性并发症的发生发展是一个长期慢性的过程，必须坚持未病先防、既病防变的中心思想。有两个措施：一是严格控制血糖；二是活血化浊通络。

The occurrence and development of chronic complications of diabetes is a long-term chronic process, so we must adhere to the central idea of preventing the occurrence before the disease occurs and preventing against deterioration when the disease exists. There are two measures: one is strictly controlling the blood sugar; the other is promoting blood circulation, resolving turbidity and unblocking the collateral.

（二）综合调控

2.2 Comprehensive regulation

糖尿病患者往往合并有高血压、高血脂、高血黏度、肥胖等，这一系列代谢障碍的问题是代谢综合征的组成成分，其相互之间存在着共同的病理基础——胰岛素抵抗。只有对胰岛素抵抗及其相关的代谢综合征进行积极治疗才能有效防治糖尿病慢性并发症。而西药在这些病症的治疗上是有效的，中药必须与之相配合，从气、血、痰、瘀、湿、食六郁的角度入手，通过散"郁"，正其气化，改善诸多代谢的异常。

Diabetes patients often have complicated diseases as hypertension, hyperlipidemia, high blood viscosity, obesity, etc. This series of metabolic disorders are the components of the metabolic syndrome, which has a common pathological basis -- insulin resistance. Only active treatment of insulin resistance and its associated metabolic syndrome can effectively prevent the occurrence of chronic complications of diabetes. Western medicine is effective in the treatment of these diseases, Chinese medicine must cooperate with western medicine to improve various kinds of metabolic disorder through dispersing "depression", restoring gasification from the perspective of six depression including qi, blood, phlegm, stasis, dampness, and food.

（三）化浊解毒

2.3 Resolving turbidity and removing toxin

浊毒内瘀是贯穿消渴病并发症始终的一条病机主线，这与现代医学认为糖尿病是以血管病变为核心的认识是一致的。虽然在不同的阶段浊毒内瘀的机制不同，但单纯通过清热、滋阴、益气、温阳等病因治疗往往疗效较差，所以必须重视化浊解毒药的使用，临床常用化浊解毒、活血化瘀之品。

Internal accumulation of turbid toxin is a dominant pathogenesis line throughout the process of diabetes complications, it agrees with modern medical science which believes that the core of diabetes is pathological change of vascular. In different stages, the mechanism of internal stasis might be different, thus simply clearing heat, enriching Yin, replenishing qi, warming Yang can not make sound effect. So we should lay stress on application of medicines of resolving turbidity and removing toxin, in clinical practice, products of turbidity resolving, toxin removing and blood circulation promoting and blood stasis resolving are generally used.

（四）中医辨证与西医分期相结合

2.4 Combination of TCM syndrome differentiation and western medicine stage differentiation

糖尿病慢性并发症是一个逐渐发展的病变，从中医学来讲，其病机及证型也是一个动态演变的过程。临床上只有抓住其病机的主要方面，掌握其基本的动态演变规律，才能知常达变，拥有治疗的主动权。

Diabetes chronic complications is a gradual development of lesions, in terms of Chinese medicine, the pathogenesis and syndrome pattern is also a dynamic evolution process. Clinically, unless grasping the main aspects of the pathogenesis, mastering the basic rule of dynamic evolution, we can learn the usual method and understand how to deal with the changes, own the initiative power of treatment.

（五）中西医结合，互补不足

2.5 Combine TCM with western medicine, inter-supplement the shortcoming of each other

在糖尿病慢性并发症的临床治疗中，必须发挥中西医各自的优势，有机结合，才能收到最好的防治效果。

In the clinical treatment of chronic complications of diabetes, the advantages of TCM and western medicine must be fully developed and organically combined in order to receive the best prevention and treatment effect.

总之，在糖尿病及其慢性并发症的中医治疗中，应始终把握浊毒这条主线，坚持预防为主、综合调控的思想，恰当运用中、西医两个治疗手段，才能真正达到防止糖尿病及其慢性并发症的发生，延缓慢性并发症进展的目的。

In short, in the TCM treatment of diabetes and its chronic complications, we should always grasp the main line of turbid toxin, adhere to the idea of preventing first and regulating comprehensively, appropriately use two measures of Chinese and western medicine, so as to truly realize the propose of preventing the occurrence of diabetes and chronic complications and delay the progress of chronic complications.

三、常用治疗方法
3. Common treatment methods

（一）化浊解毒，以治其本
3.1 Resolving turbidity and removing toxin to treat the root

血浊内瘀是糖尿病胰岛素抵抗之启动因素，现代医学认为胰岛素抵抗是多数糖尿病发病的始动原因，而血浊生成于糖尿病之始，也是胰岛素抵抗的主要启动因素，继续发展则又是持续高血糖状态并产生毒性的病理基础。

Internal stasis of blood turbidity is the initiating factor of diabetes insulin resistance. Modern medicine believes that insulin resistance is the initial cause of most diabetes, and blood turbidity occurs at the beginning of diabetes, which is also the main initiating factor of insulin resistance, and in further development is the pathological basis of continuous hyperglycemia state and generation of toxin.

李佃贵教授认为，情志、外邪或饮食等均可损伤脾胃。脾胃功能失调，则气机不畅，津液不布，水湿内生，积而成浊；水湿痰饮食积郁结体内，日久化热，蕴热入血为毒，耗伤机体气血津液，瘀阻脉络，酿生浊毒，发为消渴。浊毒蕴热，上可灼肺津，中可劫胃液，下可耗肾水；或灼伤血脉，或浊伤阳气而致阴疽之证。消渴的发病机制复杂，阴虚燥热、气阴两虚、气滞、血瘀、食积、肝风、痰湿、瘀浊、热毒等因素相夹为患，呈现出虚实错杂之证，应提早开展治疗，延缓病情进展，因此化浊解毒大法应贯穿于消渴病治疗之始终。

Professor Li Diangui believes that emotion, external evil or diet can damage the spleen and stomach. Irregular function of spleen and stomach causes abnormal operation of qi mechanism, abnormal spreading of fluid liquid, endogenous generation of water dampness, which will accumulate into turbidity; Water wet, phlegmatic retention, and food retention are stagnated in human body, will be transformed into heat with time being, accumulated heat enters blood and will turn to be toxin, consumes qi, blood, fluid, liquid, congest veins, brew turbid toxin, result in diabetes. Turbid toxin with accumulated heat, can burn lung fluid in upper energizer, can rob gastric liquid in middle energizer, can consume kidney water in lower energizer; or burn and injure blood veins, or burn and injure Yang and cause Yin gangrene. The pathogenesis of diabetes is complex, Yin deficiency, dryness and heat, dual deficiency of qi and Yin, qi stagnation, blood stasis, food retention, liver wind, phlegmatic hygrosis, turbid stasis, heat toxin and other factors inter-mixed to do evil, showing the syndrome mixed with asthenia and sthenia, should be treated in advance to delay the progress of the disease, so the big method of turbidity resolving and toxin removing should be carried out throughout the treatment of diabetes disease.

综上所述，将化浊解毒大法贯穿于糖尿病治疗的始终，排出或消散体内浊毒，促进机体新陈代谢，使浊毒去，气血畅，脾运复健，胃复和降，肝气条达，人体紊乱的内环境归于平衡，徐徐图之，效果显著。

To sum up, the method of turbidity resolving and toxin removing runs through the treatment process of diabetes to discharge or dissipate the turbid toxin from the body, promote the metabolism, make the turbid toxin disappear, make circulation qi and blood smooth, restore spleen transportation and stomach harmonizing and descending, make liver qi free and regulated, the internal environment of human disorder return to balance, and the effect will be remarkable with continous treatment.

（二）疏达气机，以畅津血

3.2 Releasing the movement to improve the circulation of fluid and blood

从无形之气到有形之痰瘀是许多疾病的共同特征，糖尿病本乃代谢性疾病，表现为糖、脂代谢失常，其形成机制包括各种致病因素作用于机体，导致气化失常从而引起气机阻滞，而致气血津液的流变障碍，精微物质不归正化而成痰、湿、浊、毒等病理产物滞留于体内，影响脏腑功能，而脏腑功能紊乱，脾胃升降失调、肝气疏泄失常、肾阳不足、三焦失常也必然能引起气化的异常，导致糖尿病。

Developing from invisible qi to tangible phlegm stasis is a common feature of many diseases, diabetes is originally a metabolic disease, manifested as sugar, lipid metabolism disorder, its pathological mechanism includes the reaction of various pathogenic factors on the body causes abnormal gasification, obstruction of qi movement, which lead to rheological obstacle of qi, blood, fluid and liquid. Cereal essence can not be normally transformed but turn to be phlegm, dampness, turbidity, toxin and other pathological products. They stranded in the body, affecting viscera function. Viscera dysfunction is manifested as abnormal operation of ascending and descending of the spleen and stomach, irregular dispersing of liver qi, deficiency of kidney Yang, abnormal work of triple energizer, which can inevitably cause abnormal gasification, lead to diabetes.

情志因素是糖尿病发展过程中不可忽视的因素。《冯氏锦囊秘录》言："七情偏胜，五脏失和，则偏害之病生矣。"情志因素导致脏腑气化失常，肝气郁结，失于疏泄而脾失健运，升降失常，气化不畅则气机郁滞，郁久则化火，聚湿生痰。故临床可予小柴胡汤寒湿并治，升降协调，疏少阳瘀滞，消胸腹蕴热，调达上下，宣通内外，和畅气机。

The emotional factor is a factor which should not be ignored in the development of diabetes. In *Feng's Secret Recor*, it says, "When the seven emotions are partially abundant, the five viscera are in disharmony, and the partial disease is born." Emotional factors lead to dysfunction of viscera gasification, depression of liver qi, dysfunction of liver dispersing and spleen transportation, abnormal operation of ascending and descending. Dysfunction of gasification causes stagnation of qi movement, prolonged stagnation turns to be fire, aggregation of dampness generates phlegm. Therefore, in clinical practice, prescription of Xiao Chaihu Decoction (the small Bupleuri soup) is used to deal with cold and dampness, regulate ascending and descending, sparse Shaoyang stasis retention, dissipate accumulated heat in thoracoabdomen, adjust the movement of up and down, diffuse and unblock the movement of inside and outside, and harmonize the operation of qi movement.

（三）益气养阴，以复其本

3.3 Replenishing qi and nourishing Yin to recover the root

糖尿病的临床表现，以口渴、多饮、多食、多尿、乏力等为其特点，一般多从燥热论治。然除滋阴清热外，补气之法亦不可忽视，盖津亏不能化气，气虚不能生津。而脾胃为气之枢纽，肺为气之主，肾为气之根，故当代中医名家多以气阴双补，重视调补肺脾肾之气以治之。

The clinical manifestations of diabetes is characterized by thirsty, more drinking, more eating, more urination, fatigue, treatment is generally made from dryness and heat. But in addition to nourishing Yin and clearing heat, method of qi tonification should not be ignored, because deficient fluid can not gasify, qi deficiency cannot generate fluid. The spleen and stomach is the hub of qi, lung, kidney is the root of the qi, so most of the contemporary TCM masters use the method of dual reinforcement of qi and Yin, pay attention to reinforcing qi of the lung, of spleen and of kidney.

（四）清热燥湿，以治其标

3.4 Clear heat and dry dampness in order to treat the tip

糖尿病多见咽燥、口干欲饮、口苦、口中黏腻、大便干结、舌苔黄腻难化等热象。《素问·奇病论》曰："有病口甘者……名曰脾瘅……此人必数食甘美而多肥也。肥者令人内热，甘者令人中满，故其气上溢，转为消渴。"疾病过程中，既可见湿热、燥热、瘀热，又可见气机不畅而成郁热、阳明热盛之结热，因而治疗糖尿病在益气、养阴、补虚的同时亦要重视多法清热。

Most of the patients of diabetes have dry throat, dry mouth with want to drink, bitter and sticky mouth, dry stool, yellow and greasy tongue moss which is difficult to resolve and other hot images. In *Simple Conversation-Discussion on Special Diseases*, it is said, "Diseases marked by sweet taste in the mouth... named Pidan (spleen heat)... patients must have frequently eaten sweet, tasty, and fat food, which produce interior heat. Sweet flavour makes people feel full in stomach, so the qi adverse flows and turns to be Xiaoke (diabetes)." In the process of disease, patients have damp heat, dry heat, stasis heat, and depressed heat when the qi movement is not smooth, stagnated heat when Yangming is excessively heat. So in the treatment of diabetes, while replenishing qi, nourishing Yin, reinforcing deficiency, attention should also be paid to multiple methods of heat clearing.

（五）活化瘀浊之血，以生新防变

3.5 Activate the turbid stasis blood to generate new blood and prevent pathological changes

《灵枢·五变》最早提出瘀血与消渴之间的关系，现代研究报道亦指出，糖尿病患者血液有高凝、高聚集、高浓度、高黏滞状态，其常见并发症有动脉硬化、中风偏瘫、冠心病、高血压、视网膜病变等，莫不与血瘀有关。瘀血既是一个致病因素，又是一个病理产物，瘀血既可引起糖尿病，病后又易产生瘀血，使病情加重，从而引发各种并发症。

Spiritual Pivot-Five Changes first points out the relationship between stasis and diabetes, it is reported also in modern research that diabetic blood has the state of high coagulation, high aggregation, high concentration, high sticky, the common complications include arteriosclerosis, stroke hemiplegia, coronary heart disease, hypertension, retinopathy, etc. which is all related to blood stasis. Blood stasis is not only a pathogenic factor, but also a pathological product. Blood stasis can cause diabetes, and diabetes can easily generate blood stasis, further aggravating the disease condition, leading to various complications.

四、常见辨证论治
4. The general syndrome differentiation treatment

中医学普遍认为糖尿病病机以阴虚为本，燥热为标，故多以清热润燥、养阴生津为本病的治疗大法。《医学心悟·三消》曰："治上消者，宜润其肺，兼清其胃"；"治中消者，宜清其胃，兼滋其肾"；"治下消者，宜滋其肾，兼补其肺"。其具体辨证论治如下。

Traditional Chinese Medicine generally believes that the root of diabetes pathogenesis is Yin deficiency, the tip is dry and heat. So the method of clearing heat and lubricating dryness, nourishing Yin and generating fluid is generally regarded as the treatment principle. *Medical Enlightenment- Sanxiao* says: "to cure Shangxiao (diabetes in upper energizer), should moisten its lungs and clear its stomach"; "to cure Zhongxiao (diabetes in the middle energizer), should clear the stomach and enrich its kidney"; "to cure Xiaxiao (diabetes in lower energizer), should nourish the kidney and tonify the lungs". The specific syndrome differentiation treatment is as follows.

（一）上消（肺热津伤证）
4.1 Shangxiao (diabetes in upper energizer), lung heat with fluid damage

1.临床表现　口渴多饮，口舌干燥，尿频量多，烦热多汗，舌边尖红，苔薄黄；脉洪数。

4.1.1 Clinical manifestations　Thirsty with more drinking, polydipsia, dry in mouth and tongue, frequent and more quantity of urination, restless hot and sweating, red edge and tip of the tongue, thin yellow moss, bounding and rapid pulse.

2.证机概要　肺脏燥热，津液失布。

4.1.2 Overview of pathogenesis　Hot and dry in lung, and dysfunction of fluid spreading.

3.治法　清热润肺，生津止渴。

4.1.3 Method of treatment　Clearing heat and moistening lung, generating fluid and stopping thirst.

4.代表方　消渴方加减。本方清热降火，生津止渴，适用于消渴肺热津伤之证。

4.1.4 Representative prescription　Xiaoke Prescription with addition and reduction. This prescription can clear heat and downbear fire, generate fluid and quench thirst, suitable for disease of Xiaoke (diabetes) manifested as lung heat and fluid damages.

5.常用药　天花粉、葛根、麦冬、生地黄、藕汁生津清热，养阴增液；黄连、黄芩、知母清热降火。

4.1.5 Medicines generally used   Tian hua fen (Radix Tricosanthis), ge gen (Radix Puerariae), mai dong (Radix Ophiopogonis), sheng di huang (Radix Rehmanniae), ou zhi (juice of Nelumbinis) to clear heat, nourish Yin and increase fluid; huang lian (Rhizoma Coptidis), huang qin (Radix Scutellariae), zhi mu (Rhizoma Anemarrhennae) to clear heat and downbear fire.

6.加减   若烦渴不止，小便频数，而脉数乏力者，为肺热津亏，气阴两伤，可选用玉泉丸或二冬汤。玉泉丸中，以人参、黄芪、茯苓益气，天花粉、葛根、麦冬、乌梅、甘草清热生津止渴。二冬汤中，重用人参益气生津，天冬、麦冬、天花粉、黄芩、知母清热生津止渴。两方同中有异，前者益气作用较强，而后者清热作用较强，可根据临床需要选用。

4.1.6 Addition and reduction   If the thirst is restless, the urination is frequent with rapid and weak pulse, the syndrome is lung heat and fluid deficient, damages in qi and Yin, can choose prescription of Yuquan Pill or Erdong Decoction (Decoction of Asparagi Radix and Ophiopogoni). In the prescription of Yuquan Pill, ren shen (Radix Ginseng), huang qi (Radix Astragali seu Hedysari), fu ling (Poria) replenish qi; tian hua fen (Radix Tricosanthis), ge gen (Radix Puerariae), mai dong (Radix Ophiopogonis), wu mei (Fructus Mume), gan cao (Radix Glycyrrhizae) are used to clear heat, produce fluit and quench thirst. The prescription of Erdong Decoction uses large dosage of ren shen (Radix Ginseng) to replenish qi and generate fluid, uses tian dong (Radix Asparagi), mai dong (Radix Ophiopogonis), tian hua fen (Radix Tricosanthis), huang qin (Radix Scutellariae), zhi mu (Rhizoma Anemarrhennae) to clear heat, generate fluid and quench thirst. The two prescriptions have differences in similarity, the former is more effective in qi replenishing, while the latter is more effective in heat clearing, can be selected properly according to clinical needs.

（二）中消

4.2 Zhongxiao (diabetes in middle energizer)

1.胃热炽盛证

4.2.1 Hot stomach with excessive fire

（1）临床表现：多食易饥，口渴，尿多，形体消瘦，大便干燥，苔黄，脉滑实有力。

4.2.1.1 Clinical manifestations: more eating, more hungry, thirsty in mouth, more urination, thin body, dry stool, yellow tongue moss, sthenia slippery strong pulse.

（2）证机概要：胃火内炽，胃热消谷，耗伤津液。

4.2.1.2 overview of pathogenesis: burning fire in stomach, stomach heat consumes grains, wearing out the body fluid.

（3）治法：清胃泻火，养阴增液。

4.2.1.3 Treatment method: to clear the stomach and purge fire, nourish Yin and increase fluid.

（4）代表方：玉女煎加减。本方清胃滋阴，适用于消渴胃热阴虚，多食易饥，口渴等症。

4.2.1.4 Representative prescription: Yunv Decoction with addition and reduction. This prescription aims at clearing stomach and enriching Yin, suitable for Xiaoke (diabetes) manifested as stomach heat and Yin deficiency, eat more and frequent hungry, thirsty in mouth and other symptoms.

（5）常用药：生石膏、知母、黄连、栀子清胃泻火；玄参、生地黄、麦冬滋肺胃之阴；川牛膝活血化瘀，引热下行。

4.2.1.5 Medicines generally used: sheng shi gao (Crude Gypsum Fibrosum), zhi mu (Rhizoma Anemarrhennae), huang lian (Rhizoma Coptidis), zhi zi (Fructus Gardeniae), clear stomach and purge fire; xuan shen (Radix Scrophulariae), sheng di huang (Radix Rehmanniae), mai dong (Radix Ophiopogonis), enrich Yin of lung and stomach; chuan niu xi (Achyranthes Bidentatae) promote blood circulation and resolve blood stasis, downbear the heat.

（6）加减：大便秘结不行，可用增液承气汤润燥通腑，"增水行舟"，待大便通后再转上方治疗。本证亦可选用白虎加人参汤。方中以生石膏、知母清肺胃，除烦热，人参益气扶正，甘草、粳米益胃护津。全方共奏益气养胃、清热生津之效。

4.2.1.6 Addition and Reduction: in case of constipation, use Zengye Chengqi Decoction to moisten dryness and unblock the fu-organ, "increase water to move boat", when the stool is normal, turn to use the upper prescription. This syndrome can also choose the Baihu Jia Renshen Decoction. In this prescription, sheng shi gao (Crude Gypsum Fibrosum), zhi mu (Rhizoma Anemarrhennae) are used to clear lung and stomach, and remove restless fever, ren shen (Radix Ginseng) is used to replenish qi and reinforce healthy qi, gan cao (Radix Glycyrrhizae), geng mi (Semen Oryzae Sativae) are used to replenish stomach and protect fluid. This prescription can collectively realize the effect of replenishing qi and nourishing stomach, clearing heat and generating fluid.

2.气阴亏虚证

4.2.2 Dual deficiency of qi and Yin

（1）临床表现：口渴引饮，能食与便溏并见，或饮食减少，精神不振，四肢乏力，体瘦，舌质淡红，苔白而干，脉弱。

4.2.2.1 Clinical manifestations: thirsty with want to drink, good appetite and loose stool, or reduced diet, depressed spirit, weak limbs, thin body, light red tongue, white and dry moss, weak pulse.

（2）证机概要：气阴不足，脾失健运。

4.2.2.2 Overview of pathogenesis: insufficient qi and Yin, dysfunction of spleen transportation.

（3）治法：益气健脾，生津止渴。

4.2.2.3 Treatment method: to replenish qi and reinforce the spleen, generate fluid and quench thirst.

（4）代表方：七味白术散加减。本方益气健脾生津，适用于消渴之津气亏虚者。《医宗金鉴》等书将本方列为治消渴的常用方之一。该方可合生脉散益气生津止渴。

4.2.2.4 Representative prescription: Qiwei Baizhu Powder with addition and reduction. This prescription can replenish qi, reinforce the spleen and generate fluid, suitable for Xiaoke (diabetes) characterized by deficiency of fluid and qi. *Golden Mirror of Medicine* and other books list this prescription as one of the commonly used prescriptions for Xiaoke (diabetes). This prescription can combine with prescription Shengmai San to replenish qi, generate fluid and quench thirst.

（5）常用药：黄芪、党参、白术、茯苓、怀山药、甘草益气健脾；木香、藿香醒脾行气散津；葛根升清生津；天冬、麦冬养阴生津。

4.2.2.5 Medicines generally used: huang qi (Radix Astragali seu Hedysari), dang shen (Radix Codonopsitis Pilosulae), bai zhu (Rhizoma Atractylodis Macrocephalae), fu ling (Poria), huai shanyao (Dioscoreae Rhizoma), gan cao (Radix Glycyrrhizae) are used to replenish qi and reinforce the spleen; mu xiang (Radix Aucklandiae), huo xiang (Herba Agastaches seu Pogostemonis) are used to invigorate spleen, promote qi circulation, and spread fluid; ge gen (Radix Puerariae) are used to ascend lucidity and generate fluid; tian dong (Radix Asparagi), mai dong (Radix Ophiopogonis) are used to nourish Yin and generate fluid.

（6）加减：肺有燥热加地骨皮、知母、黄芩清肺；口渴明显加天花粉、生地黄养阴生津；气短汗多加五味子、山茱萸敛气生津；食少腹胀加砂仁、鸡内金健脾助运。

4.2.2.6 Addition and reduction: when lungs are hot and dry, add di gu pi (Lycii Cortex), zhi mu (Rhizoma Anemarrhenae), huang qin (Radix Scutellariae) to clear lungs; in case of frequent thirsty, add tian hua fen (Radix Trichosanthis), sheng di huang (Radix Rehmanniae) to nourish Yin and generate fluid; in case of short of breath and frequent sweating, add wu wei zi (Fructus Schisandalis), shan zhu yu (Corni Fructus) to astringe qi and generate fluid; less diet with abdominal distention, add sha ren (Fructus Amomi), ji nei jin (Endothlium Corneum Gigeriae Galli) to reinforce spleen and assist transporting.

（三）下消

4.3 Xiaxiao (diabetes in lower energizer)

1.肾阴亏虚证

4.3.1 Kidney Yin deficiency syndrome

（1）临床表现：尿频量多，浑浊如脂膏，或尿甜，腰膝酸软，乏力，头晕耳鸣，口干唇燥，皮肤干燥，瘙痒，舌红苔少，脉细数。

4.3.1.1 Clinical manifestations: frequent urination with large quantity, as turbid as fat ointment, or sweet urine, lassitude in loin and knees, fatigue, dizziness, tinnitus, dry mouth and lips, dry skin, itching, red tongue with little moss, thready and rapid pulse.

（2）证机概要：肾阴亏虚，肾失固摄。

4.3.1.2 Overview of pathogenesis: kidney Yin deficiency, dysfunction of kidney sealing and storing.

（3）治法：滋阴固肾。

4.3.1.3 Treatment method: enriching the Yin and strengthening the kidney.

（4）代表方：六味地黄丸加减。本方滋养肾阴，适用于消渴肾阴亏虚之证。

4.3.1.4 Representative Prescription: Liuwei Dihuang Pill with addition or reduction. This prescription enriches Yin and nourishes kidney, is suitable for the syndrome of Xiaoke (diabetes) manifested as kidney Yin deficiency.

（5）常用药：熟地黄、山茱萸、枸杞子、五味子固肾益精；怀山药滋补脾阴，固摄精微；茯苓健脾渗湿；泽泻、牡丹皮清泄火热。

4.3.1.5 Medicines generally used: shu di huang (Radix Rehmanniae Praeparatum), shan zhu yu (Corni Fructus), gou qi zi (Lycii Fructus), wu wei zi (Fructus Schisandalis) to strengthen kidney and re-plenish essence; shan yao (Dioscoreae Rhizoma) are used to enrich spleen Yin, solid cereal essence; fu ling (Poria) to reinforce the spleen and drain the dampness; ze xie (Rhizoma Alismatis), mu dan pi (Cortex Moutan) are used to clear and discharge heat.

（6）加减：阴虚火旺而烦躁，五心烦热，盗汗，失眠者，可加知母、黄柏滋阴泻火；尿量多而浑浊者，加益智仁、桑螵蛸等益肾缩尿；气阴两虚而伴困倦，气短乏力，舌质淡红者，可加党参、黄芪、黄精益气。

4.3.1.6 Addition and reduction: in case of Yin deficiency fire flourishing and irritablity, upset and fever in heart feet and hands, night sweat, insomnia, add zhi mu (Rhizoma Anemarrhenae), huang bo (Cortex Phellodendri) to enrich Yin and purge fire; with more and turbid urine, add yi zhi ren (Alpinae Oxyphyllae Fructus) and sang piao xiao (Mantidis Ootheca), to replenish kidney and reduce urination; in case of dual deficiency of qi and Yin accompanied by drowsiness, shortness of breath, fatigue, and light red tongue, add dang shen (Radix Codonopsitis Pilosulae), huang qi (Radix Astragali seu Hedysari), huang jing (Polygonati Rhizoma) to replenish qi.

2.阴阳两虚证

4.3.2 Dual deficiency of Yin and Yang

（1）临床表现：小便频数，浑浊如膏，甚至饮一溲一，面容憔悴，耳轮干枯，腰膝酸软，四肢欠温，畏寒肢冷，阳痿或月经不调，舌苔淡白而干，脉沉细无力。

4.3.2.1 Clinical manifestations: frequent urination, as turbid as ointment, and even urinate as much as drinking, haggard face, dry earrings, lassitude in loin and knees, cold limbs, fear of coldness, impotence or irregular menstruation, pale white and dry tongue moss, sunk thready and weak pulse.

（2）证机概要：阴损及阳，肾阳衰微，肾失固摄。

4.3.2.2 Overview of pathogenesis: Yin damages Yang, kidney Yang decline, dysfunction of kidney sealing and storing.

（3）治法：滋阴温阳，补肾固涩。

4.3.2.3 Treatment method: enriching Yin and warming Yang, reinforcing kidney and sealing astringent.

（4）代表方：金匮肾气丸加减。方中以六味地黄丸滋阴补肾，并用附子、肉桂以温补肾阳，主治阴阳两虚，尿频量多，腰酸腿软，形寒，面色黧黑等症。《医贯·消渴论》对本方在消渴病中的应用进行了较好的阐述："盖因命门火衰，不能蒸腐水谷，水谷之气不能熏蒸上润乎肺，如釜底无薪，锅盖干燥，故渴。至于肺亦无所禀，不能四布水精，并行五经。其所饮之水，未经火化，直入膀胱，正谓饮一升溲一升，饮一斗溲一斗，试尝其味，甘而不成可知矣。故用附子、肉桂之辛热，壮其少火，灶底加薪，枯笼蒸溽，槁禾得雨，生意维新。"

4.3.2.4 Representative prescription: Jingui Shenqi Pill. The prescription using Liuwei rehmannia pills to enrich Yin and tonify kidney, adding fu zi (Radix Aconiti), rou gui (Cortex Cinnamomi) to warm kidney Yang, mainly deal with dual deficiency of Yin and Yang, frequent and large quantity of urination, acrid waist and soft legs, cold shape, dark face and other symptoms. *Yiguan-Discussion on Diabetes* made clear illustration on treating Xiaoke (diabetes) Disease of this prescription: "Because decay of Mingmen fire (kidney Yang) can not steam water and grain, qi of water and grain can not fumigate upto the lung, just like without wood under the bottom of the pot, the pot cover will surely be dry. Failing to receive the qi pf water and grain, the lungs can not spread water fluid through the five meridians. the water in body goes directly into the bladder without cremation, thus patients drink a litre of water, urinate a liter, drink a bucket of water, urinate a bucket. Trying the taste, it must be sweet. Therefore, adding the spicy heat of fu zi (Radix Aconiti) and rou gui (Cortex Cinnamomi), strengthen the kidney by adding small fire, like to add woods under the stove bottom, or to fumigate the water through dry steaming cage is just like to irrigate rain on withered woods, vitality is refreshed."

（5）常用药：熟地黄、山茱萸、枸杞子、五味子固肾益精；怀山药滋补脾阴，固摄精微；茯苓健脾渗湿；附子、肉桂温肾助阳。

4.3.2.5 Medicines generally used: shu di huang (Radix Rehmanniae Praeparatum), shan zhu yu (Corni Fructus), gou qi zi (Lycii Fructus), wu wei zi (Fructus Schisandalis) are used to strengthen kidney and replenish essence; shan yao (Dioscoreae Rhizoma) is used to enrich spleen Yin, solid cereal essence; fu ling (Poria) are used to reinforce the spleen and drain the dampness; fu zi (Radix Aconiti), rou gui (Cortex Cinnamomi) are used to warm warm kidney and assist Yang.

（6）加减：尿量多而浑浊者，加益智仁、桑螵蛸、覆盆子、金樱子等益肾收摄；身体困倦，气短乏力者，可加党参、黄芪、黄精补益正气；阳痿加巴戟天、淫羊藿、肉苁蓉；阳虚畏寒者，可酌加鹿茸粉0.5g，以启动元阳，助全身阳气之生化。消渴多伴有瘀血的病变，故对于上述各种证型，尤其是对于舌质紫暗，或有瘀点瘀斑，脉涩或结或代，以及兼见其他瘀血证候者，均可酌加活血化瘀的方药，如丹参、川芎、郁金、红花、泽兰、鬼箭羽、山楂等。

4.3.2.6 Addition and reduction: in case of more and turbid urine, add yi zhi ren (Alpiniae Oxypgyllae Fructus), sang piao xiao (Mantidis Ootheca), fu pen zi (Rubi Fructus), jin ying zi (Fructus Rosae Laevagatae) and other medicines to replenish kidney and astringe the sealing; in case of body drowsiness, shortness of breath and fatigue, add dang shen (Radix Codonopsitis Pilosulae), huang qi (Radix Astragali seu Hedysari), huang jing (Polygonati Rhizoma) to tonify and replenish healthy qi; in case of impotence, add ba ji tian (Morindae Officinalis Radix), yin yang huo (Epimedii Folium), rou cong rong (Cistanches Herba); in case of Yang deficiency and fear of coldness, add antler powder 0.5g, to start renal Yang, helping the generation and transformation of the whole body. Diabetes is mostly accompanied by pathological changes of blood stasis, so the above various pattern of syndromes, especially for the symptoms of purple dark tongue, or with petechia, ecchymosis, astringent, slow-irregular pulse, and other blood stasis syndromes, add blood circulation promoting and blood stasis removing medicines, such as dan shen (Salviae Miltiorrhizae), chuan xiong (Rhizoma Chuanxiong), yu jin (Radix Curcumae), hong hua (Flos Carthami), ze lan(Herba Lycopi), gui jian yu (Ramulus Euonymi), shan zha (Crataegi Fructus), etc.

糖尿病的发生、发展存在"由浊致毒"之演变规律。糖尿病的初始病机多为壅滞之气内瘀血分而成浊。早期阶段多单纯以瘀浊为主，并进而内蕴化热，耗伤人体气血阴津。随着疾病的发展，则以血浊内蕴并酿致毒性为主，且两者常相生互助为虐，不仅耗气伤阴，还可内伤肺脾肾而再生瘀浊。

The occurrence and development of diabetes has the evolution rule of "toxin caused by turbidity". The initial pathogenesis of diabetes is mostly because the abundantly stagnated qi and internal blood stasis become turbidity. In the early stage, stasis turbidity is the main syndrome, and then internal accumulated into heat, consuming the human qi, blood and Yin and fluid. Along with the development of the disease, the internal accumulation of blood turbidity is brew into toxic nature, and the two (turbidity and toxin) often help each other to do evil, not only consume qi and damage Yin, but also internally injure lung, spleen and kidney and regenerate stasis turbidity.

五、化浊解毒方药治疗
5. Treatment with prescriptions and medicines of turbidity resolving and toxin removing method

消渴病前期称为无症状期，此期多表现为脾不散精、血浊内生，患者多无明显多饮、多食、多尿，口干、消瘦等自觉症状，临床多见喜食肥甘厚味，面色晦暗，口中黏腻异味，大便黏滞不畅，舌红苔黄腻，脉弦细滑。治疗以化浊解毒大法为主，辅以疏肝理气、健脾和胃、活血化瘀。临床用芳香化浊毒之藿香、佩兰、砂仁、荷叶等化湿醒脾，健运脾胃，疏通气机，宣化中焦湿浊；苦寒解浊毒之黄连、茵陈、黄柏、黄芩、大黄、龙胆草等清热燥湿，泻火解毒；活血化瘀除浊毒之当归、丹参、赤芍、白芍、郁金、川芎、蒲黄、五灵脂等平和之品以活血化瘀，使活血而不伤正，养血而不滞血。

The early stage of diabetes is called asymptomatic period, this period is mostly manifested as dysfunction of spleen spreading essence, blood turbidity generates endogenously, patients have no obvious conscious symptoms as polydipsia, overeating, polyuria, dry mouth, emaciation and others. In clinical practice we usually see favorite of fat, sweet, thick and tasty, dark complexion, mouth sticky with abnormal smell, sticky stool, red tongue, yellow greasy moss, string thready and slippery pulse. The treatment is mainly the method of turbidity resolving and toxin removing, supplemented by method of liver dispersing and qi regulating, spleen reinforcing and stomach harmonizing, blood circulation promoting and blood stasis resolving. In clinical practice, aromatic and turbid toxin resolving medicines huo xiang (Herba Agastaches seu Pogostemonis), pei lan (Herba Eupatorii), sha ren (Fructus Amomi), he ye (Nelumbinis Folium), are used to resolve dampness and invigorate the spleen, restore the transporting function of the spleen and stomach, dredge qi mechanism, diffuse the dampness and turbidity of the midle energizer. Bitter, cold and turbid toxin removing medicines huang lian (Rhizoma Coptidis), yin chen (Artemisiae Scopariae), huang bo (Cortex Phellodendri), huang qin (Radix Scutellariae), da huang (Radix et Rhizoma Rhei), long dan cao (Gentianae Radix et Rhizoma), are used to clear heat and dry dampness, purge fire and remove toxin. Medicines of blood circulation promoting and blood stasis resolving and turbid toxin removing as dang gui (Radix Angelicae Sinensis), dan shen (Salviae Miltiorrhizae), chi shao (Radix Paeoniae Rubra), bai shao (Radix Paeoniae Alba), yu jin (Radix Curcumae), chuan xiong (Rhizoma Chuanxiong), pu huang (Pollen Typhae), wu ling zhi (Faeces Trogopterorum) and other peaceful products are used to promote blood circulation and resolving blood stasis, so as to promote blood circulation without hurting the healthy qi, nourish blood without generating stagnation.

中期多由浊转毒、浊毒内蕴，临床常见口苦黏腻，尿液浑浊，消瘦或肥胖，头身困重，神疲乏力，腰膝酸软，大便不爽或干燥，伴有口干、多饮、多食、多尿，或皮肤及外阴瘙痒，或疔疮肿痛，或潮热，或双腿胫前皮肤可见褐色斑，舌暗红，苔黄厚腻或燥，脉细数或涩。治宜化浊解毒扶正。化浊解毒方中以升降散（蝉蜕、僵蚕、姜黄、大黄）为全方之基础，方中白僵蚕、蝉蜕升阳中之清阳；姜黄、降阴中之浊阴，一升一降，内外通和，而杂气之流毒顿消矣。

In the middle stage, most of the syndrome are transforming from turbidity to toxin, internal accumulation of turbid toxin occurs. Patients see bitter and sticky mouth, urine turbidity, thin or obesity, head and body trapped, spiritually tired, lassitude in loin and knees, difficult or dry stool, accompanied by dry mouth, more drinking, more eating, and more urination, or skin and vulva itching, or malignant pain, or hot flashes, or skin in legs before tibial see brown spots, dark red tongue, yellow thick greasy or dry moss, thready rapid or astringent pulse. Treatment should be turbidity resolving, toxin removing and healthy qi strengthening. In the prescriptions of turbidity resolving and toxin removing, Shengjiang Powder (the rise and fall powder), medicines including chan tui (Cicadae Periostracum), jiang can (Bombyx Batryticatus), jiang huang (Rhizoma Curcumae Longae), da huang (Radix et Rhizoma Rhei) are the basis of the whole prescription, and chan tui (Cicadae Periostracum), jiang huang (Rhizoma Curcumae Longae) are used to rise the lucid Yang of Yang, and jiang huang (Rhizoma Curcumae Longae), da huang (Radix et Rhizoma Rhei) are used to descend the turbid Yin of Yin. Flow of miscellaneous qi is eliminated. Ascending and descending, unblock the interior and exterior, the infectious toxin are dissipated immediately.

后期多浊毒兼杂顽痰瘀血，也是引发糖尿病多种并发症的重要因素，其随浊毒所伤脏腑经络的不同而呈现诸多相关变证。此阶段的病变机制也与脾胃气机升降失常有着密切的关系，因此治疗关键在于调理脾胃气机之升降，促使阳运阴化，方可协调各脏腑，复归阴阳平衡。如治疗糖尿病周围神经病变，选用李东垣清燥汤化裁。方中黄芪、白术、人参、陈皮、茯苓、神曲健脾理气，升麻、柴胡升清，猪苓、泽泻降浊，意在恢复中气升降之枢，使气血阴阳归于和平，以通阳于四末，则诸症自解。

In the late stage, the syndrome is mixed with turbid toxin and phlegmatic retention and blood stasis, are also important factors which cause various complications of diabetes. There are many related changes due to the different degree of damages made by turbid toxin on viscera and meridians. The pathological mechanism at this stage is also closely related to the abnormal ascending and descending of the qi mechanism of the spleen and stomach, so the key of the treatment is to regulate the rise and fall of qi mechanism of the spleen and stomach. And promote Yang (spleen) transporting and Yin (stomach) digesting, so as to coordinate the viscera to restore the balance of Yin and Yang. Specifically the treatment of diabetic peripheral neuropathy can choose Li Dongyuan Qingzao Decoction (Dryness clearing Decoction). Huang qi (Radix Astragali seu Hedysari), bai zhu (Rhizoma Atractylodis Macrocephalae), ren shen (Radix Ginseng), chen pi (Pericarpium Citri Reticulatae), fu ling (Poria), shen qu (Messa Medicata Fermentata) are used to reinforce spleen and regulate qi. Sheng ma (Rhizoma Climicifugae) and chai hu (Radix Bulpleuri) are used to ascend lucidity, zhu ling (Polygorus Umbellatus) and ze xie (Rhizoma Alismatis) are used to descend turbidity, intending to restore the hub function of rise and fall of middle qi, so that qi, blood, Yin and Yang return to peace, to transport the Yang to the four end of the body, then the disease will be self-resolved.

综上所述，治疗糖尿病将化浊解毒大法贯穿治疗的始终，排出或消散体内浊毒，促进机体新陈代谢，使浊毒去，气血畅，积郁解，痰火消，脾运复健，胃复和降，肝气调达，浊毒无所生，人体紊乱的内环境归于平衡，徐徐图之，效果显著。

To sum up, the method of turbidity resolving and toxin removing should be carried out through the whole process of diabetes treatment to remove or dissipate the turbid toxin in human body, promote the body metabolism, so as to make turbid toxin disappear, smooth the circulation of qi and blood, remove the accumulation and depression, disperse the phlegmatic fire, restore spleen transportation and stomach harmonizing and descending, disperse the liver qi, turbidity toxin can never generate, the internal environment disorder of human body return to balance, to do the above gradually, the effect will be remarkable.

第三节　肥胖症浊毒论
Section 3　On Turbid Toxin of Obesity

一、中医古籍中对肥胖症治疗的认识
1. Understanding of obesity treatment in ancient works of traditional Chinese medicine

关于肥胖症的中医论述，《灵枢》云："土形之人……其为人，黄色圆面，大头，美肩背，大腹，美股胫，小手足，多肉，上下相称。"这种土形之人的体貌特征与现代之肥胖患者相似。《素问·通评虚实论》将"肥贵人则高粱之疾"的病机责之于"血黑以浊、气涩以迟"，并提出"因其重而减之"的治疗观点，与今日肥胖病治疗的中心环节——减重与保持体质。可谓不谋而合。元代朱震亨《丹溪心法》云"肥人多是湿痰"，治疗上提倡宜燥湿祛痰、行气。总之，中医学认为肥胖与饮食不节、劳逸失常、七情失调、体质禀赋、年龄、性别及地域等因素有关，各种致病因素使得人体阳气虚弱，脏腑功能失调，运化疏泄乏力，气机郁滞，升降失常，血行失畅，痰湿浊毒堆积体内，日久形成肥胖。

Regarding the discussion of obesity, *Spiritual Pivot* said: "People of earth constitution... yellow round face, big head, beautiful shoulder and back, big belly, beautiful thighs and legs, small hands and feet, more meat, symmetry up and down." The physical characteristics of such native people are similar to those of modern obese patients. *Simple Conversation-General Discussion on Deficiency and Excess* regard that pathogenesis of "the disease of sorghum of rich and fat person" is "black and turbid blood, astringent and late pulse", and put forward the treatment view of "reducing the weight of the patient", agreeing with the present treatment—the weight reduction and physical maintenance as the central link of obesity. Zhu Zhenheng of Yuan dynasty said in *What I have learned in Clinical Practice By Zhu Danxi* said: "Most of the fat people generates more dampness and phlegm." Treating the said disease, it is advocated to appropriately dry damp and dispel phlegm, promote qi circulation. In short, TCM thinks that obesity has relations with uncontrolled diet, irregular arrangement of work and rest, disorder of seven emotions, constitutional endowment, age, gender and region, different pathogenic factors make the patient weak in Yang, viscera dysfunction, short of force to transport and disperse, qi stagnation, abnormal ascending and descending, irregular blood circulation, accumulation of phlegm, dampness, turbidity and toxin in the body, leading to obesity with time being.

肥胖的中医治疗原则主要是化浊解毒、祛湿化痰、活血化瘀、健脾益气、益气补肾。

The main principles of TCM treatment of obesity are: resolving turbidity and removing toxin, removing dampness and resolving phlegm, promoting blood circulation and resolving blood stasis, reinforcing spleen and replenishing qi, replenishing qi and reinforcing kidney.

二、肥胖症的病因病机
2. The etiology and pathogenesis of obesity disease

本病的最早记载见于《黄帝内经》。《素问·异法方宜论》曰："其民华食而脂肥。"说明肥胖的发生与过食肥甘、先天禀赋等多种因素有关。后世医家在此基础上认识到肥胖的病机还与气虚、痰湿、七情及地理环境等因素有关。在治疗方面，《丹溪心法·中湿》认为肥胖应从湿热及气虚两方面论治。《石室秘录·肥治法》认为治痰须补气兼消痰，并补命火，使气足而痰消。此外，前人还认识到肥胖与其他多种病证有关，如《女科切要》指出："肥白妇人，经闭而不通者，必是湿痰与脂膜壅塞之故也。"

The earliest record of this disease is found in *The Medical Classic of the Yellow Emperor. Simple Conversation-Discussion on Different Theropeutic Methods for Different diseases* says: "People eat luxuriously and grow fat in body." It shows that the occurrence of obesity is related to excessive eating of fat and sweet food, congenital endowment and other factors. On this basis, later doctors realized that the pathogenesis of obesity is also related to qi deficiency, phlegm hygrosis, seven emotions and geographical environment. In terms of treatment, *What I have Learned in Clinical Practice By Zhu Danxi-Discussion on Middle Dampness* believes that obesity should be treated from both dampness and heat and qi deficiency. *Stone Room Secret Record-Discussion on Obesity Treatment Method* thinks that to cure phlegm must tonify qi and eliminate phlegm, and tonify renal fire, when qi is deficient, phlegm will disappear. In addition, predecessors also realized that obesity is related to a variety of other diseases, such as *Key Factors of Gynecology* points out: "Amenorrhea of fat white women must be caused by phlegmatic hygrosis and lipid membrane congestion."

李佃贵教授多年从事浊毒理论研究，通过大量的临床观察，针对肥胖症的病因病机提出了新的观点——浊毒致病。

Professor Li Diangui has been engaged in the theoretical research of turbid toxin for many years. Through a large amount of clinical observation, he put forward a new view on the pathogenesis of obesity.

浊毒是一种对人体脏腑经络和气血阴阳均能造成严重损害的致病因素，也是因脏腑功能紊乱、气血运行失常，机体内产生的代谢产物不能及时排出体外而化生的病理产物。浊与湿同源同类，湿乃浊之源，浊乃湿之重；毒与热同类，热乃毒之渐，毒乃热之极。热甚则为火，火热不解，深入血分则为毒；浊邪内蕴，阻碍气机，郁久化热，继而蕴结为毒。

故温热可转化为毒，湿浊亦可演变为毒。可见，"毒"与"浊"有着密切的联系，故而浊毒并称。

Turbid toxin is a pathogenic factor which can make serious damage to the viscera, qi, blood, Yin and Yang of the human body. It is also a pathological product transformed from the metabolites produced in the body which cannot be discharged in time due to dysfunction of the viscera and abnormal operation of qi and blood. Turbidity and dampness share the same source, belong to same category, dampness is the source of turbidity, turbidity is the severeness of dampness; toxin and heat belong to the same category, heat is the gradual progress of toxin, toxin is the extremity of heat. Severe heat is fire, Fire and heat can not be separated, when they go deeply into blood, they turn to be toxin; internal accumulation of turbidity evil hinders qi movement, if it is depressed and lingers long, it turns to be heat, and then accumulate into toxin. So warmth and heat can be transformed into toxin, dampness and turbidity can also evolved into toxin. It can be seen that "toxin" and "turbidity" have a close connection, so the word turbid toxin is generated.

浊邪为病，易阻碍气机，结滞经脉，缠绵胶着不去；毒邪伤人，性烈善变，易损害气血。浊邪常蕴于阴血之中且极易化热酿致毒邪，并常与毒邪相夹为患，浊以毒为用，毒以浊为体，胶着难愈，邪壅经络，气机不畅，邪不得散，血不得行，津不得布，化生痰浊瘀血，痰浊、瘀浊相互搏结，反复日久，耗伤脏腑气血津液，从而造成浊毒内壅，气滞络阻，脾不升清，胃失和降，阴血耗伤，气虚血郁的证机变化。肥胖症的中医病因病机如下。

When turbid evil causes disease, it will easily hinder qi movement, stagnates meridians, lingering agglutinate; when toxic evil hurt people, it will be fierce and changeable, easy to damage qi and blood. Turbid evil often accumulates in Yin blood and extremely easy to transform to heat brewing toxic evil, and often do evil together with toxic evil. Toxin is the function of turbidity, turbidity is the carrier of toxin. The two cements together and difficult to cure. The evil obstructs the meridians, thus qi mechanism operates abnormally. Evil cannot be dispersed, blood cannot circulate, fluid cannot be spread, they are transformed into phlegm, turbidity, blood stasis. Phlegm turbidity and turbid stasis fight against and agglutinate with each other, for a long time, consume and damage viscera, qi, blood, fluid and liquid, causing syndrome changes of internal accumulation of turbid toxin, qi stagnation and collateral obstruction, dysfunction of lucidity ascending of spleen, and dysfunction of stomach harmonizing and descending, consuming and damages of Yin blood, qi deficiency and blood depression. The TCM etiology and pathogenesis of obesity are as follows.

（一）年老体弱

2.1 Age

肥胖的发生与年龄有关，40岁以后明显增高。这是由于中年以后，人体的生理功能由盛转衰，脾的运化功能减退，又过食肥甘，运化不及，聚湿生痰，痰湿壅结，或肾阳虚衰，不能化气行水，酿生水湿痰浊，故而肥胖。

The occurrence of infirm obesity is related to age, it is significantly higher after age 40. This is because after middle age, the physiological function of the human body turns from prosperity to decline, the transport function of the spleen decreased, and over - taking of fat and sweet food cannot be transported in time, it aggregates with dampness and generates phlegm, phlegmatic hygrosis obstructs, or kidney Yang deficiency and decline, fails to gasify and transport water, brewing water, dampness, phlegm, and turbidity, so obesity generates.

（二）饮食不节

2.2 Irregular diet

《素问·痹论》曰：“饮食自倍，肠胃乃伤。”暴饮暴食或过饱易损伤脾胃。如饮食五味偏嗜，还会使相应的脏腑功能偏盛，久之可损伤内脏。暴饮暴食，食量过大，或过食肥甘，长期饮食不节，一方面可致水谷精微在人体内堆积成为膏脂，形成肥胖；另一方面也可损伤脾胃，不能布散水谷精微及运化水湿，致使湿浊内生，蕴酿成痰，痰湿聚集体内，日久化浊成毒，浊毒内蕴，使人体臃肿肥胖更甚。

Simple Conversation-Discussion on Bi Syndrome says: "Overeating impairs intestines and stomach." Crapulence or overloading of stomach is easy to damage the spleen and stomach. If the favorite taste is partial, it will make the corresponding viscera function partially abundant, for a long time impairs the viscera. Crapulence, eating too much, or over-taken of fat and sweet food, long-term irregular diet, on one hand, can cause cereal essence in the body accumulated into fat; on the other hand, it impairs the spleen and stomach, causes dysfunction of cereal essence spreading and water dampness transporting, results in the internal generation of dampness and turbidity, brewing of phlegm. Aggregation of phlegmatic hygrosis wil be transformed from turbidity into toxin, internal accumulation of turbid toxin make people even fatter.

（三）情志所伤

2.3 Emotional impair

中医学认为，“思伤脾”，脾伤则运化失健，水湿痰浊膏脂内生。情志抑郁，一则引起肝气不舒气机失调，津液输布失常，水湿滞留；二则肝郁“木不达土”，影响脾胃功能；三则还可引起气滞血瘀，出现血瘀的证候。

TCM believes that, "over-thinking impairs the spleen". When spleen is impaired, the function of transporting becomes abnormal, water, dampness, phlegm, turbidity, paste fat are generated endogenously. Depression of emotion firstly causes liver qi imbalance, and irregular operation of qi mechanism, abnormal spreading of fluid spreading and distribution and retaining of water dampness; Secondly, liver depression i.e "wood failing to reach earth", affects the function of the spleen and stomach; thirdly, it causes qi stagnation and blood stasis, leads to blood stasis syndrome.

（四）缺乏运动

2.4 Lack of exercise

长期喜卧好坐，缺乏运动则气血运行不畅，脾胃呆滞则运化失司，水谷精微失于输布，化为膏脂痰浊，聚于肌肤、脏腑、经络，而致肥胖。妇女在妊娠期或产后由于营养过多，活动减少，亦容易发生。

People in favor of long time sitting and lying, lack of exercise, qi and blood circulation is not smooth, spleen and stomach is sluggish, transport function does not work, the cereal essence which fails to be spread and distributed is transformed into paste, fat, phlegm and turbidity, aggregated in the skin, viscera and meridians, causes obesity. Due to excessive nutrition and reduced activity, women in pregnancy or postpartum are also easy to get obesity.

（五）劳逸损伤

2.5 Impairing from excessive labor and rest

肢体百骸为用，阳气振奋、阴精津血流畅，则气畅血运、脏腑功能协调，同时阴液为阳所动，腠理开阖而微微汗出。汗为津液所化生，"汗血同源"。《温病条辨》曰"汗者也，合阳气阴精蒸化而出者也"，可见汗液的排泄会消耗一定的"阴精"和能量。"心主血脉"，在液为汗；肺主皮毛，朝百脉，通调水道。汗出则心脉畅、肺气宣、百脉调、水道通，气血津液各为所用而不积滞为患。

Limbs and skeletons are born for use, if Yang is excited, Yin essence and fluid blood flow smoothly, qi is free and blood is transported normally, viscera function coordinates, at the same time Yin fluid invigorated by Yang is sweated slightly through opening and closing of striae. Sweat is transformed from body fluid, "sweat and blood share the same origin". *Detailed Analysis of Epidemic Warm Diseases* says: "Sweat is steamed out with cooperation of Yang qi and Yin essence", it can be seen that the excretion of sweat will consume a certain amount of "Yin essence" and energy. "Heart controls blood veins", when carrying liquid, it is sweat; lung controls fur, can reach all the veins in body, maintaining the water channels. Normal Sweating ensures the smoothness of heart pulse, diffusing of lung qi, regularity of all the veins, unblocking of water channels, qi, blood, fluid and liquid work well, without stagnation.

"脾主身之肌肉"，脾又主四肢。《素问集注·五脏生成》曰："脾主运化水谷之精，以生养肌肉，故主肌肉。"《素问·经脉别论》曰："食气入胃，散精于肝，淫气于筋。"可见，四肢肌肉筋脉的营养及功能均有赖于脾胃之水谷精微。

"The spleen controls the muscles", the spleen also controls limbs. *Collection of Explanation to Simple Conversation-Discussion on Various Relationships Concerning Five Zang - Organs* says: "The spleen transports the cereal essence to generate and nourish muscles, so it controls muscles."*Simple Conversation-Special Discussion on Channels and Vessels* says: "When food is taken into the stomach, some of the nutrient substances are transported to the liver to nourish the sinews." It can be seen that the nutrition and function of limbs and sinews depend on the cereal essence of the spleen and stomach.

（六）先天禀赋

2.6 Congenital endowment

现代已明确认识到，肥胖的发生具有家族性。阳热体质，胃热偏盛者，食欲亢进，食量过大，脾运不及，可致膏脂痰湿堆积，而成肥胖。

In modern times, it is clearly recognized that the occurrence of obesity is familial. People with Yang and heat constitution, partial stomach heat, hyperappetite, too large quantity of food for eating, spleen fails to transport in time, can cause accumulation of cream fat and phlegmatic hygrosis, and lead to obesity.

此外，肥胖的发生还与性别、地理环境等因素有关，由于女性活动量较男性少，故女性肥胖者较男性为多。

In addition, the occurrence of obesity is also related to gender, geographical environment and other factors, as the female activity is less than men, so there are more obese women than men.

肥胖症病机总属阳气虚衰、痰湿偏盛。脾气虚弱则运化转输无力，水谷精微失于输布，化为膏脂和水湿，留滞体内而致肥胖；肾阳虚衰，则血液鼓动无力，水液失于蒸腾气化，致血行迟缓，水湿内停，而成肥胖。

The general pathogenesis of obesity disease is Yang qi decline, phlegmatic hygrosis partially abundant. When the spleen qi is weak, the spleen fails to transform and transport, the cereal essence failing to be spread turns to be fat paste and water dampness, retains in the body and causes obesity; when kidney Yang is deficient, the blood agitation becomes weak, water liquid cannot be transpired and gasified, thus blood flows slowly, water dampness retains inside, and obesity is generated.

病位主要在脾与肌肉，与肾虚关系密切，亦与心肺的功能失调及肝失疏泄有关。本病多属本虚标实之候。本虚多为脾肾气虚，或兼心肺气虚；标实为痰湿膏脂内停，或兼水湿、血瘀、气滞等，临床常有偏于本虚及标实之不同。本病病变过程中常发生病机转化，一是虚实之间的转化，如食欲亢进，过食肥甘，形成肥胖，但长期饮食不节，损伤脾胃，脾虚不运，甚至脾病及肾，导致脾肾两虚，由实转虚；而脾虚日久，运化失常，湿浊内生，或土壅木郁，气滞血瘀，或脾病及肾，肾阳虚衰，不能化气行水，水湿内停，泛溢肌肤，阻滞经络，使肥胖加重，从而由虚转实或虚实夹杂。二是各种病理产物之间也可发生相互转化，主要表现为痰湿内停日久，可致气滞或血瘀。而气滞、痰湿、瘀血日久，常可化热，而成郁热、痰热、湿热、瘀热。三是肥胖病变日久，常变生他病。极度肥胖者，常易合并消渴、头痛、眩晕、胸痹、中风、胆胀、痹证等。

The disease is mainly located in the spleen and muscle, which is closely related to kidney deficiency, and is also related to cardiopulmonary dysfunction and liver dysfunction of dispersing. Most of the disease belongs to the syndrome of asthenia root and sthenia tip. Asthenia root indicates the qi deficiency of the spleen and kidney, or simultaneously qi deficiency of heart and lung; sthenia tip indicates the internal retaining of phlegmatic hygrosis and cream fat, or simultaneously with water dampness, blood stasis, qi stagnation, etc. In clinical practice, there might be differences between the syndrome partial asthenia root and partial sthenia tip. During the process of pathogenic changes, transformation of the pathogenesis often occurs. First it is the transformation between the deficiency and the excess. Such as hyperappetite and overeating of fat and sweet food causes obesity, but long-time of irregular diet damages the spleen and stomach, the spleen is deficient and fails to transport, even spleen disease affects kidney, leads to dual deficiency of the spleen and kidney, the syndrome turns from sthenia to asthenia; when spleen deficiency keeps for a long time, transportation will be abnormal, dampness and turbidity generates internally,the spleen qi will be abundantly excess, the liver qi will be depressed, qi stagnation and blood stasis, occur. Or the spleen disease affects the kidney, the kidney Yang declines, and fails to gasify qi and move water, water dampness retains internally, overfolws the skin, obstructs the meridians, and aggravate the obesity. Therefore the syndrome turns from asthenia to sthenia, or mixed with asthenia and sthenia. Second, different pathological products may inter-transform to another, manifested as long-time of internal retaining of phlegmatic hygrosis will cause qi stagnation or blood stasis. Qi stagnation, phlegmatic hygrosis and blood stasis for a long time, often can be turned into heat including depressed heat, phlegmatic heat, damp heat, blood stasis heat. Third, long course of obesity can often transforms to other diseases. Extreme obese people, are easy to get diabetes, headache, vertigo, thoracic obstruction, stroke, distention of gallbladder, arthromyodynia.

三、基本治则
3. The basic treatment principle

（一）调节整体平衡
3.1 To adjust the overall balance

治疗可以从调整阴阳入手，调节整体平衡，恢复和建立相对平衡的阴阳关系，不外乎去其有余、补其不足两个方面。去其有余，即去其阴阳之偏盛。阴盛则寒，阳盛则热，阴盛还可转化为水湿痰饮，阳盛也可转化为瘀滞燥结。故去其有余，有温、清、利、下等各种具体治法；补其不足，即补其阴阳之偏衰，有补阴与补阳之不同。

The treatment can start from adjusting Yin and Yang, to adjust the overall balance, restore and establish the relatively balanced relationship between Yin and Yang, nothing more than eliminating the excess and tonifying the deficiency. To eliminate the excess, that is, to eliminate the partial sthenia Yin and Yang. Sthenia Yin is cold, sthenia Yang is hot, sthenia Yin can also be transformed into water dampness and phlegmatic retention, sthenia Yang can also be transformed into stasis stagnation and dry binding. Therefore, to eliminate the excess, there are specific methods of warming, clearing, dissipating and purging, To tonify the deficiency is to tonify the partial declining of Yin and Yang, there is some differences between Yin and Yang reinforcing.

调节整体平衡，还要求对各种治疗措施和方药的运用都适可而止，不可矫枉过正，以防机体出现新的不平衡。

Adjusting the overall balance also requires properly using various therapeutic measures and prescriptions, knowing when and where to stop, not overdoing in righting a wrong, so as not to generate new imbalance in the body.

（二）审证求机论治
3.2 To make treatment by differentiating syndrome and detecting pathogenesis

审证求机以往一般称为审证求因，但进而言之，所谓求因实是求机，就是要从整体和动态地去分析疾病的各种复杂的征象，综合归纳推论出疾病发生发展的原因、病变的机制。这种病因观点，实际上是和病机融为一体的，而其本质仍在于求机。证与病机，都是疾病本质的反应，是疾病的主要矛盾，治疗疾病应遵从审证求机论治的原则，从疾病的本质入手，从根本上加以治疗。只要解决了疾病的主要矛盾和关键环节，一切复杂问题就会迎刃而解。

In past, it is expressed as to make treatment by differentiating syndrome and detecting the etiology. But through further consideration, so-called detecting etiology is actually to detect pathogenesis, through analyzing various complex signs of diseases entirely and dynamically, and comprehensively summarize and inference the etiology and the pathogenesis of the disease. This view of etiology is actually integrated with the pathogenesis, and its essence still lies in detecting the pathogenesis. Both syndrome and pathogenesis are the reaction of the essence of the disease as well as the main contradiction of the disease. The treatment of the disease should follow the principle of making treatment by differentiating syndrome and detecting pathogenesis, start from the essence of the disease, and treat it fundamentally. As long as the principal contradiction and key links of the disease are solved, all complex problems will be readily solved.

（三）明辨标本缓急
3.3 To make clear the root and the tip, slow and urgent

标和本是一个相对的概念，它主要说明病变过程中矛盾的主次关系。本是事物的主要矛盾，标是事物的次要矛盾。

Root and tip is a relative concept to mainly explain the contradictory primary and secondary relationship in the process of lesion. The root is the principal contradiction of things, and the tip is the secondary contradiction of things.

疾病的发生发展过程极其复杂，常常有邪正盛衰、病因病证缓急、旧病未愈新病又起、表证与里证同在等问题，在临证时必须分清疾病的标本主次、轻重缓急，而采取"急则治其标，缓则治其本"和"标本同治"的方法进行治疗，这就是明辨标本缓急的治疗原则。

The occurrence and development of the disease process is extremely complex, there are often problems as evil and healthy, excess and decline, slow and urgent of etiology and syndrome, new disease generates before recovering of the old disease, simultaneous existance of internal and external syndromes. In clinical practice, we must distinguish the root and the tip, primary and secondary, light and severe, slow and urgent, and follow the principle of "for urgent disease, treating the tip, for slow disease, curing its original" and "simultaneous treatment of the root and the tip", this is the treatment principle to deal with root and tip, slow and urgent diseases.

急则治其标，是指在疾病的发展过程中，如果出现了紧急危重的证候，影响到患者的安危时，就必须先行解决，而后再治疗其本的原则。缓则治其本，是指在病情缓和的情况下，应从根本上治疗疾病。因为标病产生于本病，本病解决了，标病自然随之而解。在标本俱急的情况下，必须采取标本同治的原则。

"Urgent disease, treating the tip", refers to in the development of the disease, if there is an emergency and critical syndrome which affects the life safety of patients, it must be treated in first priority immediately, and then cure the root of the disease. "Slow disease, curing the root", refers to in the case of moderate disease, treatment should be made fundamentally. Because the tip disease generates from the root disease, when the root disease is solved, and the tip disease will be naturally solved accordingly. In case of dual urgent of both root and tip disease, the principle of "simultaneous treatment of the root and the tip" must be adopted.

（四）把握动态变化

3.4 Grasping the dynamic changes

疾病的过程是邪正斗争，此消彼长，不断变化发展的过程。疾病的每一个阶段都有不同的病理特点，因此必须把握其动态变化，分阶段进行治疗。

The progress of disease is a process of constant change and development, the struggling between evil and healthy continues with cycle repetition of one increasing, the other decreasing. Each stage of the disease has different pathological characteristics, so we must grasp the dynamic changes and treat them according to different stages.

（五）顺应异法方宜

3.5 Adhering to the principle of different therapeutic methods for different diseases

疾病的发生、发展受多方面因素的影响，如时令气候、地理环境等，尤其是患者的个体体质因素对疾病的影响更大。因此，在治疗疾病时，必须根据季节、气候、地区及患者的体质、年龄等不同特点而选用适宜的治疗方法，这就是顺应异法方宜的治疗原则，具体包括因时制宜、因地制宜、因人制宜三个方面。

The occurrence and development of diseases is affected by many factors, such as season, climate and geographical environment, especially the individual constitutional factors of patients have a greater impact on the disease. Therefore, in the treatment of diseases, we must choose appropriate treatment methods according to different characteristics of season, climate, region, patient's constitution, age and so on. To adhere the treatment principle of different therapeutic methods for different diseases including three specific aspects as making appropriate treatment according to time, region and patients.

（六）先期治未病

3.6 Early treatment of future diseases

治未病包括未病先防和既病防变两个方面。未病先防，是指对有可能发生疾病的个体和人群及早提出预防措施，运用药物培补人体的正气，预防疾病发生的方法。既病防变，是指医者可根据疾病的传变规律，防其传变，对可能受到传变的脏腑和可能受到影响的气血津液采取预防措施，阻断和防止病变的发展和传变，把病变尽可能控制在较小的范围，以利于疾病的彻底治疗，取得最好的疗效。如《金匮要略》云："见肝之病，知肝传脾，当先实脾。"其意是说治疗肝病时，须要应用调补脾胃法，使脾气旺盛而不受邪，以防止肝病传脾。

Treatment of future diseases include two aspects: prevention before the occurrence of the disease and prevention against the deterioration of the existed disease. Prevention before the occurrence of the disease refers to provide preventing measures for the individuals and people who might be attacked by disease in near future as early as possible including cultivating and invigorating the healthy qi by using medicines and prevent the occurrence of diseases. Prevention against the transmission and deterioration of the existed disease, refers to taking preventive measures to the viscera and qi, blood, fluid, and liquid which may be affected to block and prevent the development of the lesion and transmission according to the disease transmission rule, control the lesion as far as possible, to facilitate the thorough treatment of the disease, get the best curative effect. Just as *Golden Chamber Synopsis* says: "When facing liver disease, we should know liver disease will transmit to the spleen, so we should first reinforce the spleen." It means that to treat liver disease, we should use the method of adjusting and reinforcing the spleen and stomach, to make spleen qi exuberant to defend evil in order to prevent liver disease transmitting to the spleen.

（七）重视调摄护理
3.7 Pay attention to the appropriate recuperating and nursing

恰当的调护，有利于正气的恢复、邪气的祛除和促进患者早日康复。忽视调摄护理，不仅会延误康复时间，还会出现"食复""劳复"等情况，以致病情反复。因此，必须重视调摄护理。

Recuperating and nursing is conducive to the recovery of healthy qi, the removal of evil qi and promote the early recovery of patients. Neglecting the adjusting and nursing, not only will delay the recovery time, but also cause "over-eaten relapse", "over-strained relapse" and other situations, so that the disease will be repeated. Therefore, attention must be paid to recuperating and nursing.

调摄护理的内容十分丰富，如饮食护理、生活护理、精神护理、服药护理等。这些护理措施同样是以辨证论治为指导的，因此也当辨证施护，随证而异。

The content of the recuperating and nursing is very rich, such as dietary nursing, life nursing, spiritual nursing, medication nursing and so on. These nursing measures are also guided by syndrome differentiation treatment, so they should also be implemented according to syndrome differentiation and adjust along with the changing of the syndrome.

四、中医辨证论治
4. TCM syndrome differentiation treatment

李佃贵教授经过多年临床观察，从发病机制上提出了"浊毒理论"，阐明了肥胖症病的病因病机，并以此为理论依据，制订了以"化浊解毒"为主，治疗肥胖症的一整套严谨的治则、治法，为中医药治疗肥胖症提供了一条新的思路和方法。

After years of clinical observation, professor Li Diangui pointed out "turbid toxin theory" from the pathogenic mechanism, illustrated the etiology and pathogenesis of obesity, and established a set of rigorous treatment principle and method to treat obesity on the theoretical basis, emphasizing the priority of "turbidity resolving and toxin removing", provided a new idea and method for traditional Chinese medicine in obesity treatment.

（一）浊毒内蕴
4.1 The internal accumulation of turbid toxin

1.主要症状　胃脘堵闷，嗳气，大便稀溏，不畅感，舌暗红，苔黄厚腻，脉弦滑。

4.1.1 Main symptoms　Epigastric obstruction, belching, loose and difficult stool, dark red tongue, yellow thick and greasy moss, string slippery pulse.

2.病机　浊毒内蕴。

4.1.2 Pathogenesis　Internal accumulation of turbid toxin.

3.治则　化浊解毒。

4.1.3 Treatment principle　To resolve turbidity and remove toxin.

4.方药　自拟化浊解毒方（黄芩、黄连、黄柏、砂仁、白蔻仁、蒲公英、生石膏、茵陈、藿香、佩兰）。

4.1.4 Prescription　Self-created prescription of turbidity resolving and toxin removing. Medicines: huang qin (Radix Scutellariae), huang lian (Rhizoma Coptidis), huang bo (Cortex Phellodendri), sha ren (Fructus Amomi), bai kou ren (Fructus Amomi Rotundus), pu gong ying (Herba Taraxaci cum Radice), sheng shi gao (Crude Gypsum Fibrosum), yin chen (Herba Artemisiae Scopariae), huo xiang (Herba Agastaches seu Pogostemonis), pei lan (Herba Eupatorii).

5.加减运用　伴大便不干、不溏，排便不爽，便次频数，加葛根、白芍、地榆、秦皮、白头翁；伴恶心，加紫苏叶、黄连；伴月经不调，常加川芎等。

4.1.5 Addition and reduction　Accompanied by frequent and difficult but not dry and loose stool, add ge gen (Radix Pueraiae), bai shao (Radix Paeoniae Alba), di yu (Radix et Rhizoma Sanguisorbae), qin pi (Cortex Fraxini Caulis), bai tou weng (Pulsatillae Radix); with nausea, add zi su ye (Folium Perillae), huang lian (Rhizoma Coptidis); with irregular menstruation, often add chuan xiong (Rhizoma Chuanxiong), and more.

（二）饮食积滞

4.2 Diet retention

1.主要症状　脘腹胀满，嗳腐吞酸，大便不爽或夹有不消化食物，舌质红，苔白厚腻，脉滑。

4.2.1 Main symptoms　Abdominal distension, fetid cructation and acid rigurgitation, difficult stool or with indigested food, red tongue, white thick and greasy moss, slippery pulse.

2.病机　食滞胃脘。

4.2.2 Pathogenesis　Epigastric food retention.

3.治则　健脾消食。

4.2.3 Treatment principle　Invigorate the spleen and digest food.

4.方药　保和丸加减（山楂、焦神曲、陈皮、连翘、炒莱菔子、半夏）。

4.2.4 Prescription　Baohe Pill with addition or reduction. Medicines: shan zha (Fructus Crataegi), jiao shen qu (fried Messa Medicata Fermentata), chen pi (Pericarpium Citri Reticulatae), lian qiao (Forsythiae Fructus), chao lai fu zi (fried Semen Raphani), ban xia (Rhizoma Pinelliae).

5.加减运用　胃气上逆，食入则吐，加厚朴、黄连；胃脘疼痛，加延胡索、白芷；嗳气，加石菖蒲、郁金、紫苏叶、黄连；食积滞气，嗳腐吞酸，加鸡内金、炒谷芽、炒麦芽、茵陈；呃逆，加丁香、柿蒂。

4.2.5 Addition and reduction Counterflow of stomach qi, vomiting as soon as taking - in of food, add hou po (Cortex Magnoliae Officinalis), huang lian (Rhizoma Coptidis); epigastric pain, add yan hu suo (Rhizoma Corydalis), bai zhi (Radix Angelicae Dahuricae); belching, add shi chang pu (Rhizoma Acori Graminei), yu jin (Radix Curcumae), zi su ye (Folium Perillae), huang lian (Rhizoma Coptidis); qi stagnation due to food retention, fetid cructation and acid rigurgitation, add ji nei jin (Endothlium Corneum Gigeriae Galli), chao gu ya (Setariae Fructus) and chao mai ya (Hordei Fructus Germinatus), yin chen (Herba Artemisiae Scopariae); in case of hiccups, add ding xiang (Flos Caryophylli) and shi di (Kaki Calyx).

（三）胃热炽盛

4.3 Intense stomach heat

1.主要症状 消谷善饥，口气臭秽，渴喜冷饮，小便短黄，大便秘结，舌红，苔黄，脉滑数。

4.3.1 Main symptoms Polyorexia, foul breath, thirsty with preference to cold drink, short yellow urine, constipation, red tongue, yellow moss, slippery rapid pulse.

2.病机 胃火亢盛。

4.3.2 Pathogenesis Excessive stomach fire.

3.治则 清胃泻火。

4.3.3 Treatment principle Clear the stomach and purge the fire.

4.方药 玉女煎加减（熟地黄、生石膏、麦冬、知母、牛膝）。

4.3.4 Prescription Yunv Decoction (Decoction for fair lady) with addition or reduction. Medicines: shu di huang (Radix Rehmanniae Praeparatum), sheng shi gao (Crude Gypsum Fibrosum), mai dong (Radix Ophiopogonis), zhi mu (Rhizoma Anemarrhennae), niu xi (Achyranthes Bidentatae).

5.加减运用 腹胀满，加焦槟榔、炒莱菔子、大腹皮；浊阻气机，脘痞，苔腻，加茯苓、泽泻、石菖蒲；气郁化火，胃中灼热，加黄芩、黄连、生石膏；寐差，加合欢皮、夜交藤。

4.3.5 Addition and Reduction Abdominal distention and fullness, add jiao bing lang (fried Arecae Semen), chao lai fu zi (fried Semen Raphani), da fu pi (Arecae Pericarpium); in case of turbidity resistance of qi mechanism, abdominl fullness with greasy tongue moss, add fu ling (Poria), ze xie (Rhizoma Alismatis), shi chang pu (Rhizoma Acori Graminei); When qi depression is transformed into fire with burning hot in the stomach, add huang qin (Radix Scutellariae), huang lian (Rhizoma Coptidis), sheng shi gao (Crude Gypsum Fibrosum); in case of poor sleep, add he huan pi (Albiziae Cortex) and ye jiao teng (Caulis Polygoni Multiflori).

（四）胃热湿阻

4.4 Stomach heat and dampness resistance

1.主要症状 多食善饥，渴喜冷饮，怕热，汗出较多，便秘溲赤，头晕肢体困重，倦态疲乏，口臭，舌红，苔黄腻，脉滑数。

4.4.1 Main symptoms Eat more food and easy to feel hungry, thirsty with preference to cold drink, fear of heat, sweat more, constipation, red urine, dizziness, body trapped, fatigue, halitosis, red tongue, yellow greasy moss, slippery rapid pulse.

2.病机 湿热中阻。

4.4.2 Pathogenesis Dampness and heat resistance in middle energizer.

3.治则 清热利湿。

4.4.3 Treatment principle Clear heat and dissipate dampness.

4.方药 甘露消毒饮加减（滑石、茵陈、黄芩、藿香、石菖蒲、连翘、白蔻仁、薄荷）。

4.4.4 Prescription Ganlu xiaodu Yin Decoction with addition or reduction. Medicines: hua shi (Talcum), yin chen (Artemisiae Scopariae), huang qin (Radix Scutellariae), huo xiang (Herba Agastaches seu Pogostemonis), shi chang pu (Rhizoma Acori Graminei), lian qiao (Forsythiae Radix), bai kou ren (Fructus Amomi Rotundus), bo he (Menthae Haplocalycis Herba).

5.加减运用 大便不通，加火麻仁、郁李仁；口干、口苦，加天冬、麦冬、沙参；夜寐欠安，加合欢皮、夜交藤。

4.4.5 Addition and reduction Block of stool, add huo ma ren (Semen Cannibis), yu li ren (Pruni Semen); dry and bitter mouth, add tian dong (Radix Asparagi), mai dong (Radix Ophiopogonis), sha shen (Radix Adenophorae Strictae); poor sleep at night, add he huan pi (Albiziae Cortex) and ye jiao teng (Caulis Polygoni Multiflori).

（五）肝郁气滞
4.5 Liver depression and qi stagnation

1.主要症状 胸胁胀满，胃脘痞满，月经不调甚至闭经，失眠多梦，舌质暗红，苔薄白，脉弦或弦细。

4.5.1 Main symptoms Fullness in chest and hypochondrium, epigastric ruffian, irregular menstruation or even amenorrhea, insomnia with more dreams, dark red tongue, thin white moss, string or string thready pulse.

2.病机 肝气不舒。

4.5.2 Pathogenesis Liver qi cannot be dispersed.

3.治则 疏肝理气。

4.5.3 Treatment principle Disperse the liver and regulate qi.

4.方药 柴胡疏肝散加减（柴胡、陈皮、香附、川芎、枳壳、白芍药、炙甘草）。

4.5.4 Prescription Chaihu Shugan Powder with addition or reduction. Medicines: chai hu (Radix Bulpleuri), chen pi (Pericarpium Citri Reticulatae), xiang fu (Rhizoma Cyperi) , chuan xiong (Rhizoma Chuanxiong), zhi qiao (Fructus Aurantii), bai shao (Radix Paeoniae Alba), zhi gan cao (fried Radix

Glycyrrhizae).

5.加减运用 腹胀满，加炒莱菔子、大腹皮；气机上逆，脘痞，苔腻，加茯苓、泽泻、石菖蒲；气郁化火，胃中灼热，加黄芩、黄连、生石膏；寐差，加合欢皮、夜交藤。

4.5.5 Addition and reduction Abdominal distension and fullness, add chao lai fu zi (fried Semen Raphani), da fu pi (Arecae Pericarpium); upward counterflow of qi movement, epigastric ruffian, greasy moss, add fu ling (Poria), ze xie (Rhizoma Alismatis), shi chang pu (Rhizoma Acori Graminei); when qi depression is transformed into fire with burning hot in the stomach, add huang qin (Radix Scutellariae), huang lian (Rhizoma Coptidis), sheng shi gao (Crude Gypsum Fibrosum); in case of poor sleep, add he huan pi (Albiziae Cortex) and ye jiao teng (Caulis Polygoni Multiflori).

（六）气滞血瘀

4.6 Qi stagnation and blood stasis

1.主要症状 胸胁胀满，头晕口苦，肌肤甲错，月经色暗有血块，舌紫暗，苔白，脉弦涩。

4.6.1 Main symptoms Fullness in chest and hypochondrium distension, dizziness and bitter mouth, scaly skin, dark menstruation with blood clots, purple dark tongue, white moss, string astringent pulse.

2.病机 气滞络瘀。

4.6.2 Pathogenesis Qi stagnation and blood stasis.

3.治则 行气活血通络。

4.6.3 Treatment principle Promoting qi and blood circulation and unblocking collateral.

4.方药 柴胡疏肝散合血府逐瘀汤加减（柴胡、陈皮、香附、川芎、枳壳、白芍、炙甘草、生地黄、桃仁、红花、赤芍）。

4.6.4 Prescription Chaihu Shugan Powder and Xuefu Zhuyu Decoction with addition or reduction. Medicines: chai hu (Radix Bulpleuri), chen pi (Pericarpium Citri Reticulatae), xiang fu (Rhizoma Cyperi) , chuan xiong (Rhizoma Chuanxiong), zhi qiao (Fructus Aurantii), bai shao (Radix Paeoniae Alba), zhi gan cao (fried Radix Glycyrrhizae), sheng di huang (Radix Rehmanniae), tao ren (Semen Persicae), hong hua (Flos Carthami), chi shao (Radix Paeoniae Rubra).

5.加减运用 气滞胸满，加瓜蒌、薤白；血瘀经闭、痛经，加益母草、泽兰；瘀热甚，加牡丹皮。

4.6.5 Addition and reduction Qi stagnation and chest fullness, add gua lou (Trichosanthis Fructus) and xie bai (Allii Macrostemonis Bulbus); in case of blood stasis, amenorrea, dysmenorrhea, add yi mu cao (Herba Leonuri) and ze lan (Herba Lycopi); in case of severe stagnated heat, add mu dan pi (Cortex Moutan).

（七）脾虚湿阻

4.7 Spleen deficiency and dampness resistance

1.主要症状　肢体水肿，脘腹胀满，少食，困倦嗜睡，口淡或黏腻，纳呆，舌体胖大，苔白滑腻，脉濡缓或沉细。

4.7.1 Main symptoms　Edema in limbs, abdominal distension and fullness, poor appetite, drowsiness, light or sticky mouth, anorexia, fat tongue, white slippery and greasy moss, slow weak or sunk thready pulse.

2.病机　脾虚湿盛。

4.7.2 Pathogenesis　Spleen deficiency and excessive dampness.

3.治则　健脾利湿。

4.7.3 Treatment principle　Reinforce the spleen and dissipate dampness.

4.方药　参苓白术散加减（人参、茯苓、白术、白扁豆、陈皮、山药、甘草）。

4.7.4 Prescription　Shenling Baizhu Powder with addition or reduction. Medicines: ren shen (Radix Ginseng), fu ling (Poria), bai zhu (Rhizoma Atractylodis Macrocephalae), bai bian dou (Semen Dolichoris Album), chen pi (Pericarpium Citri Reticulatae), shan yao (Dioscreae Rhizoma), gan cao (Radix Glycyrrhizae).

5.加减运用　伴中焦虚寒，可加干姜、肉桂；纳差食少，加炒麦芽、焦山楂、焦神曲；咳白痰，加半夏、陈皮等。

4.7.5 Addition and reduction　Accompanied by deficiency and cold in middle energizer, add gan jiang (Zingiberis Rhizoma) and rou gui (Cortex Cinnamomi); poor appetite, add chao mai ya (fried Hordei Fructus Germinatus), jiao shan zha (burnt Fructus Crataegi), jiao shen qu (burnt Massa Medicata Fermentata); in case of coughing white phlegm, add ban xia (Rhizoma Pinelliae), chen pi (Pericarpium Citri Reticulatae), etc.

（八）肺脾气虚

4.8 Qi deficiency of lung and spleen type

1.主要症状　咳喘痰多而稀白，腹胀，乏力，面浮足肿，大便溏，舌淡，苔白，脉弱。

4.8.1 Main symptoms　Cough with asthma, more loose and white phlegm, abdominal distension, fatigue, swelling in face and edema in feet, loose stool, light tongue, white moss, weak pulse.

2.病机　肺脾气虚。

4.8.2 Pathogenesis　Qi deficiency of lung and spleen.

3.治则　健脾益气。

4.8.3 Treatment principle　Reinforcing the spleen and replenishing qi.

4.方药　香砂六君子汤加减（人参、白术、茯苓、甘草、陈皮、半夏、砂仁、木香）。

4.8.4 Prescription　Xiangsha Liujunzi Decoction with addition or reduction. Medicines: ren shen (Radix Ginseng), bai zhu (Rhizoma Atractylodis Macrocephalae), fu ling (Poria), gan cao (Radix Glycyrrhizae), chen pi (Pericarpium Citri Reticulatae), ban xia (Rhizoma Pinelliae), sha ren (Fructus Amomi), mu xiang (Radix Aucklandiae).

5.加减运用　脾阳不振，手足不温，加附子、炮姜；气虚失运，满闷较重，加枳实、厚朴；气血两亏，心悸气短，神疲乏力，面色无华，加太子参、五味子；脾胃虚寒，加高良姜、荜茇等。

4.8.5 Addition and reduction　Sluggish spleen Yang, cool hands and feet, add fu zi (Radix Aconiti), pao jiang (prepared Ginger); qi deficiency, dysfunction of transporting, severe fullness and depression, add zhi shi (Aurantii Fructus Immaturus), hou po (Cortex Magnoliae Officinalis); dual deficiency of qi and blood, palpitation, short of breath, fatigue, dark complexion, add tai zi shen (Radix Pseudostellariae), wu wei zi (Fructus Schisandalis); spleen and stomach deficiency, add gao liang jiang (Alpiniae Officimarum Rhizoma) and bi bo (Fructus Piperis Longi), etc.

（九）脾肾阳虚型
4.9 Spleen and kidney Yang deficiency

1.主要症状　大便溏泄，腰膝酸冷，身体水肿，畏寒肢冷，舌质淡胖，苔薄白，脉缓或迟。

4.9.1 Main Symptoms　Loose stool, diarrhea, sour and cold in waist and knees, body edema, cold limbs, fear of cold, light and fat tongue, thin and white moss, slow or late pulse.

2.病机　脾肾阳虚。

4.9.2 Pathogenesis　Spleen kidney Yang deficiency.

3.治则　温补脾肾。

4.9.3 Treatment principle　Warm and tonify the spleen and kidney.

4.方药　右归丸加减（熟地黄、山药、山茱萸、枸杞子、杜仲、菟丝子、附子、肉桂）。

4.9.4 Prescription　Yougui Pill with addition or reduction. Medicines: shu di huang (Radix Rehmanniae Praeparatum), shan yao (Dioscreae rhizoma), shan zhu yu (Corni Fructus), gou qi zi (Lycii Fructus), du zhong (Cortex Eucommiae), tu si zi (Cuscutae Semen), fu zi (Radix Aconiti), rou gui (Cortex Cinnamomi).

5.加减运用　火不暖土，食少便溏，加干姜；命门火衰，飧泄、肾泄不止，加五味子、肉豆蔻；阳痿，加巴戟天、肉苁蓉等。

4.9.5 Addition and reduction　If the fire does not warm the soil, poor appetite, loose stool, add gan jiang (Zingiberis Rhizoma); if renal fire decays, undigested diarrhea, frequent midnight diarrhea, add wu wei zi (Fructus Schisandalis), rou dou kou (Semen Myristicae); impotence, add ba ji tian (Morindae Officinalis Radix), rou cong rong (Cistanches Herba), etc.

第四节　痛风病浊毒论
Section 4　On Turbid Toxin of Gout

一、病因
1. The etiology

李佃贵教授认为痛风发病分内、外因两端，有虚实标本之不同，以正气不足为本，感受外邪、浊毒瘀阻为标。

Professor Li Diangui believes that the onset of gout has etiology differences between internal and external causes, and the differences in nature of disease among asthenia and sthenia, the root and the tip, the root of the disease is the deficiency of healthy qi, the tip of the disease is being attacked by external evil, stagnation of turbid toxin.

（一）内因

1.1 Internal causes

正气不足或劳倦过度。

Lack of healthy qi or over-strained.

1.禀赋不足，肝肾亏虚　李佃贵教授认为先天禀赋不足是痛风发病之根源。肾藏精，肾主骨，肝藏血，精血互生，肝肾同源。肝属木，肾属水，肾阴不足可引起肝阴不足，肝肾阴阳，息息相通，两者一荣俱荣，一损皆损。若肝肾亏虚，精血亦亏虚，筋骨失养；肝肾之气衰弱，正气不足，易感风寒湿邪而发病。痹证日久不愈，血脉瘀阻，津聚痰凝，由经络及脏腑，导致脏腑痹。痛风病久必然导致肝肾亏损，气血不足，出现血瘀痰阻，虚实夹杂。

1.1.1 Lack of endowment and deficiency of liver and kidney　Professor Li Diangui believes that congenital endowment is the root cause of gout. Kidney stores essence, kidney controls bone, liver stores blood, essence and blood inter-promotes, liver and kidney share the same source. Liver belongs to wood category, kidney belongs to water category, kidney Yin deficiency can cause liver Yin deficiency, liver and kidney Yin and Yang, are closely linked, the two share prosperity as well as deficiency. If the liver and kidney are deficient, essence and blood will also be deficient, muscles and bones fail to be nourished; when liver and kidney qi decline, the healthy qi is deficient, patients are susceptible to wind, cold, and damp evil and fall ill. If arthromyodynia stays for a long time, the blood veins will be stagnated, fluid aggregates and phlegm will be coagulated. The disease transmits from the meridians to viscera, leads to the viscera arthromyodynia. Gout disease sustains for a long time will inevitably lead to liver and kidney deficiency, lack of qi and blood, blood stasis and phlegm resistance occurs, mixed with asthenia and sthenia.

2.气血亏虚，营卫失和　卫气主要是指功能基础——卫外、防御，而营血则主要是物质基础，两者又可相互影响，相互牵制。气为血之帅，血为气之母，血盛则气旺，气旺则血盛，气行则血行，气滞则血瘀。由上述理论可知，气血亏虚则筋脉失养；营卫失和则易感外邪，外邪入侵，易致气血运行不畅，筋脉失养。李佃贵教授认为，痛风多因浊毒之邪性热、质浊，可耗血伤气，内蕴日久气血亏损，流注经络而发病。

1.1.2 Deficiency of qi and blood, and discord of nourishing and defensive qi　The principal function of defensive qi is defending and preventing, while nutrient blood is mainly the material basis. The two can influence each other and restrict each other. Qi is the commander of blood, blood is the material source of qi. When blood is abundant, qi is sufficient, when qi is sufficient, blood will be abundant. Blood flows following the qi, blood stasis generates when qi is stagnated. It can be seen from the above theory that deficiency of qi and blood causes muscular spasm; discord of nutrient qi and defensive qi, patients will be prone to be attacked by external evil, and the invasion of external evil, leads to abnormal circulation of qi and blood, and sinews fail to be nourished. Professor Li Diangui believes that onset of gout is mostly because the nature of the turbid toxin evil is hot, but the essence of the turbid toxin evil is turbid, which can consume and impair blood and qi, after being accumulated for a long time, as qi and blood become deficient, turbid toxin flow into meridians and collateral to generate the disease.

3.脾胃虚弱，痰浊痹阻　脾为后天之本，主四肢关节肌肉，司运化之职。若先天脾胃禀赋不足，后天失养，损伤脾胃，脾胃气机不畅，运化失司，湿浊之邪内生，加之外感之邪，湿浊积聚，郁久化热，炼液成痰，痰湿痹阻，瘀血必生，痰瘀互结，滞留经络筋骨，气血运行不畅，发为本病。李佃贵教授认为，痛风是由脾虚不运，湿浊内生，湿聚成痰，日久化热瘀而成毒，浊毒内聚，注于关节，痹阻经脉而形成。

1.1.3 Weak spleen and stomach, phlegm turbidity and spasm obstruction　The spleen is the acquired foundation, controls limbs and joint muscles, is engaged in transportation. If the congenital endowment of spleen and stomach is deficient, insufficient acquired nourishment will impair the spleen and stomach. It will cause abnormal operation of qi mechanism of the spleen and stomach. Dysfunction of transporting and digesting, endogenous generation of damp and turbid evil. Coupled with external evil, wet turbidity aggregates and accumulates, and will be transformed into heat with time being, the liquid is refined into phlegm, phlegmatic hygrosis and stubborn obstruction generate blood stasis. Agglutinating of blood stasis and phlegm stranded in meridians and collateral, muscles and bones, lead to abnormal operation of qi and blood, result in the onset of gout. Professor Li Diangui believes that gout is generated because transporting dysfunction of deficient spleen causes internal generation of damp turbidity, dampness aggregates into phlegm, and then is transformed into heat, then heat is transformed into toxin, internal accumulation of turbid toxin flows into the joints and blocks the meridians.

4.脾肾两虚，浊毒内聚　脾为后天之本，肾为先天之本。脾肾两脏相互协调，主司水液代谢。脾肾两虚，则水谷运化、水液代谢失衡，继则水湿内聚，聚湿成痰，郁久化热，痰湿互结，痹阻经脉，发为痛风。李佃贵教授认为，本病病位在骨，病变脏腑归结于脾肾两脏。脾主运化，肾主水，脾肾功能失调致水液代谢失常，湿聚成痰，痰浊郁久化热成毒，浊毒随人体气之升降无处不到，游溢全身，流注于关节而发病。

1.1.4 Dual deficiency of the spleen and kidney, internal aggregation of turbid toxin   Spleen is the acquired root, kidney is the congenital root. The spleen and kidney organs coordinate with each other, mainly control metabolism of water and liquid. Dual deficiency of spleen and kidney causes abnormal transporting of water and grain, imbalance metabolism of water liquid, then water dampness aggregate into phlegm, phlegm lingering long is transformed into heat, phlegmatic dampness agglutinate, stubbornly obstruct the meridians, finally generates gout. Professor Li Diangui believes that the gout disease is located in the bone, the involved viscera are attributed to the spleen and kidney. Spleen controls transporting, kidney controls water, irregular function of spleen and kidney makes water liquid metabolism disorder, dampness aggregates into phlegm, long time depression of phlegm and turbidity will be transformed into heat then toxin, turbid toxin go everywhere of the human body along with the ascending and descending of qi movement, flow into the joints and result in the said disease.

（二）感受外邪为标

1.2 Attacked by external evil is the tip

外因风、寒、湿、热之邪侵袭人体，痹阻经络。外邪致病可以直接袭表，直接致病为患；亦可直接入里，引起脏腑失调；外邪袭表日久，可内外合邪为患。另外，个人体质、环境差异、生活饮食起居不同，所感之邪亦有别。

The external evil is of wind, cold, wet, heat attack the human body, obstruct the meridians. External evil can directly invade the surface, directly cause diseases; or directly enter the internal body, cause viscera disorder; external evil attack the surface over time, can cause diseases combining the internal and external evil. In addition, due to differences of personal constitution, environment, diet and daily life, there might be differences in category of invading evils.

（三）痰瘀浊毒互结

1.3 The Inter-binding of phlegm, stasis and turbid toxin

痰瘀浊毒的产生，是人体内外因交织的结果。

The generation of phlegm, stasis and turbid toxin is the result of the interwoven of internal and external factors of the human body.

1.内因方面   肺脾肾功能失调，水液代谢失常，痰湿内生，化生浊毒，气血运行受阻，瘀血内生，痰瘀浊毒互结，阻滞关节经络气血，气血运行不畅，则发为痛风。

1.3.1 Internal causes   Dysfunction of lung, spleen and kidney, abnormal metabolism of water and fluid, internal generation of phlegmatic hygrosis is transformed into turbid toxin, operation of qi and blood is blocked, blood stasis occurs, agglutinating of phlegm, stasis, and turbid toxin obstruct the joints, meridians, qi and blood, the abnormal operation of qi and blood lead to the onset of gout.

2.外因方面   外感湿邪，饮食不节，情志不畅等，可导致脾胃失和，进而影响肺肾功能，水湿内聚。内外因交织，错综复杂，影响疾病进程及愈后。

1.3.2 External causes   External dampness evil, irregular diet, unhealthy emotions, etc. can lead to disharmony of the spleen and stomach, and then affect the lung and kidney function, cause internal aggregation of water and dampness. Internal and external factors interweave complicatedly, affecting the progress of and recovery of the disease.

李佃贵教授认为痰瘀互结是痛风形成及反复发作的病理基础，且痰瘀贯穿于痛风的整个病程。痛风反复发作，经久不愈，符合中医"久病必瘀""久病入络"之观点。

Professor Li Diangui believes that the agglutinating of phlegm and blood stasis is the pathological basis for the formation and repeated occurrences of gout, and the phlegm and blood stasis runs throughout the whole process of gout. Frequent repetition and lingering of gout is in line with the view of "long disease generates blood stasis" and "long disease will surely get into collateral".

二、病机
2. pathogenesis

（一）湿热阻痹
2.1 Obstruction of heat and dampness

湿为阴邪，其为病多发于下肢；湿与热合，黏滞缠绵，流聚无常，故痛点常不固定，而局部肿胀灼热；湿热为有形之邪，阻遏经隧，气血不得流通，故疼痛剧烈，活动多严重受限。触之局部灼热，得凉则舒，伴发热口渴，心烦不安，溲黄，舌红苔黄腻，脉滑数，均为湿热内盛之象。

Dampness is Yin evil, it usually causes diseases in the lower limbs. Combination of dampness and heat, being sticky and lingering, with irregular state of flowing or aggregating, so the pain points are often not fixed, with local swelling and burning fever. Dampness and heat is tangible evil, which resists meridian channels obstructing qi and blood circulation, so the pain is severe and limit the freedom of activity. Patients feel locally burning hot when pressed, with want and preference to coolness, accompanied by fever and thirsty, upset, yellow urine, red tongue with yellow greasy moss, slippery rapid pulse, manifesting the image of intense excess of dampness and heat.

（二）瘀血阻络
2.2 Blood stasis resisting the collateral

湿热久羁，气血不得宣通，留而为瘀。瘀血与湿热痰浊相合，经隧阻塞更甚，故可见关节痛剧，局部肿胀变形，屈伸不利，肌肤色紫暗，按之稍硬，病灶周围或有硬结，舌质紫暗或有瘀斑，苔薄黄，脉细涩或沉弦，以及疼痛昼轻夜甚，也都是瘀血致病的特征。

Prolonged retaining of dampness and heat block the circulation of qi and blood, generating blood stasis. Combination of blood stasis, dampness, heat, phlegm and turbidity, further obstruct the meridian tunnels, patients have severe joint pain, swelling and deformation in local region of body, difficulty in flexion and extension, purple dark and slightly hard skin, or induration around the lesion, purple and dark tongue or ecchymosis, thin yellow moss, thin astringent or sunk string pulse. The pain is felt lighter at day and severe at night. All the above are the characteristics of gout caused by blood stasis.

（三）痰浊阻滞

2.3 Obstruction of phlegm and turbidity

寒湿之邪蕴于关节，日久化生痰浊，痰浊为有实而无形之品，可随气之升降无处不至。流注关节，弥漫于皮肤腠理可见关节肿胀，甚则关节周围漫肿；阻于经络可见局部酸麻疼痛；散于胸腹可见胸闷、痰多；苔黏腻、脉滑等，为痰浊素盛之象。

The evil of cold and dampness is accumulated in the joints, over time, transformed into phlegmatic turbidity. Phlegmatic turbidity is sthenia but invisible product, can reach everywhere of the body along with the ascending and descending of qi. When it flow into the joints, it diffuse in the skin and striae, causes joint swelling, even edema around the joint; When it block the meridians, local numbness pain occurs; when it is scattered in the chest and abdomen, chest tightness and more phlegm occurs; sticky greasy moss, slippery pulse is the image of usual excess of phlegmatic turbidity.

（四）浊毒阻络

2.4 Obstruction of turbid toxin in collateral

湿浊之气郁滞于关节，日久郁而化热，蕴热为毒。湿浊之气壅滞，阻滞脉络，脉络瘀阻，不通则痛，故可见关节肿痛；浊邪久蕴，化热生毒，浊毒阻滞脉络，故疼痛剧烈，甚则如刀割针刺，活动严重受限；大便秘结不通，小便短赤或黄，舌紫红，苔黄厚腻，脉滑数或弦滑数，均为浊毒壅盛之象。

Stagnation of damp turbid qi in the joints, will be transformed from depression into heat and then into toxin with time being. Abundant accumulation of damp and turbid substance obstruct the veins, pain is generated due to resistance, thus swelling and pain ofthe joint occurs; long time of accumulation of turbidity evil will be transformed into heat and toxin, turbid toxin obstructs veins, so the pain turns to be more severe, or even as painful as being knife-cutted and needled, with serious restriction of activity; constipation, short or yellow urine, purple red tongue, yellow thick and greasy moss, pulse slippery rapid or string slippery rapid pulse, are the image of intense excess of turbid toxin.

（五）肝肾阴虚

2.5 Yin deficiency of liver and kidney

痹证日久，浊毒痰瘀胶结，伤血耗气，损及肝肾，可见关节痛如被杖，局部关节变形，肌肤麻木不仁，步履艰难，筋脉拘急，屈伸不利，头晕耳鸣，颧红口干；舌红少苔，脉弦细或细数为肝肾阴虚之象。

When spasm sustains for a long time, turbid toxin and, phlegmatic stasis will be cemented, it impairs blood and consumes qi, affecting liver and kidney, patients see the joint as painful as being beaten by sticks, local joint deformation, skin numbness, difficult walking, muscular spasm, difficulty in flexion and extension, dizziness, tinnitus, red zygoma and dry mouth; red tongue less moss, string thready or thready rapid pulse are the image of liver and kidney Yin deficiency.

（六）风寒湿痹

2.6 Spasm of wind, cold and dampness

《素问·痹论》曰：　"风、寒、湿三气杂至，合而为痹。"风寒湿邪侵袭人体，流注经络，留滞关节，气血痹阻而成痹证。风气胜者，因风性善行而数变，故可见肢体、关节疼痛，或呈游走性痛；寒气胜者，因寒气凝滞，故关节剧痛遇寒加重；湿气胜者，因湿气黏滞重着，可见肢体关节重着肿痛，肌肤麻木，遇阴雨天加重；舌苔薄白，脉弦紧或濡缓为风寒湿痹之象。

Simple Conversation-Discussion on Spasm said: "Wind, cold and wet three qi joining together combine spasm." The evil of wind, cold and dampness attacks the human body, flow through meridians, stagnates in joint, obstruct the circulation of qi and blood, lead to spasm. When the wind qi is dominate, as the nature of wind is good at moving and frequent changing, patients have swelling and pain of the limbs and joints, or walking pain. When cold is dominate, as cold qi is coagulated, the pain in joint is fierce, and more fierce in case of cold attacking. When dampness is dominate, as dampness qi is sticky and heavy, patients have swelling and pain in limbs and joints, skin numbness, more severe at cloudy and raining days. Thin and white tongue moss, string tight or weak slow pulse are the image of spasm of wind, cold and dampness.

三、辨证要点
3. Syndrome differentiation points

诊断浊毒致病主要通过五个方面：①关节局部：关节局部红，肿，热，剧烈疼痛，关节迅速肿胀，以第一跖趾及拇趾关节为多见，其次为足底、踝、足跟、膝、腕、指和肘，第一次发作多在夜间。②舌质：舌质红或红绛或紫。③舌苔：苔色黄或黄白相间，苔质薄腻或厚腻。④脉象：脉滑数或弦滑。⑤分泌物、排泄物：汗液垢浊有味，大便多不爽或干结，臭秽黏腻。

Diagnosis of turbid toxin disease mainly through five aspects: a. the local part of joints: red, swelling, hot, severe pain in local part of joints, quick swelling in the joint, especially the joint of first metatarsal toe and toe joint, followed by foot bottom, foot ankle, foot heel, knees, wrist, fingers and elbow, the first onset is usually at night; b. tongue nature: red, deep red or purple tongue; c. tongue moss: yellow, or yellow and white, thin greasy, or thick greasy moss; d. pulse: slippery rapid or string slippery pulse; e. secretions, excrement: calnic and foul sweat, difficult or dry stool, foul and sticky.

（一）辨病邪

3.1 Differentiation of the disease evil

痛风的证候特征多因感受邪气的性质不同而表现各异，有风盛、寒盛、湿盛、热盛之分。

The syndrome characteristics of gout are mostly manifested differently due to the different properties of evil suffered by the patients, such as excessive wind, excessive cold, excessive dampness and excessive heat.

（二）辨急缓

3.2 Differentiation of urgent or slow disease

本病可按发作期、缓解期辨证论治。发作期，关节疼痛剧烈，症状明显，或兼恶寒发热表证，以实证为主；缓解期正虚邪恋，关节疼痛不剧烈，症状多不明显。

The disease can be treated according to the syndrome differentiation of the attacking stage or remission stage. During the attacking stage, the joint pain is severe, the symptoms are obvious, or complicated with the external syndrome of cold fearing and fever, mainly sthenia; In the remission stage, the healthy qi is deficient and the evil is lingering, the joint pain is not severe, and the symptoms are not obvious.

（三）辨虚实

3.3 Differentiation of asthenia and sthenia

一般而言，新病多实，久病多虚。实者，发病较急，正气尚能抗邪，故痛势剧，脉实有力；虚者，病程较长，多有气血不足，故疼痛绵绵，痛势较缓，脉虚无力。本病后期多见虚实夹杂，应辨明虚实，分清主次。虚证多为脾肾气阴两虚，或肝肾亏虚证。本病在早期以实证为主，缓解期则多虚实兼见，甚至以虚证为主，疼痛关节多无红肿，且疼痛不甚。

In general, new diseases are always sthenia, and long diseases are always asthenia. The sthenia disease is urgently occurred, healthy qi can still fight against evil, so pain is severe, the pulse is sthenia and powerful; the asthenia disease is usually with long course, most probably lack of qi and blood, so the pain lingers with slow tendency, pulse is weak. In the late stage of the disease, we usually see asthenia syndrome mixed with sthenia syndrome, so we should distinguish asthenia and sthenia, distinguish primary and secondary. The asthenia syndrome is mostly qi deficiency in both spleen and kidney, or deficiency both in liver and kidney. In the early stage, the disease is mainly sthenia, but in the remission stage, simultaneous asthenia and sthenia or even mainly asthenia syndromes are seen, redness and swelling can not be found in painful joints, and the pain is not serious.

（四）辨痰瘀

3.4 Differentiation of phlegm and blood stasis

各种痹证迁延不愈，症见关节漫肿，甚则强直畸形，痛如针刺，痛有定处，时轻时重，昼轻夜重，屈伸不利，舌体胖，边有齿痕，舌质紫暗，甚或可见瘀斑，脉沉弦涩。其多属正虚邪恋，瘀血阻络，痰留关节，痰瘀胶结，经络不通，关节不利，而成顽疾。

All kinds of spasm linger and difficult to recover, patients see joint swelling, even tonic deformity, as painful as being needled, fixed pain sometimes light sometimes severe, light at day and severe at night, difficulty in flexion and extension, fat tongue, with teeth mark at the edge, purple and dark tongue, or even with ecchymosis, sunk, string and astringent pulse. Most of the spasm belongs to the syndrome of deficient in healthy qi with evil lingering, blood stasis resisting the collateral, phlegm left in joints, cementing of phlegm and stasis, blocking of the meridians, and inflexible joints, consisting stubborn disease.

（五）辨兼夹

3.5 Differentiation of complex syndrome

本病之主要病因为湿热，兼夹之邪一是外邪，如起居不慎，外感风寒；二是瘀血，湿热浊毒影响气血流通而气血瘀滞。湿热浊毒与瘀血俱为有形之邪，常胶结一处，故在辨证方面须掌握其不同特征，以便了解何者为主，何者为次，而用药有所侧重。

The main etiology of the disease is dampness and heat, the complex syndrome includes external evil and blood stasis. First, external evil, for example, attacked by external evil of wind and cold due to careless daily life. The second is blood stasis, which is caused by blocking of circulation of qi and blood due to affecting of dampness, heat and turbid toxin. Dampness, heat, turbid toxin, and blood stasis are all tangible evils, usually cemented, so we must grasp its different characteristics, in order to tell the primary and the secondary and make suitable medications.

（六）望颜面五官

3.6 Observing the facial features through five sense organs

浊毒蕴结，郁蒸体内，上蒸于头面，而见面色粗黄、晦浊。若浊毒为热蒸而外溢于皮肤，则见皮肤油腻。浊毒上犯清窍而见咽部红肿，眼胞红肿、目眵增多，鼻头红肿溃烂、鼻涕多，耳屎多，咳吐黏稠之涎沫。

Internal accumulation of turbid toxin is steamed overthough the body. When the steamed turbid toxin substance reaches the head and face, patients have coarse yellow, cloudy complexion. When the turbid toxin substance reaches the skin, patients see greasy skin. When the turbid toxin substance reaches the clear orifices, patients have red and swollen throat, red and swollen eyes with more gum, nose swelling with ulceration, more nasal discharge and earwax, coughing with sticky saliva.

（七）望舌苔

3.7 Observing the tongue moss

患者以黄腻苔多见，但因感浊毒的轻重不同而有所差别。浊毒轻者舌红，苔腻、薄腻、厚腻，或黄或白或黄白相间；浊毒重者舌质紫红、红绛，苔黄腻，或中根部黄腻。因感邪脏腑不同，舌苔反映部位亦异。如浊毒中阻者，舌中部黄腻；浊毒阻于肝胆者，舌两侧黄腻。苔色、苔质根据病情的新久而变，初感浊毒、津液未伤时见黄滑腻苔，浊毒日久伤津时则为黄燥苔。

The tongue moss of most of the patients are yellow greasy, but there may be differences due to the severity of turbid toxin. Patients with light turbid toxin have red tongue, greasy moss, thin greasy, thick greasy, or yellow, or white, or yellow and white moss. Patients with severe turbid toxin have purple red, deep red tongue, yellow greasy moss, or yellow greasy moss at the middle - root of the tongue. Differences in viscera attacked by turbid toxin evil, are reflected in different part of the tongue moss. For example, obstruction of turbid toxin in middle energizer will be manifested as yellow greasy moss in the middle part of the tongue; Obstruction of turbid toxin in liver and gallbladder will be manifested as yellow greasy moss in two side edges of the tongue. The color and nature of moss will change along with the progress of the disease condition. Patients with the initial attack of turbid toxin, as the fluid and liquid has not been impaired, usually have yellow slippery greasy moss. Patients with long course of turbid toxin syndrome, as the body fluid has been impaired, usually have yellow dry moss.

（八）脉象
3.8 Pulse

浊毒证患者多见滑数脉，尤以右关脉滑数突出。临床以滑数、弦滑、弦细滑、细滑多见。病程短，浊毒盛者，可见弦滑、弦滑数脉。病程长，阴虚有浊毒者，可见细滑脉、沉细滑脉。但患者出现沉细脉时多为浊毒阻滞络瘀，而不应仅仅认为是虚或虚寒脉。

Patients with turbid toxin syndromes usually have slippery rapid pulse, especially slippery rapid pulse in right Guan pulse. In clinical practice, we usually see slippery rapid, string slippery, string slippery rapid, thready slippery pulse. If the course of the disease is short, turbid toxin is excessive, patients have string slippery, string slippery rapid pulse. Patients of turbid toxin syndrome and Yin deficiency with long course of disease, have thready slippery, sunk thready slippery pulse. However, when patients have sunk thready pulse, the syndrome is mostly obstruction of turbid toxin in collateral, and it should not only be regarded as asthenia or asthenia cold pulse.

（九）排泄物、分泌物
3.9 Excrement and secretion

浊毒内蕴，可见大便黏腻不爽，臭秽难闻，小便或浅黄或深黄或浓茶样，汗液垢浊有味。

Patients with internal accumulation of turbid toxin see difficult, sticky and foul stool, light yellow or deep yellow or thick tea-like urine, dirt and smelly sweat.

四、治疗原则
4. Principles of treatment

（一）基本治则
4.1 The basic principle of treatment

李佃贵教授从发病机制上提出"浊毒理论"，痛风为其理论中"浊毒在骨"部分，并以此为理论依据，制订了以"化浊解毒"为主治疗痛风的治则、治法，采取"急则治标，缓则治本"的法则，治疗过程中又要标本兼顾，以达到治病求本的目的，此即所谓标本先后的基本治则。

Professor Li Diangui put forward "turbid toxin theory" from the pathogenesis, in which, gout belongs to the part of "turbid toxin in bone". On the theoretical basis, he formulated the principle and method of gout treatment with "turbidity resolving and toxin removing" as the primary method, following the rule of "For urgent disease, treating from the tip. For slow disease, treating from the root". However, in the treatment process, dual attention should be paid to the tip and the root, in order to achieve the purpose of eliminating the root while curing diseases. So-called the basic principle of treatment is to distinguish the tip and the root, then decide which should be treated earlier.

李佃贵教授认为痛风当责之湿热浊毒，急性期治疗以解毒、排毒为关键，采用清热利湿、化浊解毒、通络止痛相结合的方法；缓解期病机以脾虚湿困，浊邪内蕴，肝肾亏虚为主，兼肝肾亏虚，瘀血、湿浊闭阻经络，治宜健脾除湿、通腑泻浊、补益肝肾，但亦常合用化浊法兼治其标。对久治不愈，或关节畸形者，则合用化瘀通络法。

Professor Li Diangui believes that the critical point to treat gout is to solve dampness, heat, and turbid toxin. The treatment in urgent progressing stage should focus on toxin removing, combining with the method of clearing heat and dissipating dampness, resolving turbidity and removing toxin, unblocking collateral and stopping pains. In the remission stage, the main syndrome is spleen deficiency, trap of dampness, internal accumulation of turbid evil, deficiency of liver and kidney, complicated by obstruction of blood stasis, dampness, and turbidity in the meridians. The treatment should use the method of reinforcing the spleen and removing the dampness, unblocking the fu-organ and purging the turbidity, invigorating the liver and replenishing the kidney, usually cooperating with the method of turbidity resolving to treat the tip syndrome. For long course disease which is difficult to heal, or joint deformity, the method of blood stasis resolving and collateral unblocking should be combined.

（二）常用治法

4.2 Treatment methods generally used

中医浊毒论治疗痛风病必须坚持辨证论治的原则，根据其证候表现，通常采用下列治法。

The treatment of gout disease in traditional Chinese medicine must adhere to the principle of syndrome differentiation treatment. According to its clinical manifestations, the following treatment methods are usually adopted.

1.化浊解毒法　是痛风病论治的关键，就是要把浊毒化的病理产物，通过解毒化浊，使其重新回归到生理状态，参与到人体的代谢之中去。因此，在痛风病的治疗方面，应注意适时应用芳香化浊、清热解毒法，并随症变通，从浊毒论治，以改善患者证候，逆转病势，此乃治疗痛风病的关键环节。总结起来，化浊解毒药可分为淡渗利湿之品、苦寒燥湿之品、芳香化浊之品、化瘀解毒之品、疏肝理气之品等。

4.2.1 The method of turbidity resolving and toxin removing　This method is the key to the treatment of gout. Through turbidity resolving and toxin removing, it restores the turbid toxic pathological products to the physiological state and participate in the metabolism of the human body. Therefore, in the treatment of gout, attention should be paid to the timely application of the method of turbidity resolving with aroma medicines, method of heat clearing and toxin removing, and make flexible adjustment according to syndromes. To treat according to turbid toxin theory, to improve the syndrome of the patients and reverse the disease potential, this is the key link in the treatment of gout. To sum up, the turbid toxin medicines can be divided into bland and dampness draining medicines, bitter cold and dampness drying medicines, aromatic turbidity resolving medicines, blood stasis resolving and toxin removing medicines, liver dispersing and qi regulating medicines, etc.

依据浊毒致病的特点，李佃贵教授主张治疗浊毒证应分期、分层治疗。病变早期，"浊毒"初生，以浊为主；病变中期，浊毒渐盛，胶结不去而变生百病，此阶段往往邪气盛实而正气不虚；病变后期，浊毒壅滞，以毒为主，并深入脉络，正气渐亏，病情复杂而缠绵难愈。故在临床治疗中也应根据浊毒化生的不同阶段，辨证施治，分层选药。

According to the characteristics of turbid toxin disease, professor Li Diangui advocated that the treatment of turbid toxin syndrome should be made according to different stages, and different steps. In the early stage of lesions, "turbid toxin" is generated initially, dominated by turbidity. In the middle stage of the lesion, turbid toxin gradually becomes excessive, lingers agglutinate and generates various diseases. In this stage, the evil is excessively sthenia, while the healthy qi is still not deficient. In the late stage of the lesion, turbid toxin is excessively stagnated, dominated by toxin. Turbid toxin get deep into the veins, the healthy qi gradually becomes deficient, the disease turns to be complex and difficult to heal. Therefore, the clinical treatment should also be made according to the different stages of turbid toxin progress and syndrome differentiation, medication should be provided according to the different step of treatment.

浊毒分期治疗具体治法又有祛毒、泄毒、解毒、制毒、搜毒、攻毒之不同。早期热、湿、风、寒毒邪所致之痛风，可用解、泄、祛、制之法治之；中期痰、瘀之毒邪所致痛风，则可用遏制或搜剔之法治之；对于晚期气血不足、肝肾亏虚之虚毒，则在扶正补虚损的基础上，给予攻毒之法治之。

The specific treatment measure of turbid toxin disease is different in toxin eliminating, toxin purging, detoxification, toxin restriction, toxin exorcising and toxin attacking. In the early stage the gout caused by the evil of heat, dampness, wind and cold can be solved by toxin relieving, toxin purging and toxin eliminating and toxin restricting method; in the middle stage, the gout caused by the toxic evil of phlegm and blood stasis can be solved by toxin controlling or toxin exorcising method; In the late stage, to treat the asthenia toxin syndrome due to the lack of qi and blood, the deficiency of liver and kidney, method of attacking toxin with toxin should be used on the basis of healthy qi reinforcing and deficiency reinforcing.

2.祛湿化浊法　调理脾胃、祛湿化浊，是治疗痛风病的常用方法。

4.2.2 Method of dampness dispelling and turbidity resolving　The method regulates the spleen and stomach, dispels dampness and resolves turbidity, is commonly used to treat gout.

3.调理脾胃法　中医学理论认为，先天以精气为本，后天以胃气而生，无先天而后天不立，无后天而先天不继。痛风病的形成有一个漫长的过程，本病的发生、发展及转归均与脾的功能下降有着极为密切的关系。脾失健运是痛风病形成的一个非常重要的病机，因此治疗本病的关键当以调理脾胃、健脾助运为主，同时根据临床辨证，分清虚实，并辅以益气养阴、清热解郁、化痰除湿、活血化瘀等法，做到辨病与辨证相结合，以求标本同治。

4.2.3 Method of regulating the spleen and stomach　According to TCM theory, essence qi is the congenital root of life, the stomach qi is the acquired root of life. Without the congenital root, the acquired root cannot stand. without the acquired root, the congenital root cannot sustain. The formation of gout disease has a long process, and the occurrence, development and outcome of this disease are closely related with the decline of spleen function. Dysfunction of spleen transportation is a very important pathogenesis for the formation of gout, so the key to treat the disease is to laying stress on regulating the spleen and stomach, reinforcing the spleen and assisting the transporting, at the same time, according to the clinical syndrome differentiation, distinguish asthenia and sthenia, and supplemented by the method of replenishing qi and nourishing Yin, clearing heat and releasing depression, resolving phlegm and removing dampness, promoting blood circulation and resolving blood stasis, so as to combine syndrome differentiation with disease differentiation, aiming at curing the tip as well as the root.

4.化浊祛瘀通络法　痰浊、瘀血都是疾病过程中所形成的病理产物，两者互为因果。李佃贵教授在治疗痛风时善从痰瘀论治，具体应把握以下原则：①临证时应首先辨别痰与瘀之先后、轻重，再根据辨证结果确定从痰或从瘀论治的主次：痛风早期即无症状高尿酸血症期，此时辨证以痰证为主，治疗上应注重从痰论治，组方多选用祛痰之品为主，辅以健脾祛湿之品；痛风急性期，辨证多属湿热痰瘀痹阻经络、停滞关节，此时应痰瘀并治，兼顾祛湿热，组方多选用祛痰、化瘀之品，辅以祛湿热之药；痛风慢性期，治疗上注重痰瘀并治与痰瘀互治相结合，活血以利痰消，祛痰以利血行，血活则痰化，痰化则瘀消，常用活血化瘀祛痰之品兼加搜剔通络之药。②注重调理气机以助化痰祛瘀：在治疗痛风时，运用痰瘀同治法时当注重调畅气机，临证时方中常配以益气理气之品，既可补益脾肾之气，有助于津血正常运化输布，防止痰瘀形成；又可达"气行则血行，气行则水行"之功，助祛痰化瘀之品有效地化除停滞之痰瘀。

4.2.4 Method of resolving turbidity, removing blood stasis and unblocking the collateral

phlegmatic turbidity and blood stasis are the pathological products formed in the process of disease, the two are interchangeable relations of cause and result. Professor Li Diangui is good at treating gout from phlegm and stasis. The following specific principles should be grasped: a. In clinical practice, we should first identify the priority and severity of stasis and phlegm, according to the result of syndrome differentiation, to decide whether to treat from phlegm or from stasis first: in the early stage of gout, i.e. the stage of asymptomatic hyperuricemia, at this time, the syndrome differentiation is mainly sputum syndrome, treatment should be made according to the sputum theory. The prescription should mainly choose the expectorant products, supplemented by the products of spleen reinforcing and dampness dispelling. In the acute stage of gout, syndrome differentiation is mostly dampness, heat, phlegm, and stasis obstruct the meridians, block the joints, at this time, there should dual treatment towards phlegm and blood stasis, cooperate with elimination of dampness and heat. The prescription should mainly choose medicines of removing phlegm and resolving blood stasis, with medicines of dispelling dampness and heat as auxiliaries. In the chronic stage of gout, attention should be paid to simultaneously treat phlegm and stasis and make inter-treatment of phlegm and stasis, to eliminate phlegm by promoting blood circulation, and to promote the blood circulation by eliminating the phlegm. When blood moves smoothly, the phlegm can easily be dissipated, when the phlegm is resolved, blood stasis will disappear. Generally using medicines of blood circulation promoting, blood stasis resolving, and phlegm dispelling, supplemented by evil exorcising and collateral unblocking medicines. b. focusing on the regulating qi mechanism to help resolving phlegm and removing blood stasis: when treating gout, especially when using the method of simultaneous treating phlegm and blood stasis, stress should be laid on regulating the qi movement, in clinical practice, products of replenishing and regulating qi are often equipped. It can both replenish the spleen and kidney qi, assist the normal transporting and distribution of fluid and blood, prevent the formation of sputum and blood stasis; at the same time, can prove that "when qi moves, blood flows, when qi moves, water follows", helping the product for dispelling phlegm and removing blood stasis to effectively remove the stagnant phlegm and blood stasis.

从上述病因病理看，本病主要是脾肾功能失调，痰浊瘀滞血中而成，故治疗应以化痰泄浊为主，兼以调理脾肾，佐以活血化瘀通络止痛。在痛风病的治疗中，从脾论治，可以更好地提高临床疗效。

Observing from the above etiology and pathology, this disease is mainly caused by spleen and kidney dysfunction, and stagnation of phlegm and turbidity in blood, so the treatment should mainly resolve phlegm and purge turbidity, simultaneously regulate the spleen and kidney, and auxiliarily promote blood circulation, resolve blood stasis, unblock collateral and relieve pain. To treat the gout disease from the spleen can better improve the clinical efficacy.

五、从浊毒论治痛风病
5. To treat gout disease according to turbid toxin theory

李佃贵教授主张痛风病宜根据临床表现分期进行辨证治疗，即急性发作期、慢性缓解期、间歇期三个阶段。

Professor Li Diangui advocated that gout disease should be treated by syndrome differentiation according to clinical manifestations in different stage: acute onset stage, chronic remission stage and interval stage.

（一）急性发作期（浊毒炽盛期）
5.1 Acute attack stage (stage of intense excess of turbid toxin)

本期多由热毒炽盛，瘀滞血脉，闭阻经络关节所致。临床表现多为起病急骤，关节红肿发热，痛如刀割或咬噬样剧烈，口干口渴，面红目赤，大便干，小便黄赤，舌质红，脉数。故该期治疗以解毒、排毒为关键。排毒则重视利小便、通大便，使浊毒从二便而下，以达到洁净脏腑之作用。治宜清热解毒、利湿通络，方用五味消毒饮合四妙散加减。常用药物：金银花、蒲公英、紫花地丁、苍术、薏苡仁、牛膝、黄柏、虎杖、大黄、土茯苓、山慈菇、苦参、猪苓、泽泻、车前草、滑石、竹叶等。现代药理研究证实：大黄有抗感染、解热、降血脂、调节免疫的作用；黄柏中的小檗碱等生物碱有解热、抗感染、抗血小板聚集及提高免疫的作用；苍术能改善脾虚动物的代谢功能，提高红细胞的功能，有抗缺氧的作用；牛膝提取物有提高机体免疫功能、镇痛、利尿、解热、抗感染、消肿、稳定感染细胞作用，总皂苷呈现较好的镇痛及活血止痛作用，多糖类可增强体液免疫。二妙丸能燥湿清热，显著抑制小鼠接触性皮炎，两者配合有增强趋势，并能抑制超敏反应，生品急性抗感染作用最强。四妙丸中，黄柏合苍术通治上下湿气，有抗菌与显著排盐作用；薏苡仁解热镇痛的强度与氨基比林相似。金银花、黄柏可消除感染反应，缓解关节红肿疼痛症状；山慈菇具有较好的促进尿酸排出、降低血尿酸、止痛的作用，其内含秋水仙碱，可在几个小时内使关节的红肿热痛消失。另外山慈菇、滑石等还具有碱化尿液的作用，可起到一箭双雕之效。该期的主要治疗目的是缓解症状，迅速控制急性感染反应。嘱患者卧床休息，抬高患肢，避免受累关节负重，一般在关节疼痛缓解72小时后开始恢复活动；避免高嘌呤的食物，禁饮酒；鼓励多饮水，以促进尿酸的排泄；注意患肢保温，避免受凉。

In this stage the syndrome is mostly caused as the intense excess of hot toxin is stagnated in blood and veins, blocks the meridians and joints. The clinical manifestations are acute onset, redness and fever in joints, the pain is as severe as being knife-cut, or bitten by animals, dry and thirsty mouth, red eyes and faces, dry stool, yellow red urine, red tongue, rapid pulse. Therefore, the key of treatment in this period is mainly toxin removing. To remove toxin, we should attache importance to dissipate urine, unblock stool, so that turbid toxin can be discharged along with defecation and urination, in order to achieve the purpose of cleaning the viscera. The treatment method is clearing heat and removing toxin, dissipating the dampness and unblocking the collateral. The prescription is Wuwei Xiaodu Decoction (five disinfection drink), combined with Simiao Powder (powder of four wonderful drugs) with addition or reduction. Medicines generally used are: jin yinhua (Loniceriae Japonicae Flos), pu gong ying (Herba Taraxaci cum Radice), zi hua di ding (Herba Violae), cang zhu (Rhizoma Atractylodis), yi yi ren (Semen Coisis), niu xi (Radix Achyranthis BidenTatae), huang bo (Cortex Phellodendri), hu zhang (Rhizoma Polygoni Cuspidati), da huang (Radix et Rhizoma Rhei), tu fu ling (Rhizoma Smilacis Glabrae), shan ci gu (Pseudobulbus Cremastrae Variabilis), ku shen (Sophorae Flavescentis Radix), zhu ling (Polygorus Umbellatus), ze xie (Rhizoma Alismatis), che qian cao (Herba Plantaginis), hua shi (Talcum), zhu ye (Folium Phillostachydis Nigrae), etc. Modern pharmacological research proves that da huang (Radix et Rhizoma Rhei) has the function of anti-infection, anti-pyretic, reducing blood lipid, and regulating immunity; the berberine extracted from huang bo (Cortex Phellodendri) has function of antipyretic, anti-infection, anti-platelet aggregation and the function of improving immunity; cang zhu (Rhizoma Atractylodis) can improve metabolic function of spleen deficiency animals, improve red cell function, anti-hypoxia; niu xi (Radix Achyranthis BidenTatae) can improve immune function, analgesia, diuresis, antipyretic, anti-infection, swelling and stable infected cells, polysaccharides can enhance humoral immunity. Ermian Pill can dry dampness and heat, significantly inhibit contact dermatitis in mice, the two have an enhancement trend, and can inhibit hypersensitivity reaction, the acute anti-infection effect is the strongest. In Simiao Wan, huang bo (Cortex Phellodendri) combining with cang zhu (Rhizoma Atractylodis) has antibacterial and significant salt discharge effect in treatment of the upper and lower moisture. The antipyretic and analgesic strength of yi yi ren (Semen Coisis) is similar to that of amino bilin. jin yin hua (Flos Lonicerae Japonicae Flos) and huang bo (Cortex Phellodendri) can eliminate infection reaction and relieve joint swelling and pain symptoms; shan ci gu (Pseudobulbus Cremastrae Variabilis) can promote the discharge of uric acid, reduce blood uric acid and relieve pain. It contains colchicine and can disappear within a few hours. In addition, shan ci gu (Pseudobulbus Cremastrae Variabilis), hua shi (Talcum) also have the role of alkaline urine, can play the effect of killing two birds with one stone. The primary treatment objective in this phase is to relieve symptoms and rapidly control the acute infection response. Tell patients to rest in bed, raise the affected limb, avoid weight bearing on affected joints, and resume activity 72 hours after joint pain relief; avoid high purine foods and avoid alcohol; encourage the patients to drink more water to promote the excretion of uric acid; pay attention to keep warm of the affected limb to avoid catching cold.

（二）慢性缓解期（浊毒潜伏期）

5.2 Chronic remission stage (turbidity poison incubation period)

缓解期热毒之邪虽解，但湿热之邪仍缠绵。临床表现：关节红肿热痛症状明显缓解，但某些关节仍肿痛不适，舌质略红，苔薄黄，脉弦细。治宜清热利湿，方选萆薢分清饮（《医学心悟》）加减。常用药物：萆薢、石菖蒲、黄柏、白术、茯苓、车前子、丹参、薏苡仁、土茯苓等。现代药理研究证实：萆薢、土茯苓有利尿作用，能增加尿素、尿酸和氮化物的排泄；黄柏、薏苡仁能增强血流量及血尿酸排泄。诸药合用，能促进尿酸排泄，使关节肿痛进一步缓解。

Although the evil of heat toxin is solved, but the evil of dampness and heat is still lingering. Clinical manifestations are: symptom of red, swelling, hot and painful joint is obviously relieved, but some joints are still swollen and uncomfortable, slightly red tongue, thin yellow moss, and string thready pulse. To treat the syndrome, use the method of clearing heat and dissipate dampness, the proper prescription is Bixie Fenqing Decoction (Medical Enlightenment). Medicines generally used: bi xie (Rhizoma Dioscrea), shi chang pu (Rhizoma Acori Graminei), huang bo (Cortex Phellodendri), cang zhu (Rhizoma Atractylodis), fu ling (Poria), che qian zi (Semen Plantaginis), dan shen (Salviae Miltiorrhizae), yi yi ren (Semen Coisis), tu fu ling (Rhizoma Smilacis Glabrae), etc. Modern pharmacological studies confirm that bi xie (Rhizoma Dioscrea) and tu fu ling (Rhizoma Smilacis Glabrae) have diuretic effect and can increase the excretion of urea, uric acid and nitride, while huang bo (Cortex Phellodendri) and yi yi ren (Semen Coisis) can enhance blood flow and blood uric acid excretion. Combined drugs can promote the excretion of uric acid, further relieving the symptom of joint swelling and pain.

（三）间歇期（浊毒留恋期）

5.3 Intermittent stage (stage of turbid toxin lingering)

李佃贵教授认为本期的病机以脾虚湿困为主，兼肝肾亏虚，瘀血、湿浊闭阻经络，故治疗上以防止痛风急性发作、纠正高尿酸血症、预防尿酸盐沉积造成关节破坏及肾脏损害为主要目标。治宜健脾除湿，通腑泻浊，补益肝肾。常用药物：党参、白术、薏苡仁、土茯苓、制大黄、萆薢、猪苓、泽泻、车前子、滑石、牛膝、地龙、苍术等。车前子、土茯苓、地龙等有一定的排尿酸作用。若痰毒为著，关节畸形、结石者，治宜活血化瘀、软坚散结，常选药物穿山甲、白芥子、皂角刺、夏枯草、王不留行、山慈菇、两头尖、牡蛎、牡丹皮、赤芍、红花、牛膝、鸡血藤、当归、生地黄、川芎等。其中，牡丹皮、赤芍、红花、牛膝可扩张血管，改善局部微循环。

Professor Li Diangui believes that the pathogenesis in this period is mainly spleen deficiency and trapping of dampness, accompanied by liver and kidney deficiency, blood stasis and damp turbidity obstructing the meridians, so the main goal of treatment in this stage is to prevent acute attack of gout, correct hyperuricemia, prevent joint damage caused by uric and urinate deposition and damages of kidney. The treatment method is reinforcing the spleen and removing dampness, unblocking the fu-organ and purging turbidity, and tonifying and replenishing the liver and kidney. Medicines generally used are: dang shen (Radix Codonopsitis Pilosulae), bai zhu (Rhizoma Atractylodis Macrocephalae), yi yi ren (Semen Coisis), tu fu ling (Rhizoma Smilacis Glabrae), zhi da huang (prepared Radix et Rhizoma Rhei), bi xie (Rhizoma Dioscrea), zhu ling (Polygorus Umbellatus), ze xie (Rhizoma Alismatis), che qian zi

(Semen Plantaginis), hua shi (Talcum), niu xi (Radix Achyranthis BidenTatae), di long (Lumbricus), cang zhu (Rhizoma Atractylodis), etc. Che qian zi (Semen Plantaginis), tu fu ling (Rhizoma Smilacis Glabrae), di long (Lumbricus), have certain effect to remove urine acid. If phlegmatic toxin is obvious, joint deformity, calculus occur, treatment should promote blood circulation and resolve blood stasis, soften hardness and dissipate binds, medicines generally used are: chuan shan jia (Squanma Manitis), bai jie zi (Semen Snapis Albae), zao jiao ci (Gleditsiae Spina), xia ku cao (Spica Prunellae), wang bu liu xing (Vaccariae Semen), shan ci gu (Pseudobulbus Cremastrae Variabilis), liang tou jian (Anemones Raddeanae Rhizoma), mu li (Ostreae Concha), mu dan pi (Cortex Moutan), chi shao (Radix Paeoniae Rubra,) hong hua (Flos Carthami), niu xi (Radix Achysanthis Bidentatae), ji xue teng (Caulis Spatholobi), dang gui (Radix Angelicae Sinensis), sheng di huang (Radix Rehmanniae), chuan xiong (Rhizoma Chuanxiong), etc. Among them, mu dan pi (Cortex Moutan), chi shao (Radix Paeoniae Rubra), hong hua (Flos Carthami), and niu xi (Radix Achyranthis Bidentatae) can dilate blood vessels and improve local microcirculation.

第十一章　眼病浊毒论
Chapter 11　On Turbid Toxin of Eye Disease

第一节　五轮浊毒辨证
Section 1　Five Rounds of Turbid Toxin Syndrome Differentiation

　　五轮学说是中医眼科的独特理论，把眼分为五个部分，分属五脏，对应五行。眼由外至内分为五个部分，即眼睑、两眦、白睛、黑睛和瞳神，并分别分属于脾、心、肺、肝和肾五脏，命名为肉轮、血轮、气轮、风轮、水轮，用于说明眼的解剖、生理、病理及其与脏腑的关系，并用于指导临床辨证治疗。由于五脏的相互关系、五行的生克乘侮，五轮之间亦存在着密切关系，轮脏相关的理论是中医眼科特有的辨证方法。

　　The five-round theory is a unique theory of ophthalmology in traditional Chinese medicine. The eye is divided into five parts, belonging to the five viscera, corresponding to the five elements. Eye from outside to inside is divided into five parts: eyelid, canthus, eyes, black eyes and pupil, and respectively belong to the spleen, heart, lung, liver, and kidney, named meat wheel, blood wheel, air wheel, wind wheel, water wheel, to illustrate eye anatomy, physiology, pathology and its relationship with viscera, and used to guide clinical differentiation treatment. Due to the inter-relationship of five zang - organs, the generating, restraining, over - restraint and counter - restraint relations of five elements, five rounds also has a close relationship, wheel and viscera related theory is traditional Chinese medicine eye differentiation method.

　　五轮辨证为眼科独特的辨证方法，因浊毒感邪的轻重不同而有不同的临床表现。将浊毒理论与五轮辨证相结合用于临床实践，对于疾病的诊断及治疗具有重要的指导作用。

　　Five - round syndrome differentiation is a unique syndrome differentiation method of ophthalmology, which has different clinical manifestations due to the different severity of attacking of turbid toxin evil. Combining turbid toxin theory with five-round syndrome differentiation in clinical practice has an important guiding role in the diagnosis and treatment of ophthalmology diseases.

一、肉轮辨证
1. Meat wheel syndrome differentiation

　　浊毒初犯胞睑可见胞睑红肿、疼痛，压痛明显，胞睑皮肤可见红赤、糜烂、水疱、渗出。浊毒日久，阻滞经络气血，胞睑失养可见胞睑皮肤干枯、皱缩、无光泽，胞睑提升无力可见胞睑下垂，气血不荣筋脉可见胞睑蠕动。浊毒初犯胞睑可见睑内颗粒大而红，浊毒日久可见睑内颗粒扁平，颜色污浊。

When turbid toxin initially attacks the internal eyelid, patients have redness, swelling, pain and obvious tenderness. Redness, erosion, blisters, exudation can be seen in eyelid skin. When turbid toxin stays for a long time, The eyelid fails to be nourished, the skin becomes dry, wrinkled, lustreless; when the eyelid is difficult to be lifted, thus the eyelid is dropped; as the blood qi does not nourish the sinews, the eyelid peristalsis. When the turbid toxin first attacks the eyelid, patients have the large and red eyelid particles. When turbid toxin stays for a long time, the particles in the eyelid becomes flat with filthy color.

二、血轮辨证
2. Blood wheel syndrome differentiation

浊毒初犯两眦可见硬结，红赤、疼痛、压痛明显。眦角皮肤红赤，糜烂，渗出。两眦赤脉粗大，颜色鲜红。眦部胬肉红赤，发展迅速，眼珠磨涩不适。浊毒日久，可见两眦部红黄夹杂，颜色污浊，眦部皮肤干枯，无光泽。两眦赤脉迂曲扩张，颜色发暗。

When turbid toxin initially attacks two canthus, patients have induration, redness, pain and obvious tenderness. The skin in canthal corner is red, erosive and oozing. The hyperemia of the two canthus is coarse and large, with bright red color. The pterygium is red and develops rapidly. The eyeballs are uncomfortable with sense of whet and astringent. When turbid toxin stays for a long time, the canthus of patients are mixed with red and yellow, filthy, the canthal skin is dry and dull. The hyperemia of the two canthus are circuitous and expand around, and the color is dark.

三、气轮辨证
3. Qi wheel syndrome differentiation

浊毒初犯白睛可见白睛红赤，颜色鲜红，或白睛混赤，或局限性红赤，眼珠疼痛拒按，白睛赤脉粗大，颜色鲜红。白睛表层可见浮肿，眵泪增多，分泌物黏稠，有热感。浊毒日久，白睛可见颜色污浊、枯涩、无光泽，白睛赤脉迂曲，白睛可遗留片状高低不平、颜色污浊或青蓝色结节。

When turbid toxin initially attacks the white eyes, patients have red white eyes, with bright red color, or white mixed with red eyes, or limited red eyes, the eyeballs are painful and refused to be pressed. The hyperemia of white eyes are thick, with bright red color. Patients have edema in white eye surface, more tears and gum, sticky secretion with sense of heat. When turbid toxin stays for a long time, white eyes can be seen filthy, dry, dull, the hyperemia of white eyes are winding, white eyes can leave uneven pieces of filthy blue nodules.

四、风轮辨证
4. Wind wheel syndrome differentiation

浊毒初犯黑睛可见黑睛混浊，黑睛生翳，翳大或溃陷，赤脉伸入黑睛，赤脉颜色鲜红，排列稠密，眵泪增多，分泌物黏稠，有热感。浊毒日久，可见黑睛污浊，遗留斑片状，或斑点状云翳，云翳颜色灰白或瓷白，黑睛周边赤脉颜色污浊。

When turbid toxin first attacks the black eyes, patients have cloudy black eyes generating nebula, which grows and collapse. The hyperemia gets into the black eyes, with bright red colour, densely arranged, with More tears and gum, sticky secretion with sense of heat. When turbid toxin stays for a long time, patients have filthy black eyes, leaving patches, or spot-shaped nebula with gray white or porcelain white colour, the hyperemia around the black eyes are muddy.

五、水轮辨证
5. Water wheel syndrome differentiation

浊毒初犯瞳神可见瞳神散大，眼胀眼疼，眼硬如石，或瞳神缩小，神水混浊，黑睛后壁有沉着物，黄液上冲，视力骤减。浊毒日久，可见瞳神歪斜不正，或干缺不圆，或瞳神紧缩不开，或内结白色圆翳，视物模糊。

When turbid toxin initially attacks the pupil, patients have pupil platycoria, distension and pain in eyes, the eyes are as hard as stone, or contracted pupil, with cloudy pupil water, deposition in the back wall of eyes, with yellow fluid flushing upward, the vision sharply reduces. When turbid toxin stays over time, patients have aslant pupil, or dry but not round pupil, or pupil contracted, or internally generates white circle nebula, with obscure vision.

浊毒初犯神膏可见尘状、片状、条状或团块状混浊；目系水肿，充血隆起，颜色鲜红，边缘模糊；视衣血管迂曲扩张，或呈串珠样；视衣火焰状或点片状出血，颜色鲜红；视衣弥漫性或局限性水肿，视衣色素沉着较少见。浊毒日久，神膏可见絮状或线状混浊；目系色淡，或色白或苍白；视衣血管动脉细，或动静脉均细；视衣污浊，可见暗红色点片状出血，或黄白色渗出或萎缩灶，黄斑区污浊，可有局限性水肿；视衣色素紊乱或色素堆积。

When turbid toxin initially attacks the vitreous body, patients have dust-like, pieces of, strips of, or mass state vitreum; edema in eyes, congestion of bright red color, and obscure edges; retina vessels dilated, or just like a string of beads; retina bleeding like flame or spot with bright red colour; retina with diffused or localized edema, retina pigmentation is scarcely seen. When turbid toxin stays over time, the vitreous body have flocculent or linear turbidity; the colour of eyes color are light, or white or pale; retina vessel artery is thready, or both the retina vessels and veins are thready; retina is filthy, with dark red spots or pieces of bleeding, or yellow white leakage or atrophy, muscular area is muddy, may have localized edema; retina pigment disorder or pigment accumulation.

第二节　结膜炎浊毒论
Section 2 On Turbid Toxin of Conjunctivitis

一、结膜炎的中医学概述
1. Overview of conjunctivitis in Traditional Chinese Medicine

结膜炎是眼科最常见的疾病，是指球结膜和睑结膜的病变。中医学的白睛包括了球结膜，所以说结膜炎的病变部位在白睛。白睛属肺，病变脏腑与肺有关。结膜炎在中医学有详细的论述，归属于多个疾病，如"暴风客热""赤丝虬脉""天行赤眼""时复症"等。

Conjunctivitis is the most common disease of ophthalmology, which refers to the lesions of the ball conjunctiva and eyelid conjunctiva. As the white eyes in traditional Chinese medicine includes the ball conjunctiva, so the lesions of conjunctivitis are in the white eyes. The white eye belongs to the lung, and the diseased viscera is related to the lung. Conjunctivitis has been discussed in detail in traditional Chinese medicine, belonging to a number of diseases, such as "fulminant wind and retained heat", "hyperemia of ocular conjunctiva", "epidemic red eye", "recurrent diseases" and so on.

二、结膜炎的病因病机
2. The etiology and pathogenesis of conjunctivitis

结膜炎的病因病机与天、地、人之浊毒有关。结膜炎最常见的病因为外感风热之邪或疫疠浊毒之气，或是体内素有蕴热或湿热，复受外邪，内外合邪，上犯于目。

The etiology and pathogenesis of conjunctivitis is associated with the turbid toxin of heaven, earth and man. The most common disease of conjunctivitis is because of the evil of external wind heat or epidemic turbid toxin, or internal accumulated heat or damp heat in body is attacked by external evil, the combination of internal and external evil invade the eyes.

天之浊毒方面，最常见的致病因素为微生物感染，随着全球气候变暖，生态环境恶化，致病微生物大量繁殖，气候变化还会使人的抵抗能力和免疫能力下降，增加结膜感染的概率。另外，空气中污染物增加，包括悬浮颗粒物、粉尘、二氧化硫、一氧化碳、碳氢化物、氮氧化物等。眼部结膜与空气直接接触后，这些物质产生的物理性刺激与化学性的损伤可增加结膜感染的概率，而且影响泪膜的稳定性，使结膜炎的发病率大大增加，病变迁延不愈，往往反复发作。

In terms of heaven turbid toxin, the most common pathogenic factor is microbial infection. Along with the global warming, the deterioration of ecological environment and the proliferation of pathogenic microorganisms, and the climate changes will reduce people's ability of resistance and immunity, increases the probability of conjunctive infection. In addition, increasing of the pollutants in the air including suspended particular, dust, sulfur dioxide, carbon monoxide, hydrocarbons, nitrogen oxides and so on. When the eye conjunctiva contacts air directly, the physical stimulation and chemical damage produced by the above substances increases the probability of conjunctive infection, and affect the stability of the tear film, so the incidence of conjunctivitis greatly increased, the lesions lingers and difficult to heal, often repeat again and again.

地之浊毒方面，主要是指受污染的水和食物。水是一切生命赖以生存的基础，被污染的水一方面与眼部结膜直接接触，增加结膜感染的概率，且长期的水污染易使结膜炎迁延不愈或反复发作；另一方面，水污染使食物的质量安全难以得到保障，被污染的水和食物首先经口进入人体的消化系统，损伤脾胃，使后天之本受损，变生浊毒，脏腑功能紊乱而致百病丛生，眼部受累而病。

The turbid toxin of the earth mainly refers to the polluted water and food. Water is the fundamental substance to survive people's life, on one hand, the contaminated water which direct ly contact with the ocular conjunctiva will increase the possibility of conjunctive infection, and the chronic water pollution make conjunctivitis linger and difficult to heal; on the or the hand, water pollution affect the quality safety of food, the contaminated water and food first enter the digestive system of the human body, damaging the spleen and stomach,i.e damaging the acquired root of life, producing turbid toxin, causes disorder of viscera function and various diseases, involving eyes and lead to the said disease.

人之浊毒方面，主要与生活方式的改变及心之浊毒有关。眼部疾病与情志关系密切，情志不畅，肝气不疏，复受外邪，内外合邪，蕴积为浊毒上犯于目；另一方面，过食膏粱厚味，脾胃受损，体内蕴热变生浊毒而上犯于目。另外，现代人生活方式及生活节奏的改变，长期使用电脑、手机等视频终端，经常熬夜，工作压力大、紧张、劳累等，均可使眼部抵抗力下降，增加结膜炎感染的概率。

Human turbid toxin, it is mainly related with lifestyle changes and the turbid toxin of mind. Eye diseases are closely related with emotions. When the emotion state is abnormal, the liver qi is not sparse, once suffering from the attack of external evil, the combination of internal and external evil will be accumulated into turbid toxin which invade the eyes. On the other hand, over-taking of the greasy food impairs the spleen and stomach, the undigested substances are transformed into heat and then turbid toxin, invading the eyes. In addition, the changes of modern lifestyle and life pace including long-term use of computers, mobile phones and other video terminals, often staying up late, working pressure, tension, fatigue, etc. can reduce the eye resistance, increase the probability of conjunctivitis infection.

三、浊毒辨证论治
3. Turbid toxin syndrome differentiation treatment

结膜炎辨证应分辨虚实，实者还应辨清内外之邪。外邪见于外感浊毒之邪，浊毒上犯；内邪见于脏腑浊毒内蕴，与脾胃、肝胆、心关系密切。虚者多为浊毒伤阴及浊毒伤气，与肺脾气虚关系密切。

The conjunctivitis syndrome differentiation treatment should distinguish the asthenia and sthenia, and for sthenia syndrome we should further distinguish the internal and external evil. The external evil is usually the external turbid toxin evil, which attacks the eyes. The internal evil is usually seen as internal accumulation of viscera turbid toxin, closely related with the spleen, stomach, liver, gallbladder and heart. The asthenia syndromes are usually impair of Yin and qi by turbid toxin, which is closely related with qi deficiency of lung and spleen.

（一）外感浊毒

3.1 Suffering from external turbid toxin

1.证候　白睛红赤，痛痒兼作，胞睑肿胀，眵多胶结。头痛鼻塞，口渴思饮，小便黄，甚或大便秘结，舌红，舌苔薄黄，脉数或浮数。

3.1.1 Symptoms　Red white eyes, pain and itching, eyelid swelling, cemented gum.Headache, nasal congestion, thirsty with want to drink, yellow urine, or even constipation, red tongue, thin yellow tongue moss, rapid or floating rapid pulse.

2.病机　外感浊毒上犯白睛，故白睛红赤，痛痒兼作，眵多胶结；浊毒壅于胞睑则胞睑肿胀；浊毒上犯头目则头痛鼻塞；浊毒伤津则口渴思饮，小便黄、大便秘结。

3.1.2 Pathogenesis　The external turbid toxin attacks the white eyes.

3.治则　疏风清热解毒。

3.1.3 Treatment principle　Dispersing wind, clearing heat and removing toxin.

4.主方　自拟疏风清热解毒汤加减。

3.1.4 Main prescription　Self-proposed prescription of wind dispersing, heat clearing and toxin removing decoction with addition or reduction.

5.药物　柴胡、荆芥、防风、薄荷、黄芩、桔梗、甘草等。

3.1.5 Medicines　Chai hu (Radix Bulpleuri), jing jie (Herba Schizonepetae), fang feng (Radix Saposhnikoviae), bo he (Menthae Haplocalycis Herba), huang qin (Radix Scutellariae), jie geng (Radix Platycodi), gan cao (Radix Glycyrrhizae), etc.

6.加减　浊毒重症可加用金银花、连翘、野菊花以疏风清热解毒；大便秘结者，加大黄、芒硝以泻火通便。

3.1.6 Addition and reduction　Severe turbid toxin disease, add jin yin hua (Lonicerae Japonicae Flos), lian qiao (Forsythia Radix), ye ju hua (Herba et Radix Chrysanthemi) to clear heat and remove toxin; in case of constipation, increase da huang (Radix et Rhizoma Rhei), mang xiao (Natrii Sulfas) to purge fire and unblock the defecation.

（二）浊毒内蕴

3.2 Internal accumulation of turbid toxin

1.证候　白睛红赤或混赤、肿胀，焮热疼痛，刺痒交作，胞睑红肿，眵多黏稠色黄。头痛头晕，口干口苦，喜饮，小便黄赤短少，大便秘结，舌质红，舌苔黄或黄腻，脉数或滑数。

3.2.1 Symptoms   Red or mixed red white eyes, swelling, burning hot and painful, alternative acantha and itching, red and swollen eyelid, sticky and yellow gum. Headache, dizziness, dry and bitter mouth, like to drink, yellow red and short little urine, constipation, red tongue, yellow or yellow greasy tongue moss, rapid or slippery rapid pulse.

2.病机　患者体内素有浊毒内蕴，上熏白睛则白睛红赤、刺痒交作、眵黄黏稠，浊毒重症可见白睛混赤、肿胀、甚或焮热疼痛；浊毒壅于胞睑则胞睑红肿；浊毒上犯头目可见头痛头晕；浊毒伤津耗液可见口干口苦、小便黄赤短少、大便秘结。

3.2.2 Pathogenesis   Internal accumulated turbid toxin attacks the white eyes.

3.治则　清热化浊解毒。

3.2.3 Treatment principle   Clearing heat, resolving turbidity and removing toxin.

4.主方　自拟清热化浊解毒汤加减。

3.2.4 Main prescription   Self-intended prescription of clearing heat and resolving turbidity and removing soup with addition or reduction.

5.药物　黄连、黄芩、夏枯草、栀子、决明子、荆芥、防风、大黄等。

3.2.5 Medicines   Huang lian (Rhizoma Coptidis), huang qin (Radix Scutellariae), xia ku cao (Spica Prunellae), zhi zi (Fructus Gardeniae), jue ming zi (Semen Cassiae), jing jie (Herba Schizonepetae), fang feng (Radix Saposhnikoviae), da huang (Radix et Rhizoma Rhei), etc.

6.加减　白睛溢血广泛可加用生地黄、牡丹皮以凉血清热；眼睛奇痒可加用蝉蜕、木贼、乌梅以祛风止痒。

3.2.6 Addition and reduction   Overflow of blood in white eyes, add sheng di huang (Radix Rehmanniae), mu dan pi (Cortex Moutan) to cool serum heat; itchy eyes, add chan tui (Cicadae Periostracum), mu zei (Scouring Rush), wu mei (Fructus Mume) to dispel wind and stop itching.

（三）浊毒伤阴

3.3 Turbid toxin impairing Yin

1.证候　白睛微红或不红，赤脉迂曲细小，眼涩，不耐久视，灼热感，时轻时重，眵少质稀。口干咽干，头晕耳鸣，舌红少津，脉细。

3.3.1 Symptoms   White eyes slightly red or not red, the hyperemia is winding and small, astringent eyes impatient for long-time watching, with sense of burning hot sometimes light sometimes severe, less and loose gum. Dry mouth and pharynx, dizziness, tinnitus, red tongue with little fluid, fine pulse.

2.病机　浊毒日久不祛，浊毒伤阴，白睛红赤不明显，营血暗伤，赤脉细小；阴津不足，津不上承，故眼干涩不适、不耐久视；阴虚火旺，则有灼热感；口干咽干，头晕耳鸣为阴虚之象。

3.3.2 Pathogenesis   Turbid toxin will impair Yin if it stays for a long time, the white of eye is slightly red, blood is impaired silently, conjunctival congestion occurs. Yin liquid is insufficient and cannot be transferred upward therefore the eyes of the patient become dry, astringent and cannot concentrate. Burning heat sensation occurs due to Yin deficiency with blood-heat. Dry mouth and throat, dizziness and tinnitus are the image of Yin deficiency.

3.治则 养阴清热解毒。

3.3.3 Treatment principle Nourish Yin, clear heat and remove toxin.

4.主方 自拟养阴清热解毒汤加减。

3.3.4 main prescription Self-intended prescription of Decoction of Nourishing Yin, Clearing Heat and Removing Toxin with addition or reduction.

5.药物 生地黄、知母、玄参、黄芩、泽泻、牡丹皮、甘草等。

3.3.5 Medicines Sheng di huang (Rehmannia), zhi mu (Rhizoma Anemarrhennae), xuan shen (Radix Scrophulariae), huang qin (Radix Scutellariae), ze xie (Rhizoma Alismatis), mu dan pi (Cortex Moutan), gan cao (Radix Glycyrrhizae), etc.

6.加减 若心烦失眠，加酸枣仁、茯神以养心安神；若津少便结，加决明子、火麻仁以润肠通便。若偏于肺阴伤，加沙参、麦冬以滋养肺阴。

3.3.6 Addition and reduction If upset and insomnia, add suan zao ren (Semen Zizyphi Jujubae), fu shen (Parasita Poriae) to nourish the mind; in case of less fluid, constipation, add jue ming zi (Semen Cassiae), huo ma ren (Semen Cannibis) to moisten the intestines and unblock the defecation. If partial to lung Yin impairing, add sha shen (Radix Adenophorae Strictae), mai dong (Radix Ophiopogonis) to nourish lung Yin.

（四）浊毒久滞，肺脾两虚

3.4 Pro-longed stagnation of turbid toxin, dual deficiency of lung and spleen

1.证候 白睛微红或不红，赤脉淡红，日久难愈，或反复发作。精神倦怠，气短乏力，食欲不振，大便溏薄，舌淡，舌苔薄白，脉缓无力。

3.4.1 Symptoms White eyes slightly red or not red, the hyperemia is light red, difficult to heal, or with repeated attacks. Spiritually fatigue, short of breath, poor appetite, loose and thin stool, light tongue, thin and white tongue moss, slow and weak pulse.

2.病机 浊毒日久不祛，损伤肺脾，正虚不足，故白睛微红或不红，赤脉淡红；土不生金，卫外不固，故病久难愈，或反复发作；精神倦怠、气短乏力、食欲不振、大便溏薄为肺脾两虚之象。

3.4.2 Pathogenesis Turbid toxin damaging the lung and spleen, deficiency of healthy qi. So white eyes are slightly red or not red, the hyperemia is light red; soil promotes metal, the exterior defensive qi is not solid, thus the disease is difficult to heal, or will reoccur again and again; spiritually fatigue, short of breath, poor appetite, loose and thin stool, are the appearance of double dificiency of lung and spleen.

3.治则 健脾补肺祛浊。

3.4.3 Treatment principle　Strengthen the spleen and replenish the lung to dispel turbidity.

4.主方　参苓白术散加减。

3.4.4 Main prescription　Shenling Baizhu Powder with addition or reduction.

5.药物　党参、白术、茯苓、山药、桔梗、陈皮、甘草等。

3.4.5 Medicines　Dang shen (Radix Codonopsitis Pilosulae), bai zhu (Rhizoma Atractylodis Macrocephalae), fu ling (Poria), shan yao (Chinese yam), jie geng (Platycodon Grandiflorum), chen pi (Pericarpium Citri Reticulatae), gan cao (Radix Glycyrrhizae), etc.

6.加减　若偏于肺气虚，可加黄芪以补肺益气。

3.4.6 Addition and reduction　If the lung qi partially deficient, add huang qi (Radix Astragali seu Hedysari) to tonify the lung and replenish qi.

第三节　角膜炎浊毒论
Section 3　On Turbid Toxin of Keratitis

一、角膜炎的中医学概述
1. Overview of keratitis in Traditional Chinese Medicine

角膜炎属于中医学"聚星障""银星独见""湿翳""凝脂翳"等范畴。"聚星障"是指黑睛浅层骤生多个细小星翳，其形或连缀，或团聚，伴有沙涩疼痛，羞明流泪的眼病。"银星独见"是指黑睛独生一翳，色白如银，形状如星的眼病。"湿翳"病程长，可反复发作，严重者会引起黑睛毁坏而失明。"凝脂翳"是指黑睛生翳，状若凝脂，多伴有黄液上冲的急重眼病。

Keratitis belongs to the category of "clustered star nebula", "silvery star nebula", "wet nebula", "fat coagealing nebula" and so on. "Clustered Star Nebula" refers to a few small thin star - like union, or re-union nebula are suddenly generated over the shallow layer of the black part of the eyes accompanied by astringent pain, shy tears of eye diseases. "Silvery star Nebula" refers to one star- like silver white nebula disease generated over the black part of eye. "Wet nebula" has long course, will reoccur repeatedly, the serious syndrome might cause black eye damage and blindness. "Fat coagealing nebula" refers to the sudden onset fat coagulation like nebula disease over the black part of eyes accompanied by yellow liquid flowing upwards.

二、角膜炎的病因病机
2. The etiology and pathogenesis of keratitis

角膜炎属外障眼病范围，其发病与外邪关系密切。肝开窍于目，目为肝之外候，五轮学说中角膜属风轮，与肝相应。《兰室秘藏》云："夫五脏六腑之精气，皆禀受于脾，上贯于目。脾者诸阴之首也，目者血脉之宗也，故脾虚则五脏之精气皆失所司，不能归明于目也。"根据以上理论及临床观察，浊毒学说认为角膜炎反复发作的病机为脾虚则清阳不升、浊阴不降。清气不升可致眼部炎症反复发作，重者可出现角膜溃疡，日久不敛。角膜炎急性发作的病机除单纯外邪侵袭外，更多为肝火上炎或肝胆浊毒内蕴，复感外邪而发病。

Keratitis belongs to the scope of external eye diseases, and its incidence is closely related to external evil. The liver opens orifices as eyes, and the eye is external manifestation of the liver. In the five rounds of theory, the cornea belongs to the wind wheel, corresponding to the liver. *The Secret Collection of the Orchid Room* says: "The essence qi of the viscera are transported by the spleen, and will be sent up to the eyes, thus the spleen is the head of the Yin, the eye is the collection of the blood vessels. So the spleen deficiency will cause dysfunction of all the essence of the viscera, failing to create the brightness of eyes." According to the above theory and clinical observation, the theory of turbid toxin believes that the pathogenesis of recurrent keratitis is spleen deficiency. The Spleen fails to ascend the lucid Yang and descend turbid Yin due to spleen deficiency. Abnormal ascending of lucid qi can cause repeated onset of eye inflammation, if severe, corneal ulcer occurs, lingers for a long time without recovering. In addition to the simple attack of external evil, the pathogenesis of acute onset of keratitis is that hepatic fire inflammation or internal accumulation of liver and gallbladder turbid toxin combines with external evil and generates diseases.

三、浊毒辨证论治
3. Turbid toxin syndrome differentiation treatment

角膜炎辨证应分辨虚实，实者应辨内邪与外邪，虚者与脾关系密切。

Keratitis syndrome differentiation should distinguish asthenia and sthenia, the sthenia syndrome should further distinguish the internal and external evil, and the deficiency is closely related to the spleen.

（一）外感热毒
3.1 Suffering from external heat toxin

1.证候　黑睛浅层骤生细小星翳，羞明流泪，沙涩不适，抱轮红赤，伴口干咽痛，大便干，小便黄，甚或大便秘结，舌红，舌苔薄黄，脉数或浮数。

3.1.1 Symptoms　A few small thin star-like union, or reunion nebula are suddenly generated over the shallow layer of the black part of the eyes, photophobia with tears, discomfort with trachoma astringent, ciliary congestion, with dry mouth and sore throat, dry stool, yellow urine, or constipation, red tongue, thin and yellow tongue coating, rapid or floating rapid pulse.

2.病机　外感毒邪，上犯清窍，经气不利，故沙涩不适，羞明流泪，抱轮红赤；毒邪上犯，则口干咽痛。

3.1.2 Pathogenesis　External toxic evil attacks eyes , inhibitted flow of meridian qi, photophobia with tears, discomfort with trachoma astringent, ciliary congestion, with dry mouth and sore throat.

3.治则　解毒疏风退翳。

3.1.3 Treatment principle　Remove toxin, disperse wind and retreat the nebula.

4.主方　解毒祛风汤加减。

3.1.4 Main prescription　Jiedu Qufeng Decoction with addition or reduction.

5.药物　金银花、连翘、蒲公英、栀子、射干、蔓荆子、木贼、玄参、赤芍、甘草。

3.1.5 Medicines　Jin yin hua (Lonicerae Japonicae Flos), lian qiao (Forsythiae Fructus), pu gong ying (Herba Taraxaci cum Radice), zhi zi (Fructus Gardeniae), she gan (Belamcandae Rhizoma), man jing zi (viticis Fructus), mu zei (Scouring Rush), xuan shen (Radix Scrophulariae), chi shao (Radix Paeoniae Rubra), gan cao (Radix Glycyrrhizae).

6.加减　抱轮红赤明显者加大青叶、板蓝根、紫草以清热凉血退翳。

3.1.6 Addition and reduction　With obvious ciliary congestion, add da qing ye (Folium Isatidis), ban lan gen (Radix Isatidis), zi cao (Radix Arnebiae) to clear heat and cool blood and retreat nebula.

（二）浊毒内蕴

3.2 Internal accumulation of turbid toxin

1.证候　黑睛生翳溃腐，或黑睛肿胀增厚，混浊不清，抱轮红赤，反复发作，病情缠绵，头重胸闷，舌质红，舌苔黄或黄腻，脉数或滑数。

3.2.1 Symptoms　Nebula generated over the ulcerated black part of eyes, or swelling in black part of eyes becomes thicker, cloudy, ciliary congestion, repeatedly occurs, lingering, heaviness of head and tightness of chest, red tongue, yellow or yellow greasy moss, rapid or slippery rapid pulse.

2.病机　患者体内素有浊毒内蕴，上熏黑睛则黑睛生翳、病情反复，重者可见生翳溃腐，黑睛浑浊不清，形如圆盘，浊毒上犯可见头重胸闷。

3.2.2 Pathogenesis　Internal accumulation of turbid toxin fumigate the black part of eyes with repeated attacks, for severe patients, nebula and ulceration occur, the black part of eyes is turbid as a round plate. When turbid toxin attacks upward, head heaviness and chest tightness occur.

3.治则　化浊解毒退翳。

3.2.3 Treatment principle　Resolve turbidity, remove toxin and retreat the nebula.

4.主方　化浊解毒退翳汤。

3.2.4 Main prescription　Decoction of turbidity resolving, toxin removing and nebula retreating.

5.药物　龙胆草、黄芩、车前子、草决明、钩藤、金银花、蒲公英、天花粉、菊花、蒺藜、木贼、赤芍、牡丹皮。

3.2.5 Medicines　Long dan cao (Gentianae Radix et Rhizoma), huang qin (Radix Scutellariae), che qian zi (Semen Plantaginis), cao jue ming (Semen Cassiae), gou teng (Uncariae Ramulus Cum Unicis), jin yin hua (Lonicerae Japonicae Flos), pu gong ying (Herba Taraxaci cum Radice), tian hua fen (Radix Tricosansthis), ju hua (Chrysanthemi Flos), ji li (Fructus Tribuli), mu zei (Scouring Rush), chi shao (Radix Paeoniae Rubra), mu dan pi (Cortex Moutan).

6.加减　便秘或口渴加生石膏、知母以清热泻火滋阴；伤胃者加茯苓、枳壳调理脾胃。

3.2.6 Addition and reduction　Constipation or thirsty in mouth, add sheng shi gao (Crude Gypsum Fibrosum), zhi mu (Rhizoma Anemarrhennae) to clear heat, purge fire and enrich Yin; in case of stomach impairing, add fu ling (Poria), zhi qiao (Fructus Aurantii) to regulate the spleen and stomach.

（三）脾虚生浊，清阳不升
3.3 Spleen deficiency generates turbidity, qing Yang does not ascend

1.证候　黑睛浅层点状星翳，白睛微红或不红，赤脉淡红，日久难愈，或反复发作。精神倦怠，气短乏力，食欲不振，大便溏薄，舌淡，边有齿痕，舌苔薄白，脉缓无力。

3.3.1 Symptoms　Light dotted star - like nebula generate in shallow layer of the black part of eyes, white part of eyes slightly red or not red, the hyperemia is lightly red, difficult to heal, or repeatedly attacks. Spiritually fatigue, short of breath, poor appetite, loose stool, light tongue, marginal teeth mark, thin and white tongue moss, slow and weak pulse.

2.病机　脾虚运化水谷精微失常，正虚不足，不能抵御外邪，故病情迁延不愈；黑睛浅层点状星翳，白睛微红或不红均为余邪难祛的表现；精神倦怠、气短乏力、食欲不振、大便溏薄为脾运化失常之象。

3.3.2 Pathogenesis　Spleen deficiency causes abnormal transporting of cereal essence, healthy qi deficiency, unable to resist external evil, so the disease is lingering; light dotted star-like nebulas generate in shallow layer of the black part of eyes, white part of eyes slightly red or not red is the manifestation of the lingering remaining evil; spiritual fatigue, shortness of breath, lack of appetite, thin and loose stool manifest the transporting disorder of the spleen.

3.治则　健脾益气化浊，升清退翳。

3.3.3 Treatment principle　Reinforce the spleen, replenish qi, resolve turbidity, ascend the lucidity and retreat the nebula.

4.主方　健脾化浊退翳汤。

3.3.4 Main prescription　Decoction of reinforcing the spleen, resolving turbidity and retreating nebula.

5.药物　黄芪、白术、苍术、薏苡仁、茯苓、赤芍、防风、木贼、丹参、蝉蜕。

3.3.5 Medicines　Huang qi (Radix Astragali seu Hedysari), bai zhu (Rhizoma Atractylodis Macrocephalae), cang zhu (Rhizoma Atractylodis), yi yi ren (Semen Coisis), fu ling (Poria), chi shao (Radix Paeoniae Rubra), fang feng (Radix Saposhnikoviae), mu zei (Scouring Rush), dan shen (Salviae

Miltiorrhizae), chan tui (Cicadae Peristracum).

6.**加减**　偏于气虚者加太子参；头部不适明显者加升麻、柴胡以升清，加陈皮以健脾化浊理气。

3.3.6 Addition and reduction　Patients partial to qi deficiency, add tai zi shen (Radix Pseudostellariae); obvious head discomfort, add sheng ma (Rhizoma Climicifugae), chai hu (Radix Bulpleuri) to ascend the lucidity, add chen pi (Pericarpium Citri Reticulatae) to strengthen the spleen, resolve turbidity and regulate qi.

第四节　葡萄膜炎浊毒论
Section 4　On Turbid Toxin of Uveitis

一、葡萄膜炎的中医学概述
1. Overview of uveitis in Traditional Chinese Medicine

葡萄膜炎属于中医学"瞳神紧小"及"瞳神干缺"范畴，前葡萄膜炎伴有前房积脓，属"黄液上冲"范畴。瞳神紧小是指黄仁受邪，以瞳神持续缩小，展缩不灵，多伴有抱轮红赤、黑睛内壁沉着物、神水混浊及视力下降为主要临床症状的眼病。本病若失治、误治，特别是不及时散瞳，极易造成黄仁后粘连，导致瞳神干缺或其他眼病，引起失明。瞳神干缺是指瞳神紧小症失治、误治，导致黄仁与其后晶珠发生粘连，瞳神失去正圆，边缘参差不齐，形如锯齿或花瓣，且伴有视力下降的内障眼病。

Uveitis belongs to the category of "contracted pupil" and "pupilliary metamorphosis" in traditional Chinese medicine, and anterior uveitis is accompanied by hypopyon, which belongs to the category of "flushing on yellow fluid". Contracted pupil refers to the eye disease caused by yellow sclera being attacked by evil, with clinical symptoms as pupil continues to contract, inflexible to enlarge and shrink, accompanied by ciliary congestion, deposited substances in the inner wall of black part of eyes, turbid aqueous fluid and diminution of vision. If this disease is not treated in time, or treated by mistake, especially mydrasis cannot be made in time, it will cause yellow sclera adhesion, lead to pupilliary metamorphosis or other eye diseases, even causing blindness. The pupilliary metamorphosis refers to internal barrier eye disease caused by the delayed or mistake treatment of contracted pupil which leads to adhesion of sclera and the posterior crystal bead, incomplete pupil circle, saw-teeth or petals shape uneven edges, accompanied by diminution of vision.

二、葡萄膜炎的病因病机
2. The etiology and pathogenesis of uveitis

由于现代生活水平的提高，生活压力的增加，加之恣食肥甘厚味、饮酒过度，结合情志等因素，该病常见病因有肝失疏泄，肝气郁结，日久火毒内生，郁久生风，体内的肝火与肝风同气相求，易招引风热之邪而诱发本病；肝胆火盛，日久转为毒邪，黄仁受灼，或因浊毒内蕴，熏蒸黄仁；湿致病者，因恣食肥甘厚味、情志因素致湿热浊毒内蕴，浊毒内蕴困着体内，胃气上逆，肺气不降，清阳不升，浊阴不降，气机不畅，肝气郁滞，诱发本病。因湿热之邪难速去，故病情多缠绵，加之这类患者发病急，眼部症状较重，病久伤及肝肾，肝肾阴虚，或因热毒伤阴，虚火上炎再则病程缠绵，耗伤气血，浊毒留滞，正虚邪实，乃致脾肾阳虚。

The onset of uveitis is due to the improvement of modern living standards, the increase of life pressure, over-taking of greasy food, excessive drinking, combined with emotional factors. The general causes of the disease are dysfunction of liver dispersing, long-time depression of liver qi generates internal fire toxin and wind, the liver fire and wind in body like attracts like, are easy to attract the evil of wind and heat to generate the said disease; the fire of liver and gallbladder is excessive, will turns to be toxic evil over time, the yellow sclera is burnt, or the internal accumulation of turbid toxin fumulate the yellow sclera; disease caused by dampness, over - taking of greasy food and emotional factors causes internal accumulation of turbid toxin of dampness and heat, stomach qi counterflows, the lung qi does not descend, lucid Yang does not rise, the turbid Yin does not descend, the qi movement cannot operate normally, lead to liver qi stagnation, induce the generation of the said disease. Because the evil of dampness and heat cannot be quickly removed, so the disease is usually lingering. In addition, as the disease of these patients often attacks acutely with severe eye symptoms, long course disease impairs liver and kidney, the liver and kidney Yin becomes deficient. Or because heat toxin injures Yin, the deficiency fire generates inflammation, so the course of disease is long, consuming qi and blood. Turbid toxin retains, healthy qi is deficient and evil is excessive, and even the spleen and kidney Yang becomes deficient.

三、浊毒辨证论治
3. Turbidity poison syndrome differentiation on treatment

中医学认为本病主要是由于浊毒内蕴，病邪由少阳、三焦内归肝胆；或嗜食肥甘厚味，酿成脾胃湿热，浊毒内蕴或外感风湿，郁久化热，风湿与热相搏，循肝经上犯清窍所致。本病为瞳神疾病，瞳神属肾，而本病主要病变部位为黄仁，黄仁位于眼底中央主土，黄仁色黄，故黄仁属脾，因此本病与肝、脾、肾关系密切。

Traditional Chinese medicine believes that the disease is mainly caused by internal accumulation of turbid toxin. The disease evil attacks shao yang, triple energizer and invades liver and gallbladder; or being addicted to greasy food results dampness and heat in the spleen and stomach, internal accumulation of turbid toxin or exogenous rheumatism, long time of depression turns to be heat, rheumatism and heat fight against each other, attacks the clear orifice i.e. eye along with the liver meridian. This disease is pupil disease, pupil belongs to the kidney. The main lesion is in yellow sclera located in the bottom centre of eyes which belongs soil. The yellow sclera is in yellow colour, so yellow sclera reflects the spleen, so this disease is closely related with the liver, spleen and kidney.

　　将中医学与浊毒理论相结合，本病辨证的重点为辨虚实，急性起病者多为实证，以外感风热之邪、肝经风热及浊毒上犯多见，起病较缓或反复发作者多为虚证，以浊毒内蕴伤阴多见。临证应辨清病因，分清虚实。

Combining the turbid toxin theory with traditional Chinese medicine, the focus of the syndrome differentiation is to identify asthenia and sthenia. The disease of acute onset is mostly sthenia, generally caused by the external evil of wind heat, attack of wind heat through the liver meridian, and upward-attack of turbid toxin. If the onset of the disease is slow or repeated, it is usually asthenia, generally caused by internal accumulation impairing Yin. Clinical treatment should make clear the cause, and distinguish the asthenia and the sthenia.

（一）肝经风热，毒邪上犯

3.1 The upward attack of the wind and heat evil in liver meridian

1.全身症状　头痛发热，口干舌红，苔薄白或薄黄，脉浮数。

3.1.1 Systemic symptoms　Headache and fever, dry mouth, red tongue, thin white or thin yellow moss, floating and rapid pulse.

2.眼部症状　起病较急，瞳神紧小，眼珠坠痛，视物模糊，抱轮红赤，神水混浊，黄仁晦暗，纹理不清。

3.1.2 Ocular symptoms　Urgent onset, small and tight pupil, dropping painful of eyeballs, blurred vision, ciliary congestion, muddy aqueous fluid, dark yellow sclera, unclear texture.

3.病机　风热毒邪循经上犯清窍。

3.1.3 Pathogenesis　Wind, heat and toxin evil attack eyes along with the channels.

4.治则　疏风清热解毒。

3.1.4 Treatment principle　Dredging wind, clear heat and detoxification.

5.主方　自拟清热解毒疏风汤。

3.1.5 Main prescription　Self-prepared decoction of dispersing wind, clearing heat and removing toxin.

6.药物　金银花、蒲公英、柴胡、黄芩、钩藤、防风、蝉蜕、木贼、桑白皮、桑叶、桔梗、甘草。

3.1.6 Medicines　Jin yin hua (Lonicerae Japonicae Flos), pu gong ying (Herba Taraxaci cum Radice), chai hu (Radix Bulpleuri), huang qin (Radix Scutellariae), gou teng (Uncariae Ramulus Cum Unicis), fang feng (Radix Saposhnikoviae), chan tui (Cicadae Peristracum), mu zei (Scouring Rush), sang bai pi (Cortex Mori), sang ye (Folium Mori), jie geng (Platycodon Grandiflorum), gan cao (Radix Glycyrrhizae).

（二）浊毒内蕴，风热外袭

3.2 Internal accumulation of turbid toxin and external attack of wind heat evil

1.全身症状　头重胸闷，肢节酸痛，口渴，汗出，心烦，尿赤，或口苦，胁痛，舌质红，苔黄腻，脉弦滑数。

3.2.1 Systemic symptoms　Head heaviness and chest tightness, acrid pain in limbs, thirsty, sweat, upset, red urine, or bitter mouth, pain in hypochondrium, red tongue, yellow and greasy moss, string slippery rapid pulse.

2.眼部症状　发病或急或缓，眼红赤、眼痛、怕光、流泪，瞳神紧小或偏缺不圆，目赤痛，眉棱痛，视物昏蒙，神水混浊。

3.2.2 Ocular symptoms　Urgent or slow onset, red eyes, pain in eyes, fear of light, tears, pupil tight and small or incompletely round, red eyes with pain, pain in eyebrow, dizzy vision, turbid aqueous fluid.

3.病机　风热浊毒上犯清窍。

3.2.3 Pathogenesis　Upward attack of wind heat turbid toxin on the clear orifice.

4.治法　化浊解毒祛风。

3.2.4 Treatment principle　To resolve turbidity, remove toxin and dispel wind.

5.主方　自拟祛风解毒汤。

3.2.5 Prescription　Self-prepared decoction of wind dispelling and toxin removing.

6.药物　黄柏、黄连、薏苡仁、生石膏、知母、防风、秦艽、决明子、茯苓。

3.2.6 Medicines　Huang bo (Cortex Phellodendri), huang lian (Rhizoma Coptidis), yi yi ren (Semen Coisis), sheng shi gao (Crude Gypsum Fibrosum), zhi mu (Rhizoma Anemarrhennae), fang feng (Radix Saposhnikoviae), qin jiao (Radix Gentianae Macrophyllae), jue ming zi (Semen Cassiae), fu ling (Poria).

（三）浊毒内蕴

3.3 Internal accumulation of turbid toxin

1.全身症状　胁肋灼热胀痛，厌食腹胀，口苦，干呕，大便不调，小便短赤，或见寒热往来，身目发黄，或阴部瘙痒，或带下色黄秽臭，舌质红，苔黄腻，脉弦数或滑数。

3.3.1 Systemic symptoms　Hypochondrium burning and distension pain, anorexia, abdominal distension, bitter mouth, retching, irregular stool, short red urine, or alternative attack of coldness and heat, yellow eyes and body, or genital itching, or with yellow and foul leukorrahea, red tongue, yellow and greasy moss, string rapid or slippery rapid pulse.

2.眼部症状　视物模糊，瞳神甚小，珠痛拒按，痛连眉棱骨，抱轮红甚，神水混浊，黄液上冲。

3.3.2 Ocular symptoms　Blurred vision, smaller pupil, pain in eyeball refused to press, pain even involves supra-orbital ridge, ciliary congestion, muddy aqueous fluid, upward rushing of yellow liquid.

3.病机　浊毒内蕴，上蒙清窍。

3.3.3 Pathogenesis Internal accumulation of turbid toxin hoodwinking the clear orifice.

4.治则 化浊解毒，祛风开窍。

3.3.4 Treatment principle Turbidity resolving, toxin removing, wind dispelling and orifice opening.

5.主方 自拟解毒化浊祛风汤。

3.3.5 Main prescription Self-proposed decoction of toxin removing, turbidity resolving and wind dispelling.

6.药物 龙胆草、栀子、黄芩、柴胡、生地黄、车前子、泽泻、木通、甘草、当归、荆芥、防风。

3.3.6 Medicines Long dan cao (Gentianae Radix et Rhizoma), zhi zi (Fructus Gardeniae), huang qin (Radix Scutellariae), chai hu (Radix Bulpleuri), sheng di huang (Radix Rehmanniae), che qian zi (Semen Plantaginis), ze xie (Rhizoma Alismatis), mu tong (Akebiae Caulis), gan cao (Radix Glycyrrhizae), dang gui (Radix Angelicae Sinensis), jing jie (Herba Schizonepetae), fang feng (Radix Saposhnikoviae).

（四）浊毒伤阴

3.4 Turbid toxin impairing Yin

1.全身症状 虚烦少寐，寐则汗出，醒则汗止，形体消瘦，午后潮热，五心烦热，女子月经不调，男子梦遗，口苦咽干，舌红少苔，脉细而数。

3.4.1 Systemic symptoms Insomnia with deficient restlessness, sweating while sleeping, stop sweating as soon as awakening, thin body, hectic fever in the afternoon, upset fever in five centres, women's menstrual disorder, men's nocturnal emission, bitter mouth and dry throat, red tongue less moss, thready and rapid pulse.

2.眼部症状 病势较缓或病至后期，眼干涩不适，视物昏花，赤痛时轻时重，反复发作，瞳神多见干缺不圆。

3.4.2 Ocular symptoms The disease is gradual or in late stage, eyes are dry and uncomfortable, dizziness, red pain sometimes light sometimes severe, repeated attacks, pupil usually dry and not round.

3.病机 浊毒伤阴，阴虚内热。

3.4.3 Pathogenesis Turbid toxin impairing Yin, Yin deficiency with internal heat.

4.治则 滋阴解毒。

3.4.4 Treatment principle Enriching Yin and removing toxin.

5.主方 自拟滋阴解毒汤。

3.4.5 Main prescription Self-prepared decoction of enriching Yin and removing toxin.

6.药物 生石膏、知母、玄参、麦冬、天花粉、生地黄、黄柏、荆芥、防风。

3.4.6 Medicines Sheng shi gao (Crude Gypsum Fibrosum), zhi mu (Rhizoma Anemarrhennae), xuan shen (Radix Scrophulariae), mai dong (Radix Ophiopogonis), tian hua fen (Radix Tricosanthis), sheng di huang (Radix Rehmanniae), huang bo (Cortex Phellodendri), jing jie (Herba Schizonepetae), fang feng (Radix Saposhnikoviae).

第五节　糖尿病视网膜病变浊毒论
Section 5　On Turbid Toxin of Diabetic Retinopathy

一、糖尿病视网膜病变的中医学概述
1. Overview of diabetic retinopathy in Traditional Chinese Medicine

糖尿病视网膜病变为中医"消渴目病"，是糖尿病的眼部严重并发症，其特点为"外不见症从内而蔽之"。糖尿病属于中医"消渴""消瘅"范畴，病名首见于《黄帝内经》，刘完素在《三消论》中指出："夫消渴者，多变聋盲。"然而对于糖尿病视网膜病变，在古代中医文献中，没有关于本病病名的明确记载。但是对于其原发病消渴所引起的视力障碍则早有记载，并对其病因病机提出了各种见解。由于古代文献中没有明确的病名记载，根据视力的损害程度及自觉症状，应属于中医眼科"视瞻昏渺""云雾移睛""血灌瞳神""暴盲"等范畴。

Diabetic retinopathy, "Xiaoke disease" in Traditional Chinese Medicine, is a serious complication in eyes of diabetes characterized by "invisible from outside, but obstructing the view from the inside". Diabetes belongs to "Xiaoke", "Xiaoyang" category of TCM, the name first seen in *The medical Classic of the Yellow Emperor*. Liu Wansu pointed out in *Three Elimination*: "Diabetes patients will most probably become deaf and blind." Although there is no clear record of the disease name as "diabetic retinopathy" in the ancient Traditional Chinese Medicine literature. But the visual impairment caused by the original onset of diabetes has been recorded earlier, and various insights on the etiology and pathogenesis of the disease have been put forward. Because there is no clear disease name recorded in ancient literature, according to the degree of visual impairment and conscious symptoms, it should belong to the categories of "blurred vision", "cloud-foggy moving before the eyes", "blood pouring in the pupil" and "sudden blindness".

二、糖尿病视网膜病变的病因病机
2. The etiology and pathogenesis of diabetic retinopathy

随着人们生活水平的不断提高，传统的饮食习惯已被打破，高热量、高蛋白、高脂饮食及强食过饮现象非常普遍。我国糖尿病患者日渐增多，总数每年至少增加100万，我国糖尿病患者中糖尿病视网膜病变的患病率为44%～51.3%。究其原因，一是过食强食，损伤脾胃，一是运动减少，气血阻滞。两者导致血中浊毒积聚，浊毒瘀阻于目络而为病。

Along with the continuous improvement of people's living standards, the traditional diet habits have been broken, high calories, high protein, high fat diet and excessive eating and drinking phenomenon is very popular. The number of diabetes patients in China is constantly increasing, the total number of diabetes patients increases at least 1 million per year, the prevalence of diabetic retinopathy in diabetes patients is 44% to 51.3%. One of the reason is over - eating, which impairs the spleen and stomach. The other reason is decreasing of movement causes obstruction of qi and blood. The two reasons lead to aggregation of turbid toxin in the blood, stagnation of turbid toxin in eye collateral, resulting in the said disease.

糖尿病视网膜病变的重要病因病机是过食强食导致浊毒瘀阻于目络。一方面现代人饮食失节，过食肥甘厚味，损伤脾胃运化功能，导致湿聚食积，化为痰饮，蕴郁日久，化为浊毒之邪；另一方面，现代人生活方式的改变，长年伏案，以车代步，室外活动减少，不仅可以导致气血亏虚，而且还可以使气机阻滞，津液运化、布散失常，从而浊毒之邪滋生。《张氏医通·诸血门》亦曰："人饮食起居，一失其节，皆能使血瘀滞不行也。"血瘀久则成毒，百病乃变化而生。

The important etiology and pathogenesis of diabetic retinopathy is that excessive eating food leads to obstruction of turbid toxin in the collateral of eyes. On the one hand, modern diet, over - taking of greasy food, damages the function of transportation and digesting of spleen and stomach. Wet aggregation and food retention turns to be phlegmatic retention, and then will be transformed into turbid toxin evil with time passes. On the other hand, the life style changes of modern people, years of over - desk work, out - going in cars instead of walking, decreasing of outdoor activities, can not only lead to deficiency of qi and blood, but also can make qi block, disorder of fluid transporting and spreading, thus the evil of turbid toxin generates. *Zhang's Medical Pass-All Blood Gate* also says: "Irregular diet and daily life all can make blood stasis." Blood stasis for a long time will turn to be toxin, generates all kinds of diseases.

浊毒瘀阻于目络，血行不畅，目络瘀滞，导致视网膜静脉迂曲扩张，微血管瘤形成；血行失其常道，血溢脉外，可见视网膜出血；血不利则为水，浊邪上犯，可见视网膜水肿混浊；血行瘀阻可见棉絮斑。浊邪日久耗伤津液，阴液亏虚，阴亏火旺，迫血妄行，致视网膜出血或玻璃体积血。病程久者，气血亏虚或气阴两虚，气虚无力摄血，导致视网膜反复出血。随着病程的发展，血浊日盛，精血日亏，视网膜失养，可见视网膜脱离而严重影响视力。

Turbid toxin obstructs the eye collateral, blood circulation is unsmooth in the eye collateral, causes winding enlargement of retinal veins and microhemangioma; abnormal blood circulation, blood overflow the vessel, retinal bleeding occurs; abnormal blood flow generates water, turbidity evil attacks upwards, retinal edema and turbidity occurs; obstruction of blood circulation causes cotton wool patches. Long turbidity evil consumes body fluid and liquid, Yin liquid deficiency, Yin deficiency and fire flourishing, forced blood to move rashly, causing retinal hemorrhage or vitreous blood accumulation. Patients with long disease course are deficient in qi and blood or dual deficient in qi and Yin, they are too deficient in qi to nourish blood, thus repeated retinal bleeding occurs. Along with the progress of the the disease course, blood turbidity is gradually increased, while the essence and blood decline, the retina is lack of nourishment, patients see retinal detachment which seriously affect vision.

三、浊毒辨证论治
3. Turbidity poison syndrome differentiation on treatment

糖尿病视网膜病变为中医消渴目病，是消渴的并发症，因此首先应由内科配合治疗，控制好血糖，只有全身症状得到好转，本病才能得到控制。辨证论治以内科消渴为基础，结合患者体质及眼局部出血、渗出、水肿等几方面综合辨证。

Diabetic retinopathy is a disease of Xiaoke in traditional Chinese medicine, which is a complication of diabetes. Therefore, it should be treated in cooperation with internal disease to control blood sugar. Only when the systemic symptoms are improved can the disease be controlled. The syndrome differentiation treatment should be made comprehensively combining the patient's constitution with local bleeding, exudation, edema of eyes and other aspects on the basis of Xiaoke in the internal disease.

（一）浊毒伤阴
3.1 Turbid Toxin impairing Yin

1.全身症状　五心烦热，口干欲饮，手足心热，腹胀纳差，大便干，舌质红，舌苔少，脉弦细数。

3.1.1 Systemic symptoms　Upset fever in five centres, dry mouth with want to drink, poor appetite, abdominal distension, dry stool, red tongue, less tongue moss, string thready and rapid pulse.

2.眼部症状　视物模糊，目睛干涩，视网膜可见散在出血，颜色新鲜，血管瘤，少量渗出。

3.1.2 Ocular symptoms　Blurred vision, dry eyes, scattered bleeding over retinas, with fresh color, hemangioma, a small amount of exudation.

3.病机　浊毒伤阴，阴虚火旺。

3.1.3 Pathogenesis　Turbid toxin impairing Yin, Yin deficiency and fire flourishing.

4.治则　解毒滋阴，凉血解郁。

3.1.4 Treatment principle　Detoxification and nourishing Yin, cool blood and relieve depression.

5.主方　自拟滋阴解毒通脉汤。

3.1.5 Main prescription　Self-prepared prescription of removing toxin, enriching Yin, cooling blood and dispersing depression.

6.药物　生地黄、黄芩、知母、天花粉、白芍、黄柏、赤芍、牡丹皮、白茅根、茜草。

3.1.6 Medicines　Sheng di huang (Rehmanniae Radix), huang qin (Radix Scutellariae), zhi mu (Rhizoma Anemarrhennae), tian hua fen (Radix Tricosanthis), bai shao (Radix Paeoniae Alba), huang bo (Cortex Phellodendri), chi shao (Radix Paeoniae Rubra), mu dan pi (Cortex Moutan), bai mao gen (Rhizoma Imperatae), qian cao (Rubiae Radix et Rhizoma).

7.加减　毒邪盛者可加栀子；阴虚明显者可加玄参；新鲜出血较多者可加大蓟、小蓟、仙鹤草；肝郁气滞明显者可加郁金、夏枯草、柴胡、枳壳。

3.1.7 Addition and reducion　For patients with excessive toxin evil, zhi zi (Fructus Gardeniae) is added; for patients with obvious syndrom of Yin deficiency, xuan shen (Radix Scrophulariae) is added; for patients with more fresh bleeding, da ji (Herba seu Radix Cirsii Japoniei), xiao ji (Herba seu Radix Cephalanoploris), xian he cao (Herba Agrimoniae) are added; for patients with syndrome of liver depression and qi stagnation, yu jin (Radix Curcumae), xia ku cao (Spica Prunellae), chai hu (Radix Buplueri), zhi qiao (Fructus Aurantii) are added.

（二）脾虚浊毒内蕴
3.2 Spleen deficiency and internal accumulation of turbid toxin

1.全身症状　体倦神疲，乏力健忘，下肢浮肿，饮食减少，面色少华，大便溏，舌质淡，苔厚腻或黄厚腻。

3.2.1 Systemic symptoms　Physically and spiritually fatigue, forgetfulness, swollen lower limbs, reduced diet, dull complexion, loose stool, light tongue, greasy moss or greasy yellow thick moss.

2.眼部症状　视物模糊或不见或暴盲，视网膜散在出血，颜色暗，或玻璃体积血，血管瘤，大量渗出及棉绒斑，黄斑区可见水肿。

3.2.2 Ocular symptoms　Blurred or invisible or sudden blindness, scattered bleeding in retina, dark color, or vitreous hemorrhage, hemangioma, massive exudation and cotton villi patches, edema in the macular area.

3.病机　脾失运化，浊毒内蕴上犯清窍。

3.2.3 Pathogenesis　Dysfunction of spleen transporting, turbid toxin attacking the clear orifice upwards.

4.治则　健脾利湿，化浊解毒。

3.2.4 Treatment principle　Reinforce the spleen and disinhibit dampness, resolve turbidity and remove toxin.

5.主方　自拟健脾化浊解毒汤。

3.2.5 Main prescription　Self-prepared prescription of reinforcing spleen, resolving turbidity and remove toxin.

6.药物　白术、茯苓、车前子、猪苓、半夏。

3.2.6 Medicines　Bai zhu (Rhizoma Atractylodis Macrocephalae), fu ling (Poria), che qian zi (Semen Plantaginis), zhu ling (Polygorus Umbellatus), ban xia (Rhizoma Pinelliae).

7.加减　瘀浊明显者加昆布、夏枯草、浙贝母；视网膜水肿明显者加益母草、泽兰。

3.2.7 Addition and reduction　Obvious stasis turbidity, add kun bu (Thallus Laminariae seu Eckloniae), xia ku cao (Spica Prunellae), zhe bei mu (Bulbus Fritillariae Thunbergii); with obvious retinal edema, add yi mu cao (Herba Leonuri), ze lan (Herba Lycopi).

（三）气阴两虚，血浊瘀阻

3.3 Dual deficiency of qi and Yin, obstruction of blood turbidity

1.全身症状　口渴欲饮，能食善饥，神疲乏力，面色不华，或口干不欲饮，或头晕多梦，手足心热，舌质红，苔少，脉细数。

3.3.1 Systemic symptoms　Thirsty with want to drink, good appetite and easy to feel hungry, fatigue in body and spirit, dull complexion, or dry mouth with no want to drink, or dizziness, more dream, fever in hands and feet, red tongue, little moss, and thready rapid pulse.

2.眼部症状　视物模糊病程较长，眼底出血不多，色暗红，散在微血管瘤，视网膜水肿混浊。

3.3.2 Ocular symptoms　A long course of blurred vision, little bleeding at the bottom of eyes, dark red color, scattered microhemangioma, retinal edema and opacity.

3.病机　气不摄血，阴虚毒蕴，血溢脉外。

3.3.3 Pathogenesis　Qi does not nourish blood, Yin deficiency and toxin accumulation, blood overflow out of the veins.

4.治则　益气养阴，活血通脉。

3.3.4 Treatment principle　Qi replenishing, Yin nourishing, blood circulation promoting and veins unblocking.

5.主方　自拟益气养阴通脉汤。

3.3.5 Main prescription　Self-prepared prescription of qi replenishing, Yin nourishing and veins unblocking.

6.药物　人参、麦冬、五味子、生地黄、黄芪、茯苓、赤芍、三七、当归。

3.3.6 Medicines　Ren shen (Radix Ginseng), mai dong (Radix Ophiopogonis), wu wei zi (Fructus Schisandalis), sheng di huang (Radix Rehmanniae), huang qi (Radix Astragali seu Hedysari), fu ling (Poria), chi shao (Radix Paeoniae Rubra), san qi (Radix Notoginseng), dang gui (Radix Angelicae Sinensis).

7.加减　陈旧性出血明显者可加桃仁、红花、川芎；新鲜出血多，加白茅根、蒲黄。

3.3.7 Addition and reduction　Obvious bleeding with history can add tao ren (Semen Persicae), hong hua (Flos Carthami), chuan xiong (Rhizoma Chuanxiong); fresh bleeding, add bai mao gen (Rhizoma Imperatae) and pu huang (Pollen Typhae).

（四）痰浊瘀血互结

3.4 Inter-binding of phlegmatic turbidity and blood stasis

1.全身症状　体倦神疲，乏力健忘，腰酸肢冷，手足凉麻，阳痿早泄，下肢浮肿，大便溏结交替，舌质淡胖少津，有齿痕，或唇舌紫暗，脉沉细无力。

3.4.1 Systemic symptoms　Physical and spiritual tiredness, fatigue, amnesia, acrid waist and cold limbs, cold and numbness of hands and feet, impotence and premature ejaculation, lower limb edema, alternatively loose and dry stool, light and fat tongue with little fluid, teeth marks, or dark purple lips and tongue, sunk thready and weak pulse.

2.眼部症状　视物模糊，病程较长，眼底反复出血，视网膜水肿混浊明显及棉絮状斑较多。

3.4.2 Ocular symptoms　Blurred vision, long course of disease, repeated fundus bleeding, obvious retinal edema and opacity and more cotton wool patches.

3.病机　脾肾双虚，浊毒与瘀血互结。

3.4.3 Pathogenesis　Dual deficiency in spleen and kidney, inter-binding of turbid toxin and blood stasis.

4.治则　补脾益肾，化浊逐瘀通络。

3.4.4 Treatment principle　Tonifying spleen, replenishing kidney, resolving turbidity, removing blood stasis and unblocking collateral.

5.主方　自拟健脾补肾通脉汤。

3.4.5 Prescription　Self-prepared prescription of reinforcing spleen, tonifying kidney and unblocking veins.

6.药物　黄芪、茯苓、山药、生地黄、玄参、陈皮、浙贝母、鸡内金、三七、赤芍。

3.4.6 Medicines　Huang qi (Radix Astragali seu Hedysari), fu ling (Poria), shan yao (Dioscreae Rhizoma), sheng di huang (Radix Rehmanniae), xuan shen(Radix Scrophulariae), chen pi (Pericarpium Citri Reticulatae), zhe bei mu (Bulbus Fritillariae Thunbergii), ji nei jin (Endothlium Corneum Gigeriae Galli), san qi (Radix Notoginseng), chi shao (Radix Paeoniae Rubra).

7.加减　脾虚痰浊明显者加党参、猪苓、泽泻、车前子；瘀血明显者加桃仁、红花、川芎等；肾虚明显者加山茱萸、杜仲、菟丝子。

3.4.7 Addition and reduction　For obvious spleen deficiency, add dang shen (Radix Codonopsitis Pilosulae), zhu ling (Polygorus Umbellatus), ze xie (Rhizoma Alismatis), and che qian zi (Semen Plantaginis); for obvious blood stasis, add tao ren (Semen Persicae), hong hua (Flos Carthami) and chuan xiong (Rhizoma Chuanxiong); for obvious kidney deficiency, add shan zhu yu (Corni Fructus), du zhong (Cortex Eucommiae) and tu si zi (Cuscutae Semen).

第六节　视网膜静脉阻塞浊毒论
Section 6　On Turbid Toxin of Retinal Vein Obstruction

一、视网膜静脉阻塞的中医概述
1. Overview of retinal vein obstruction in Traditional Chinese Medicine

视网膜静脉阻塞属于中医眼科"暴盲"范畴。"暴盲"是指眼外观正常而视力骤然下降，甚至盲无所见的内障眼病。该病名首见于《证治准绳·杂病》，书中对暴盲进行了详细论述，指出了本病的临床特点："暴盲，平日素无他病，外不伤轮廓，内不损瞳神，倏然盲而不见也。"《审视瑶函》及《目经大成》都沿用此名。《抄本眼科》名其曰落气眼，指出："落气眼不害疾，忽然眼目黑暗，不能视见，白日如夜，此症乃元气下陷，阴气上升。"

Retinal vein obstruction belongs to the category of "sudden blindness" in ophthalmology of Traditional Chinese Medicine. "Sudden blindness" refers to the internal impaired eye disease with normal eye appearance and sudden decline of vision, or even blindness. The name of the disease was first seen in *Zhengzhi Zhunsheng (Evidence Treatment Criteria)-Miscellaneous Diseases*, The book makes a detailed discussion of sudden blindness, points out the clinical characteristics of the disease: "Patients of sudden blindness, usually have no other disease, neither hurt in the outline of the eyes, nor damage on the pupil inside, suddenly blindness occurs, seing nothing." *Yao Han Review* and *Mujing Dacheng* continuously uses this disease name. Chaoben Yanke (Codex Ophthalmology) calls it Luoqi Yan, pointed out: "Luoqi Yan patients do not have any other diseases, suddenly the eyes become dark, fail to see anything, spending days like nights, this is because renal qi sinks, Yin qi rises."

二、视网膜静脉阻塞的病因病机
2. The etiology and pathogenesis of retinal vein obstruction

由于现代人饮食结构和生活方式的改变，以及情绪的影响等都可使人体内产生浊毒。《格致余论·涩脉论》曰："或因忧郁，或因浓味，或因无汗，或因补剂，气腾血沸，清化为浊。"

The changes of modern diet structure and lifestyle, as well as the influence of emotion can make human body generate turbid toxin. *Ge Zhi Yu Lun-Discussion on Astringent Pulse* says: "Melancholy, or thick taste, or no sweat, or improper using of supplements, cause qi steaming and blood boiling, turn lucidity into turbidity."

《素问·举痛论》曰"百病生于气也"。情志不畅可使人体气机失调，气血运行失常，津液水湿不化，痰浊瘀血内停，日久蕴化浊毒，玄府不利，神光发越障碍，故视物昏蒙。情志抑郁，肝失调达，肝郁气滞，气滞血瘀，玄府不利，或暴怒伤肝，肝火上炎，日久为毒邪灼伤目络。

Simple Conversation-Discussion On Pains says: "All diseases are born from qi." Abnormal state of mood can make irregular operation of qi mechanism, abnormal blood circulation, fluid, liquid, water, dampness do not gasify, phlegmatic turbidity and blood stasis retain internally, over time which will be accumulated into turbid toxin. Sweat pores blocked, incapacity of divine light, so blurred vision occurs. Emotional depression, liver dysfunction of dispersing, liver depression, qi stagnation, and blood stasis, sweat pores are blocked. Or fierce rages injure liver, liver fire upward rushing generating inflammation, turbidity evil burns eye collaterals.

现代人生活水平不断提高，饮食习惯也在发生变化，多见嗜食肥甘厚腻及辛辣炙煿之品，伤于脾胃，运化失司，湿浊内生，久而化生浊毒。正如《素问·奇病论》中所说："肥者令人内热，甘者令人中满。"《医方论》中说："多食浓厚，则痰湿俱生。"饮食伤于脾胃，运化失司，湿浊内生，久而化生浊毒，浊毒上犯，壅滞目窍。

Along with the constant improving of modern people's living standards, diet habits are simultaneously changing, more and more people are in favour of fat, sweet, thick and greasy food, or hot, spicy and fried and roasted products, which impair the spleen and stomach, lead to transporting dysfunction, generate wet turbidity endogenously, then being transformed into turbid toxin with time being. Just as *Simple Conversation-Qibing Lun* says: "Fat causes internal hot, sweet generates fullness in middle energizer." *Discussion on Medical Prescriptions* says: "More taking of greasy food, phlegm and dampness generate together." Diet impairs the spleen and stomach, causes transport dysfunction and endogenous generation of dampness and turbidity, and the turbidity will be transformed into turbid toxin over time, attack upwards to obstruct eyes.

故本病最常见的病因为浊毒内蕴，困着于脾，日久脾虚失运，浊毒损伤津液，日久阴津耗损而阴虚火旺，迫血妄行。本病初期主要病机为肝郁气滞、血瘀；或浊毒迫血妄行，损伤脉络；或浊毒久蕴，上犯目窍。病程日久后脾虚加重，导致脾不统血，或浊毒致津液耗损，故肝肾阴虚及虚火上炎为本病后期的主要病机。

Therefore, the most common etiology of the disease is internal accumulation of turbid toxin, which traps the spleen, causes spleen deficiency over time, impairs body fluid, over time lead to exhaustion of Yin and fluid, Yin deficiency and fire flourishing, forcing the blood to move rashly. The main pathogenesis in the initial stage of the disease is liver depression, qi stagnation and blood stasis, or turbid toxin forces the blood to move rashly, impairs veins and collateral; or prolonged accumulation of turbid toxin upward attacks the eye orifice. The spleen deficiency aggravates after a long course of disease, which leads to failure of spleen to control the blood circulation, or turbid toxin causes exhaustion of fluid and liquid. Therefore, Yin deficiency of liver and kidney and deficiency fire generates upper inflammation are the main pathogenesis in the later stage of the disease.

三、浊毒辨证论治
3. Turbid toxin syndrome differentiation treatment

本病的关键是静脉阻塞而致出血，阻塞属瘀，离经之血亦是瘀，故为血瘀之证。瘀久浊毒内生，阴虚火旺，因此化瘀解毒、通脉应贯穿始终。出血早期应凉血解毒、通脉，中晚期可活血解毒、通脉、养阴清热。

The key of this disease is venous obstruction causes bleeding, obstruction belongs to stasis, blood out of the veins is also stasis, so it is a syndrome of blood stasis. Long time of blood stasis will generate internal turbid toxin, Yin deficiency and fire flourishing, so the principle of resolving blood stasis, removing toxin and unblock the veins should be carried out through the process of the treatment. In early stage of bleeding, doctors should cool blood, remove toxin and unblock the veins; in middle and late stage of the disease, doctors should promote blood circulation, remove toxin, unblock the veins and nourish the Yin and clear heat.

（一）肝郁化火

3.1 Liver depression turns to be fire

1.全身症状　眼胀头痛，胸胁胀痛，情志抑郁，食少嗳气，或愤怒、烦躁失眠，或乳房胀痛，月经不调。舌质红，有瘀斑，脉弦数、涩。

3.1.1 Systematic symptoms　Eye distension and headache, chest and hypochondrium distension pain, emotional depression, poor appetite and belching, or anger, irritability, insomnia, or breast distension and pain, irregular menstruation. Red tongue, with ecchymosis, string rapid and astringent pulse.

2.眼部症状　视力突然下降，视网膜静脉粗大迂曲，隐没于出血之中，视网膜火焰状出血及水肿，或可见视盘出血、水肿。

3.1.2 Ocular symptoms　Sudden decline of vision, retinal veins thick and circuitous, hidden in bleeding, retinal flame - like hemorrhage and edema, or optic disc bleeding, edema.

3.病机　肝郁化火，迫血妄行。

3.1.3 Pathogenesis　Liver depression turns to be fire, forces blood to move rashly.

4.治则　清肝解郁、凉血解毒止血。

3.1.4 Treatment principle　Clear liver, resolve depression, cool blood, remove toxin and stop bleeding.

5.主方　自拟凉血解毒汤。

3.1.5 Main prescription　Self-prepared prescription of decoction of cooling blood and removing toxin.

6.药物　生地黄、知母、龙胆草、黄芩、赤芍、木贼、蝉蜕。

3.1.6 Medicines　Sheng di huang (Radix Rehmanniae), zhi mu (Rhizoma Anemarrhennae), long dan cao (Gentianae Radix et Rhizoma), huang qin (Radix Scutellariae), chi shao (Radix Paeoniae Rubra), mu zei (Scouring Rush), chan tui (Cicadae Peristracum).

7.加减　出血量多而较新鲜者加牡丹皮、侧柏叶、槐花、白茅根以凉血止血；视盘或黄斑区水肿明显者加车前子、茯苓、泽兰以活血利水；眼底出血较多，血色紫暗，加蒲黄、茜草、三七以化瘀止血；肝气郁滞明显者加枳壳以疏肝理气；失眠多梦者加珍珠母、夜交藤镇静安神。

3.1.7 Addition and reduction　In case of fresh and large amount of bleeding add mu dan pi (moutain Cortex), ce bai ye (Platycladi Cacumen), huai hua (Sophorae Flos), bai mao gen (Rhizoma Imperatae) to cool blood and stop bleeding; obvious edema in visual disc or macular area, add che qian zi (Semen Plantaginis), fu ling (Poria), ze lan (Herba Lycopi) to promote blood circulation and disinhibit water; more fundus bleeding in purple dark colour, add pu huang (Pollen Typhae), qian cao (Rubiae Radix Et Rhizoma), and san qi (Radix Notoginseng) to resolve stasis and stop bleeding; obvious depression of liver qi, add zhi qiao (Fructus Aurantii) to soothe liver and regulate qi; in case of insomnia and more dreams, add zhen zhu mu (Margaritifera Concha), ye jiao teng (Caulis Polygoni Multiflori).

（二）浊毒瘀血互结
3.2 Inter-binding of turbid toxin and blood stasis

1.全身症状　头重眩晕，形体肥胖，食少纳呆，精神疲乏，胸闷脘胀，肢体倦怠，舌苔白腻，舌有瘀点，脉弦或弦滑。

3.2.1 Systemic symptoms　Head heavy, dizziness, body obesity, eating less food and anorexia, spiritually fatigue, chest tightness and gastric distension, limb burnout, white and greasy tongue coating, with tongue petechia, string or string slippery pulse.

2.眼部症状　视物昏蒙，视网膜静脉粗大迂曲，视盘充血、水肿，有黄白色硬性渗出或棉絮状白斑，或黄斑囊样水肿，视网膜动脉可有反光增强，有增生膜形成等硬化征象。

3.2.2 Ocular symptoms　Blurred vision, retinal vein thick and circuitous, optic disc congestion, edema, yellow and white hard exudation or cotton flocculent white spot, or muscular cystic edema, retinal artery might have reflective enhancement, hyperplasia membrane formation and other sclerosis signs.

3.病机　浊毒内蕴，瘀血阻络。

3.2.3 Pathogenesis　Internal accumulation of turbid toxin and blood stasis obstructing the collaterals.

4.治则　化浊解毒，活血通脉。

3.2.4 Treatment principle　Resolve turbidity, remove toxin, promote blood circulation and unblock the veins.

5.主方　自拟化浊解毒通脉方。

3.2.5 Main prescription　Self-drafted prescription of resolving turbidity, removing toxin and unblocking the veins.

6.药物　茯苓、泽泻、白术、赤芍、牡丹皮、木贼、防风。

3.2.6 Medicines　Fu ling (Poria), ze xie (Rhizoma Alismatis), bai zhu (Rhizoma Atractylodis Macrocephalae), chi shao (Radix Paeoniae Rubra), mu dan pi (Cortex Moutan), mu zei (Scouring Rush), fang feng (Radix Saposhnikoviae).

7.加减　视网膜渗出、水肿明显者，可加益母草、泽兰以利水化瘀消肿；脾虚痰浊明显者加半夏、胆南星、陈皮以化痰祛浊；对于浊毒明显者加黄芩、薏苡仁、猪苓、泽泻、车前子以清热利湿化浊；对于机化膜明显者加浙贝母、海藻、昆布以软坚散结。

3.2.7 Addition and reduction For obvious retinal exudation and edema, add yi mu cao (Herba Leonuri) and ze lan (Herba Lycopi), to disinhibit water, resolve stasis and dissipate edema; in case of obvious spleen deficiency and phlegmatic turbidity, add ban xia (Rhizoma Pinelliae), dan nan xing (Arisaema Cumbile), chen pi (Pericarpium Citri Reticulatae), to resolve phlegm and remove turbidity; for obvious turbid toxin, add huang qin (Radix Scutellariae), yi yi ren (Semen Coisis), zhu ling (Polygorus Umbellatus), ze xie (Rhizoma Alismatis), che qian zi (Semen Plantaginis) to clear heat, disinhibit dampness and resolve turbidity; for obvious organic membrane, add zhe bei mu (Bulbus Fritillariae Thunbergii), hai zao (Sargassum), kun bu (Thallus Laminariae seu Eckloniae) to soften the hardness and dissipate binds.

（三）虚火上炎

3.3 Hyperactivity of deficient fire

1.全身症状　头晕耳鸣，唇红颧赤，五心烦热，口干，舌红苔少，脉弦细数。

3.3.1 Systemic symptoms Dizziness and tinnitus, red lips and zygomatic red, upset fever in five centers, dry mouth, red tongue less moss, string thready rapid pulse.

2.眼部症状　视力骤降或云雾移睛，眼前有红色阴影或絮状混浊，视网膜静脉暗红色出血、迂曲，有黄白色硬性渗出，或黄斑囊样水肿，视网膜动脉变窄。

3.3.2 Ocular symptoms Sudden decline of vision or cloud - fog moving before the eyes, red shadow or flocculent opacity in front of eyes, dark red circuitous bleeding of retinal veins, yellow and white hard exudation, or macular cystic edema, retinal artery is narrowing.

3.病机　浊毒伤阴，阴虚火旺。

3.3.3 Pathogenesis Turbid toxin impairing Yin, Yin deficiency and fire flourishing.

4.治则　养阴清热解毒，凉血通脉。

3.3.4 Treatment principle Nourishing Yin, clearing heat, removing toxin, cooling blood and unblocking the veins.

5.主方　自拟养阴清热汤。

3.3.5 Prescription Self-prepared prescription of nourishing Yin and clearing heat.

6.药物　生地黄、知母、天花粉、牡丹皮、赤芍、当归、木贼、防风、蝉蜕。

3.3.6 Medicines Sheng di huang (Radix Rehmanniae), zhi mu (Rhizoma Anemarrhennae), tian hua fen (Radix Tricosanthis), mu dan pi (Cortex Moutan), chi shao (Radix Paeoniae Rubra), dang gui (Radix Angelicae Sinensis), mu zei (Scouring Rush), fang feng (Radix Saposhnikoviae), chan tui (Cicadae Peristracum).

7.加减　阴虚明显者加女贞子、墨旱莲以养阴凉血；加银柴胡以疏肝解郁，益阴明目；虚热明显者加玄参、知母以养阴清热；血瘀明显者加丹参、白芍活血祛瘀，养血敛阴安神。

3.3.7 Addition and reduction　For obvious Yin deficiency, add nv zhen zi (Fructus Ligustri) and mo han lian (Herba Ecliptae) to nourish Yin and cool blood; add yin chai hu (Radix Stellariae) to disperse liver and remove depression, replenish Yin and bright eyes; with obvious deficient heat, add xuan shen (Radix Scrophulariae) and zhi mu (Rhizoma Anemarrhennae) to nourish Yin and clear heat; with obvious blood stasis, add dan shen (Salviae Miltiorrhizae), bai shao (Radix Paeoniae Alba) to promote blood circulation and remove blood stasis, and nourish blood, astringe Yin and relieve mind.

（四）肝肾阴虚

3.4 Liver and kidney Yin deficiency

1.全身症状　头晕耳鸣，腰膝酸软，舌淡苔少，脉细。

3.4.1 Systematic symptoms　Dizziness and tinnitus, lassitude loin and knees, light tongue less moss, thready pulse.

2.眼部症状　视物昏蒙、视物变形，眼底出血，视网膜色泽变淡或污秽，血管呈白线状，边缘可见异常扩张的血管及点状出血，静脉白鞘、纤维增生膜形成、视网膜前出血，黄斑区继发性视网膜前膜，异常扩张的毛细血管。

3.4.2 Ocular symptoms　Poor vision, visual distortion, fundus bleeding, retinal color pale or foul, white thread - state of blood vessels, abnormally dilated blood vessels and dotted bleeding, venous white sheath, formation of fibro - hyperplastic membrane, preretinal bleeding, retinitis in secondary macular area, abnormally dilated capillaries.

3.病机　肝肾阴虚，目失所养。

3.4.3 Pathogenesis　Liver and kidney Yin deficiency, the eyes are lack of nourishment.

4.治则　补益肝肾。

3.4.4 Treatment principle　Tonifying and replenishing the liver and kidney.

5.主方　自拟益肾明目汤。

3.4.5 Prescription　Self - prepared prescription of decoction of replenishing kidney and Brightening the eyes.

6.药物　熟地黄、山药、山茱萸、茯苓、女贞子、墨旱莲、枸杞子、泽泻、牡丹皮、赤芍、柴胡、当归、五味子。

3.4.6 Medicines　Shu di huang (Radix Rehmanniae Praeparatum), shan yao (Dioscreae Rhizoma), shan zhu yu (Corni Fructus), fu ling (Poria), nv zhen zi (Fructus Ligustri), mo han lian (Herba Ecliptae), gou qi zi(Lycii Fructus), ze xie (Rhizoma Alismatis), mu dan pi (Cortex Moutan), chi shao (Radix Paeoniae Rubra), chai hu (Radix Bulpleuri), dang gui (Radix Angelicae Sinensis), wu wei zi (Fructus Schisandalis).

7.加减　眼底有机化瘢痕共存者加陈皮、半夏、浙贝母、牡蛎以软坚散结；失眠多梦者加酸枣仁、夜交藤以养心安神。

3.4.7 Addition and reduction　Coexistence of fundus organic scar, add chen pi (Pericarpium Citri

Reticulatae), ban xia (Rhizoma Pinelliae), zhe bei mu (Bulbus Fritillariae Thunbergii), mu li (Ostreae Concha) to soften the hardenss and dissipate the binding; in case of insomnia and more dreams, add suan zao ren (Semen Zizyphi Jujubae), ye jiao teng (Caulis Polygoni Multiflori) to nourish heart and comfort the spirit.

第十二章　新冠病毒感染浊毒论
Chapter 12 On Turbid Toxin of COVID-19

第一节　病因病机
Section 1 Etiology and Pathogenesis

一、病因
1. The etiology

新冠病毒感染的病因为"浊毒疫疠之气"，该病为"浊毒疫"。

COVID-19 is caused by "pestilence qi of turbid toxin", which is "turbid toxin pestilence".

新冠病毒感染是一种烈性传染病，它属于中医学"疫病"范畴。它的侵入途径是不是自肌表，而是自口鼻。《素问·刺法论》曰："避其毒气，天牝从来。"在对于病因的认识上，古人已知疫病"不可以年岁四时为拘，盖非五运六气所能定"，也非"四时不正之气"引起。《温疫论》明确指出"夫温疫之为病，非风、非寒、非暑、非湿，乃天地之间别有一种异气所感"，强调"异气"为六淫之外的特殊邪气。那么，这个"异气"究竟是什么气呢?

COVID-19 is a serious infectious disease, which belongs to the category of "epidemic disease" in Traditional Chinese Medicine. Its invasion way is from the mouth and nose, not from the muscle surface. *Simple Conversations-Discussion on Acupuncture Methods* says: "(when the pestilence has occurred, cares should be taken to) avoid its toxic substance. Evil (epidemic) qi usually gets into and out of the body through the nose." In the understanding of the cause of the disease, the ancients have known that diseases "is neither detained by four seasons of years, nor determined by five movements and six climates", it is also not caused by "improper qi of four seasons". *Discussion On The Warm Epidemic* clearly points out that "the warm epidemic is generated, not form wind, cold, heat, and wet, but there is infected by special different substance between heaven and earth", emphasizing that "different substance" is a special evil beyond the six excessive evils. Now, what is the "different substance"?

该病初期，舌苔变化不大，但是到中期，舌苔多厚腻，并有身热不扬、渴不欲饮、胸闷脘痞、大便溏滞不爽等，所以多数医家认为本病病因属性以"湿"为主，不无道理。但是深究之，则知该病病因"类湿而非湿"。原因有三：一则湿邪为六淫之一，本身不具有传染性，吴又可明确指出瘟疫之为病，"非湿"所感；二则湿邪为病，多起病隐袭，病程缠绵，而本病发病迅猛；三者湿邪多受之卫表肌腠，性趋下而易伤阴位，该病从口鼻而入，首犯华盖，似与之不符。

In the early stage of the disease, the tongue moss does not change much, but in the middle stage, the tongue moss is thick and greasy, and the body is hiding fever, thirsty in mouth but with no want to drink, chest tightness and epigastric fullness, loose and difficult stool, so most doctors think that the etiology of the disease is mainly "dampness", not unreasonable. But in further investigation, the cause of the disease is "similarly damp but not damp". There are three reasons: first, damp evil is one of the six excess evils, itself is not infectious, Wu Youke clearly indicates that the plague is a disease infected "not by wetness"; second, when wet evil generates diseases, the onset are usually vague, with lingering disease course, but the onset of COVID-19 is abrupt and fierce; third, The damp evil usually attacks defensive qi, skin surface, and striae, from lower part of the body, impairing the Yin, the COVID-19 gets into the body through mouth and nose, first attacking the lungs, not agreeing with the above.

中医多将湿浊并称，而深究之，则有不同。浊者，《说文解字注》谓清之反也。湿从水，有清浊之分，湿之秽者为浊。吴鞠通《温病条辨》云："疫者，疠气流行，多兼秽浊。"《伤寒指掌》称："六气之外，另有一种疠气，乃天地秽恶之气，都从口鼻吸入。"清代雷丰在《时病论》中专列"芳香化浊法"，以治"梅湿"，并治"秽浊之气"。且历代医家多认为疫气为感天地秽浊之气而致，晋唐时期侧重于祛邪辟秽药物；随着经验的不断积累，明清时期医家认为，"治法要当辟散疫气、扶正气为主"，且认为芳香药物具有增强正气的作用，故明清除继承晋唐大量驱邪避疫方药外，更集中和侧重于芳香辟秽药物的使用，均以辟秽浊为防治要义。而疫之为气，本为毒气。何秀山云："疫必有毒，毒必传染。"《素问·刺法论》曰："避其毒气，天牝从来。"所以此次新冠病毒感染的病因应该是外感"浊毒疫疠之气"，为"浊毒疫"。

Traditional Chinese Medicine usually call dampness and turbidity as "damp turbidity", but there are differences through further consideration. According to the illustration of *Annotation On Shuowen Jiezi* turbidity is the antonym of "lucid". Dampness following water are divided into clear and turbid, the filthy dampness is turbidity. Wu Jutong said in *Detailed Analysis of Epidemic Warm Diseases*, "Epidemic diseases are epidemic pestilence, usually accompanied by filthy turbidity." *Shanghan Zhizhang* says: "Beyond the six excess evil, there is special kind of qi, named pestilence, which is the filthy and evil qi of heaven and earth breathed into human body through nose and mouth." In the Qing dynasty, Lei Feng used a special method of "turbidity resolving by aromatic medicines" to treat the "plum dampness" and the "filthy turbid qi" in *Discussion On Seasonal Diseases*. Most of the doctors of different dynasties agrees that pestilence is infected by filthy turbid qi of heaven and earth. In the dynasty of Jin and Tang, the treatment partially depends on the the medicines of evil eliminating and filth resolving. Benefited from the increasing experience, doctors of the Ming and Qing dynasties think that "the treatment method should principally dissipate the pestilence and reinforce the healthy qi", and also believes that the aromatic medicines are effective in strengthening the healthy qi. So while inheriting the prescription and medicines of evil dispelling and epidemic avoiding, the doctors of Ming and Qing dynasties emphasizes on the application of aromatic medicines of filth dispelling, believes that preventing filth and turbidity is the key idea of the treatment. And the epidemic is qi, originally is poison qi. He Xiushan said: "Epidemic must be toxic, toxic epidemics must be infectious." *Simple Conversation-Discussion on Acupuncture Methods* says: "(when the pestilence has occurred, cares should be taken to) avoid its toxic qi. Evil (epidemic) qi usually gets into and out of the body through the nose."

So the etiology of COVID-19 should be "turbid toxin epidemic", i.e "externally infected by the turbid toxin pestilence qi".

二、病机
2. Pathogenesis

新冠病毒感染的病机是"浊毒化"。具体就该病而言，浊毒的病机特征可以归纳为以下六点。

The pathogenesis of COVID-19 is "turbid toxin changing". Specifically, the pathogenesis characteristics of turbid toxin diseases can be summarized as the following six points.

（一）传变速，易散行诸经
2.1 Transmit in high speed, easy to spread through all the meridians

新冠病毒感染属"疫病"，传染性强，如《素问·刺法论》曰："五疫之至，皆相染易，无问大小，病状相似。"且其传变迅速，无规律可循，既非典型的六经传变，又非典型的三焦及卫气营血传变。有以发热咳嗽为主症者，有以脘痞呕恶为主症者，有兼尿浊（蛋白尿）者。诚如王九思在《难经集注》中所说："散行诸经，不知何经虚而传受此邪，故随其所在取其病邪也。"

COVID-19 belongs to epidemic diseases, which is highly infectious. Just as the description in *Simple Conversation-Discussion on Acupuncture Methods* "Patients attacked by the five kinds of epidemics, will infect other people, no matter children or adults, the symptoms are similar." And the transmission is rapid, irregular, neither transmitted according to transmission rule of six channels, nor transmitted according to the transmitting rule of triple energizer and the transmitting rule of Wei-defence, qi, Ying nutrients and blood. The main syndrome of the patients might be fever and coughing, epigastric fullness, nausea, and vomiting, or complicated by turbid urine. Just as Wang Jiusi said in *Explanation to Nanjing*: "The evil can scatter to any meridian. It is unclear which channel will be next deficient one to be transmitted. Therefore, we have to treat the disease wherever the evil occurs."

（二）毒性强，易直中脏腑
2.2 Strong toxicity, easy to get into the viscera straightly

该病病情凶险，可直中脏腑，多侵及肺胃，出现咳喘、呼吸困难、咯血。肺失宣肃加之阳明腑实，使浊毒郁闭，直传心包，所以有些重症患者在1周之后出现呼吸困难，甚至进展为急性呼吸窘迫综合征、脓毒症休克、难以纠正的代谢性酸中毒和凝血功能障碍等，甚至出现多器官功能障碍综合征（MODS），危重症患者多需要呼吸机辅助通气，甚至应用体外膜氧合（ECMO）。

The disease is fierce and dangerous, can get into the viscera straightly, most probably invade and lung and stomach, generating coughing and asthma, dyspnea, hemoptysis. Dysfunction of Lung diffusing and sthenia fu-organ of Yangming, make the turbid toxin depressively obstructed, directly get into the pericardium, so some severe patients see dyspnea after one week, even progress to acute respiratory distress syndrome, septic shock, metabolic acidosis and coagulation dysfunction difficult to correct, and even multiple organ dysfunction syndrome (MODS). Patients of severe and critical disease need ventilator to assist ventilation, or even apply ECMO.

（三）遏气机，易化热伤津

2.3 Blocking the qi movement, easy to be transformed into heat and impair fluid

浊毒之邪，其性类湿，易阻遏气机，吴又可谓"时疫初起，邪气盘踞于中，表里阻隔，里气滞而为闷，表气滞而为头身疼痛"，所以气机郁滞是疫病的关键因素。此次新冠病毒感染患者早期乏力明显，但虚象不明显，应该为浊毒阻遏气机，精微失于输部而致。而气郁则易化热，况疫病多为热邪。王士雄曰："疫证皆属热毒，不过有微甚之分耳。"吴又可曰："夫疫乃热病也，邪气内郁，阳气不得宣布，积阳为火，阴血每为热搏，暴解之后，余焰尚在，阴血未复。"所以浊毒为病，一是容易阻遏气机，二是由于其性多热，容易伤津，日久则气阴两伤。

The evil of turbid and toxin, its nature is similar to dampness, easy to block the qi movement, Wu Youke said that "at the beginning of the epidemic, evil qi entrenched in the middle part of the body, obstructed the normal qi interflow between the external to the internal. The internal qi stagnation generates sulks, external qi stagnation generates pains in head and body", so the depression and stagnation of qi mechanism is the key factor of the disease. In the early stage of COVID-19, patients have obvious fatigue, but the deficiency is not obvious, which should be caused by turbid toxin obstruction of qi mechanism and the transporting and distribution failure of essence. While qi depression is easy to be transformed into heat, and most epidemic diseases are heat evil. Wang Shixiong said: "Epidemic syndromes are all heat toxin, but there are differences of light and severe." Wu Youke said: "Epidemic is heat disease, internal depression of evil qi, Yang qi can not be diffused, Yang is accumulated into fire, Yin blood is frequently attacked by heat, after the attacking, the remaining fire is still burning, but the Yin blood is not recovered." So when turbid toxin generates diseases, one characteristic is easy to restrain the qi movement, the other is easy to impair fluid and impair both qi and Yin with time passes due to the nature of heat.

（四）性秽腻，易生瘀生痰

2.4 Filthy and greasy, easy to generate stasis and phlegm

浊毒性秽腻，阻遏气机，气郁则血瘀，加之疫本热毒，热毒壅于血分亦可生瘀。且肺朝百脉，为水之上源，肺部受邪，则气、血、水三者运行失常，既可生瘀，又易生痰湿浊毒。从新冠病毒感染患者的CT表现来看，进展期双肺实变影增多，病变周围小叶间隔可因为间质水肿而增厚，重症期可因为双肺弥漫性病变而出现"白肺"，说明了水肿与瘀血并见的病理改变。从尸体解剖来看，新冠病毒感染患者的肺组织没有严重纤维化，肺泡还存在，但是炎症很厉害，有大量的黏液，非常黏，导致患者的通气不通顺。

The nature of turbid toxin is filthy and greasy, it restrains qi movement, causes qi depression and blood stasis, the epidemic is originally heat toxin, heat toxin choked in the blood can also generate blood stasis. The lung is connected with all vessels, is the upper source of water. When lung is attacked by evil, the operation of qi, blood, water is abnormal. It can generate blood stasis, and easy to generate phlegmatic hygrosis and turbid toxin. From the perspective of CT manifestations of COVID-19 patients, the solid lesions of double lungs increased in the progressive period, the lobular interval around the lesion is thickened due to interstitial edema. The "white lung" appears due to the diffusing lesions in the critical stage of double lungs. This indicates the simultaneous pathological changes of edema and blood stasis. From the autopsy, the lung tissue of COVID-19 patients is not severe fibrosis, the alveoli still exists, but the inflammation is very severe, there is a lot of mucus, very sticky, resulting in poor ventilation of the patient.

（五）浊害清，易蒙蔽清窍
2.5 Turbidity impairs lucidity, easy to hoodwink the clear orifices

叶天士在《外感温热篇》中提出："湿与温和，蒸郁而蒙蔽于上，清窍为之壅塞，浊邪害清也。"湿为重浊之邪气，与热相合，湿热蕴积而上蒸，以致孔窍壅塞，出现头昏目胀、耳聋、鼻塞等症状。所谓清窍，头目也，其实是脑，脑为元神之府，浊毒之邪上犯，则易蒙蔽清窍而出现神昏、烦躁之症。

Ye Tianshi put forward in *Discussion On External Warm and Heat Diseases*: "wet and warm combine, steame and hoodwink the upper part of the body, clear orifices are obstructed, turbidity evil impairs clear orifices." Because dampness is the evil of severe turbidity, when it combines with heat, damp and heat are accumulated and steamed upward, the orifices are obstructed, generating dizziness, deafness, nasal congestion and other symptoms. The so-called clear orifices refer to head and eyes, in fact, refer to the brain, which is the house of the renal spirit. When turbid toxin evil attacks upwards, it is easy to hoodwink the clear orifices and generate dizziness, irritability disease.

（六）同气求，易引动宿疾
2.6 Birds of a feather flies together, evil of COVID-19 is easy to activate chronic disease

《周易》曰："同声相应，同气相求，水流湿，火就燥。"作为中医学的特色理论之一，"同气相求"是指人体内的某种因素与外界的致病因素相对应而形成一定类型的疾病而言。浊毒有内外之分，若人体内素有浊毒蕴结，则更容易患病，且预后不佳。据统计，该病死亡患者80%为60岁以上的老年患者，75%以上是有一种或一种以上的基础病，大多有心脑血管疾病、糖尿病和肿瘤等基础病。

Zhou Yi said: "the same voice corresponds, the birds of a feather flies together, wet is generated from water flowing, the fire is produced due to dry of environment." As one of the characteristic theories of traditional Chinese medicine, "Tongqi Xiangqiu" refers to certain factors in human body corresponds with the external pathogenic factors, generating certain type of diseases. Turbid toxin are divided into internal and external turbid toxin. If a person has internal accumulation of turbid toxin, will easily be affected by COVID-19, and the prognosis is poor. According to statistics, 80% of the dead patients are elderly patients over 60 years old, more than 75% of the dead patients have one or more than one kind of basic disease most probably related with cardiovascular and cerebrovascular diseases, diabetes and cancer and others.

第二节 治疗原则
Section 2 Principles of Treatment

一、化浊解毒，以物制气
1. To resolve turbidity and remove toxin, to restrict qi with things

疫气为病，虽然肉眼不能见，但是"物者气之化也，气者物之变也"。气可以制约物体，物体也可以制约气。"夫物之可以制气者，药物也。"清代雷丰在《时病论》中专列"芳香化浊法"，以治"梅湿"，并治"秽浊之气"。且历代医家多认为疫气为感天地秽浊之气而致。晋唐时期，其侧重于祛邪辟秽药物。随着经验的不断积累，明清时期医家认为，"治法要当辟散疫气、扶正气为主"，且认为芳香药物具有增强正气的作用，故明清除继承晋唐大量驱邪避疫方药外，更集中和侧重于芳香辟秽药物的使用，均以辟秽浊为防治要义。如喻嘉言认为："（瘟疫）治法，未病前，预饮芳香正气药……此为上也；邪既入，急以逐秽为第一义。"

Epidemic qi is a disease, although the naked eye can not see, but "the things are transformed from qi, qi is changed from the thing". Qi can restrict things, and things can also restrict qi. "Things which can restrict qi are medicines." In the Qing dynasty, Lei Feng specially listed in *Discussion on Seasonal Diseases* "resolving turbidity with aroma" method to treat the "plum dampness" and treat the "filthy and turbid qi". Most of the doctors of different dynasties agrees that pestilence is generated by filthy turbid qi of heaven and earth. In the dynasty of Jin and Tang, the treatment partially depends on the the medicines of evil eliminating and filth resolving. Benefited from the increasing experience, doctors of the Ming and Qing dynasties think that "the treatment method should principally dissipate the pestilence and reinforce the healthy qi", and also believes that the aromatic medicines are effective in strengthening the healthy qi. So while inheriting the prescription and medicines of evil dispelling and epidemic avoiding, the doctors of Ming and Qing dynasties emphasizes on the application of aromatic medicines of filth dispelling, believes that preventing filth and turbidity is the key idea of the treatment. As Yu Jiayan said: "To treat pestilence, the best way is to use aromatic and healthy qi reinforcing medicine to prevent it before the disease; when the disease evil has get into the body, to remove the filth urgently is most important."

此次新冠病毒感染的治疗，国家和各省均出台了多版诊疗方案，虽然不尽相同，但是有一点却基本取得共识，就是芳香化浊类药物的应用，比如广藿香等，国家中医药管理局推荐的"三方"均有广藿香。广藿香味辛，性微温，归脾、胃、肺经，行于上中二焦。《本经逢原》曰："凡时行疫疠，山岚瘴疟，用此醒脾健胃，则邪气自无容而愈矣。"

In the treatment of COVID-19, Chinese government and the government of different provinces have issued multi-versions of diagnosis and treatment solutions. Although there exists some differences among the soltions, but there is a basic consensus on the application of aromatic turbidity resolving medicines, such as Guang huo xiang (Herba Pogostemonis). The "three prescriptions" recommended by the State Administration of Traditional Chinese Medicine have guang huo xiang (Herba Pogostemonis). Guang huo xiang (Herba Pogostemonis) with spicy taste and slight warm nature, belongs to the meridian of the spleen, stomach, lung, moves in the upper and middle energizers. *Ben Jing Feng Yuan (Enrichment and Explanation to Shennong's Classic of Materia Medica)* said: "In case of epidemic pestilence, mountain haze miasma malaria, with this Herba Pogostemonis to invigorate the spleen and reinforce the stomach, then the evil qi will be dippelled and the disease recovers."

程钟龄在《医学心悟》中指出"时疫之证，来路两条，去路三条，治法五条"，还总结出了"发散、解秽、清中、攻下，补虚"的治疫五大原则。其所说的来路两条包括在天之疫与在人之疫，与浊毒理论的"天之浊毒""人之浊毒"高度契合。去路三条与浊毒理论的"透表化浊解毒""通腑泄浊解毒"和"渗湿化浊解毒"异曲同工。而其总结的上述五大治疫原则概括来讲不外乎就是扶正排毒，结合新冠病毒感染的特点，我们认为化浊解毒、扶正祛邪当贯穿防治始终，为其基本治则。我们在临床上经实践证明，疗效显著。

Cheng Zhongling pointed out in *Medical Enlightenment*: "For epidemic diseases, there are two ways to come, three ways to go, five principles of treatment to be used." It also summarizes the five principles as "dispersing (the superficial exopathogens), removing filth, clearing the middle energizer, attacking the lower energizer, and tonifying the deficiency". "The two ways to come", refers to the epidemic of the heaven and the human epidemic, which are highly consistent with the "turbid toxin of the heaven" and "the turbid toxin of human" of the turbid toxin theory. "The three ways to go", are similar to the methods of "resolving turbidity and removing toxin through outthrusting the external", "unblocking the fu-organ, purging turbidity and removing toxin" and "draining dampness, resolving turbidity and removing toxin". The five treatment principles summarized above are nothing more than strengthening the healthy qi and discharging toxin. Considering the characteristics of COVID-19 epidemic, we believe that resolving turbidity and removing toxin, reinforcing the healthy qi and removing evil as the basic treatment principle should be carried out through the whole process of the disease it has been proved to be remarkably effective in clinical practices.

二、化浊解毒、镇惊开窍为该病的关键治法
2. Resolving turbidity and removing toxin, relieving convulsion and resuscitation is the key treatment method of the disease

中医谓"浊邪害清"，浊毒之邪，性黏腻秽浊，容易蒙蔽清窍。窍为何意？《说文解字注》曰："穴也，空也。"《黄帝内经》说"人有九窍"，即耳、目、口、鼻和前后二阴，以与天地相通。但是仔细思之，五脏六腑均当有窍，以连经络而通气血。肺主气司呼吸，肺窍闭则宣肃失司，发为咳嗽、喘憋，动辄益甚，患者血氧饱和度下降；又肺为储痰之器，肺病则内生痰浊。患者之所以出现呼吸困难，综合分析来看，主要是由于肺组织内黏液分泌过多，且质黏稠（痰栓），不易排出，而这也是浊毒内闭肺窍的病理基础。心主血脉，疫毒之邪可犯肺而逆传心包，造成心功能下降、心律失常、循环不稳定、血压下降，形成心阳暴脱之变。脑为元神之府，浊邪害清，清窍为之壅塞，则出现神昏、烦躁等症，变生脓毒性脑病。鉴于疫毒之邪，性多炽热，且多兼秽浊，而客邪贵乎早逐，所以疾病初期应该及早运用安宫牛黄丸或至宝丹等解毒化浊，镇惊开窍。热度偏盛，毒重于浊者，宜安宫牛黄丸；痰浊壅盛，浊重于毒者，宜至宝丹。其总以开窍为要，及早截断病

势，防治病情恶化。

So-called "turbid evil impairs the lucidity" in Traditional Chinese Medicine indicates that the evil of turbid toxin with nature of greasy and filthy can easily hoodwink the clear orifices. What does qiao (orifice) mean? *Annotation On Shuowen Jiezi* explains: "It means cave, hole." *The Medical Classic of the Yellow Emperor* says that "people have nine orifices", including double ears, double eyes, double nasal holes, mouth, front and back Yin (urethra and anus), to connect with heaven and earth. But think carefully, there should be orifice for each of the viscera, to connect the meridians and transport qi and blood. Lung controls qi serving breathing, if the lung orifice is closed, the function of diffusing and cleaning will be abnormal, cough, asthma occurs, which might be more severe when moving, the oxygen saturation of patients will decrease; besides, the lung is the organ to store sputum, if lung is ill, it will endogenously generate phlegmatic turbidity. The reason why patients have dyspnea is mainly due to the excessive secretion of mucus in the lung tissue, which is thick and sticky (sputum plug), difficult to be discharged, this is also the pathological basis of obstruction of turbid toxin in lung orifice. The heart controls the blood vessels, the evil of epidemic toxin can invade the lung and reversely transmitted into the pericardium, resulting in the decline of heart function, arrhythmia, circulation instability, blood pressure decline, forming sudden collapse of heart Yang. The brain is the house of the renal spirit, when turbid evil impairs the clear orifice, the clear orifice of brain will be obstructed, dizziness, irritability and other diseases occur, which might be turned into septic encephalopathy. As the evil of the disease is usually burning hot, and filthy, and it is better to remove evil as early as possible, so it is advocated to use Angong Niuhuang Pill or Zhibao Dan in the early stage of the disease to remove toxin, resolve turbidity, settle fright and open the orifice. Intensively hot with more severe turbid toxin, it is proper to use Angong Niuhuang Pill; phlegm and turbidity congestion, turbidity is more severe than toxin, it is proper to use Zhibao Dan. Opening the orifice is most important, so as to cut off the disease potential quickly, and prevent the deterioration of the disease.

第三节　分期论治
Section 3　Treatment by Stages

一、无症状感染者（包括密切接触者），治以扶正化浊解毒
1. Asymptomatic infected persons (including close contacts) should be treated to strengthen healthy qi, resolve turbidity and remove toxin

新冠病毒无症状感染指的是没有新冠病毒感染的临床表现，但是在新型冠状病毒核酸检测中核酸检测是阳性。对于无症状感染者，包括密切接触者，我们认为当以扶正固表为主，及时截断病势，避免病情发展，正如《医学心悟》所言："大抵邪之所凑其气必虚，体虚受邪，必须以补法驾驭其间，始能收效万全。"治以玉屏风散加藿香、贯众。玉屏风散益气固表。藿香辛温，理气和中，芳香辟秽，兼治表里。贯众苦寒，《会约医镜》谓其

"解时行疫气"。

COVID-19 asymptomatic infection refers to the absence of clinical manifestations of COVID-19, but the nucleic acid test is positive in the novel coronavirus nucleic acid test. Asymptomatic infected people with new pneumonia may also become the source of COVID-19 infection, so the management of asymptomatic COVID-19 infections is the focus of the current epidemic prevention and control. For asymptomatic infected persons, including close contacts, the author believes that the treatment should be reinforcing the healthy qi and strengthening the surface, timely cut off the tendency of the disease to avoid the development of the disease, just as *Medical Enlightenment* says: "Wherever the evil attacks, there must be qi deficiency. For patients being attacked by evil due to physical deficiency, we must use tonifying method to control the progress, so as to to achieve full effect." The prescription is Yupingfeng Powder adding huo xiang (Herba Agastaches seu Pogostemonis), guan zhong (Rhizoma Dryopteris Gassirhizomae). Yupingfeng Powder can replenish qi and strengthen the surface. Huo xiang (Herba Agastaches seu Pogostemonis) spicy and warm, can regulate qi and harmonize the middle energizer, fragrant to dispel the filth, treat both internal and external. Guan zhong (Rhizoma Dryopteris Gassirhizomae) is bitter and cold, can "remove the epidemic pestilence" according to *Huiyue Medical Mirror*.

二、轻型患者，治以升清降浊，表里双清
2. To treat the mild patients, ascend the lucidity and descend the turbidity, clear both the internal and the external

轻型患者，邪尚轻浅，当以发散透表、清热解毒为主要治则。然而疫之为病，传变迅速，既要清病邪已犯之地，又要安病邪未犯之所。《温疫论》曰："夫疫者胃家事也，盖疫邪传胃十常八九，既传入胃，必从下解，疫邪不能自出，必藉大肠之气传送而下，而疫方愈。"已故国医大师朱良春教授深谙吴氏之旨，更提出治温病不必拘于卫气营血的传变规律，起病初期可表里双解、破除"温病三禁"，提出"通下岂止夺实，更重在存阴保津，既能泄无形之邪热，又能除有形之秽滞"的学术思想。蒲辅周也认为："温病最怕表气郁闭，热不得越；更怕里气郁结，秽浊阻塞。"方邦江教授创"三通疗法"，通过发汗、通利大小便以泄热。病之初起邪在表而不从外解，必致热结阳明，邪热蕴结，化燥伤阴，就应及早运用下法，表里双解，内外并调，迅速排泄邪热疫毒从大小便排出。所以此时应该表里双清，方用升降散合宣白承气汤加减。方中僵蚕、蝉蜕，升阳中之清阳；姜黄、大黄，降阴中之浊阴，一升一降，内外通和，而杂气之流毒顿消矣。生石膏清泄肺热，苦杏仁宣肺止咳，瓜蒌皮润肺化痰。升麻，《神农本草经》谓其"主解百毒⋯⋯辟温疾、瘴邪。"，《本草纲目》谓其"行瘀血"，既可以化浊解毒，又可以活血化瘀，改善血液循环，一药两用。全方共奏表里双清之功效。

For mild patients, as the evil is still light and shallow, the principal treatment principle should be dispersing the evil by outthrusting the external, clearing heat and removing toxin. However, the epidemic disease transmits rapidly, we should not only clear the place where the disease evil has invaded, but also protect the place where the disease evil has not invaded. *Discussion on Plague Diseases* says: "The epidemic diseases are stomach affairs, because 80% to 90% of the epidemic disease will surely transmit into the stomach, as the disease has got into the stomach, the disease evil will be discharged from the lower part of the body, and the disease evil will not leave itself, it should be discharged by the intestinal qi, then the epidemic disease recovers." The late National Master of TCM Zhu Liangchun is well versed in Wu's idea, further put forward that the treatment of seasonal febrile disease does not have to be confined to the transmission rule of wei-defence, qi, ying, nutrients and blood. At the beginning of the disease, method of dual removing of internal and external disease evil can be used, breaking the "three bans of the seasonal febrile diseases", put forward the academic thought "to unblock the lower energizer can not only remove the sthenia, more important, it can store Yin and protect fluid. It can discharge the invisible evil and heat, as well as purging the filthy stagnation". Pu Fuzhou also said: "Seasonal febrile disease is most afraid of depression of external qi which can not be bypassed by heat; more afraid of stagnation of internal qi and obstruction of filth and turbidity." Professor Fang Bangjiang created the "triple-unblocking therapy", to relieve heat through sweating, defecation and urination. At the beginning of the disease, as evil is in the surface of the body, if we do not remove the evil from the external surface, it will cause heat stagnation in Yangming meridian. The accumulated bind of evil and heat will turns to be dryness impairing Yin. The purging method should be used as early as possible to realize the dual clearing of surface and inner, dual regulation of internal and external, to purge excretion of evil heat and epidemic toxin rapidly along with the urine and feces. So at this time, we should clear both the surface and inner evil, using the prescription of Shengjiang Powder (the rise and fall powder), combined with Xuanbai Chengqi Decoction with addition or reduction. In this prescription, jiang can (Bombyx Batryticatus), chan tui (Cicadae Periostracum), are used to rise lucid Yang in the Yang; jiang huang (Rhizoma Curcumae Longae), da huang (Radix et Rhizoma Rhei) are used to descend the turbid Yin in the Yin. The combination of ascending and descending unblocks and harmonizes the internal and external, and the pernicious influence of miscellaneous qi are removed thoroughly. Sheng shi gao (Crude Gypsum Fibrosum) can clear and discharge the lung heat, xing ren (Semen Armeniacae Amarum) diffuses the lung and stops cough; gua lou pi (Trichosanthis Cortex) lubricates the lung and resolves phlegm. Sheng ma (Rhizoma Climicifugae), as *Shennong's Classic of Materia Medica* said: "it can remove various kinds of toxin... prevent seasonal febrile disease, miasma, and evil qi", *Compendium of Materia Medica* says "it can resolve the blood stasis". Therefore, it can not only resolve turbidity and remove toxin, but also promote blood circulation and resolve blood stasis, improve blood circulation, one medicine, two functions. The whole prescription makes the effect of dual clearing of both the surface and the internal.

三、重型患者，治以清浊解毒，开窍镇惊
3. Severe patients should be treated by clearing turbidity, removing toxin,opening the orifices and settling the frightness

　　浊毒内闭于肺，肺不宣肃，则胸闷气促；或入里化热，变为热毒，结于阳明，故身热不退，腹胀便秘；或热毒内盛，气壅血凝；或灼伤血络，而瘀血内生；或水道不通，邪陷心包，惕惕不安。治以清浊解毒，开窍镇惊。方用时疫丹加生石膏、大黄，方中重用生甘草和生石膏。生甘草清热解毒兼散表邪，《药品化义》谓其"生用凉而泻火，主散表邪，消痈肿，利咽痛。"《神农本草经》谓其尚可以"主五脏六腑寒热邪气，坚筋骨，长肌肉，倍气力……解毒。"生甘草扶正祛邪，清热解毒，一药多用。生石膏，张锡纯谓其

"凉而能散，有透表解肌之力"，善清瘟疹、咽喉、头面之热。二者共为君药。佩兰、藿香，芳香化浊，透表和中；白芷辛香温散，入阳明，胜湿安脾胃；薄荷芳香走窜，可清头痛及鼻、咽、喉痛等症；大黄涤荡肠胃，活血化瘀，泄浊解毒；冰片开窍辟秽；麝香通关透窍；朱砂镇惊安神。全方以重剂生甘草、生石膏为主，辅以走窜通下之品，是浊毒之邪无藏匿之处，佐以开窍镇惊之品，使神明不乱，先安未受邪之地，共奏清浊解毒、开窍镇惊之功效。

As turbid toxin is obstructed in the lung, the lung cannot diffuse, patients feel chest tightness and rapid breath; or turbid toxin get into the viscera, turns to be heat, then into heat toxin, stagnated in Yangming, so the fever in body does not retreat, abdominal distension and constipation occur; or heat toxin is excessively abundant inside, thus qi obstruction and blood coagulation occur; or burn the blood collateral, and blood stasis generates endogenously; or waterway obstruction, evil sunk in pericardium, restlessly frightened. The treatment method is clearing turbidity, removing toxin, opening the orifices and settling the fright. Prescription of Shiyi Dan is used adding sheng shi gao (Crude Gypsum Fibrosum), da huang (Radix et Rhizoma Rhei). Sheng gan cao (Radix Glycyrrhizae) and sheng shi gao (Crude Gypsum Fibrosum) are used in large amount. Raw licorice is used to clear heat, remove toxin and disperse the surface evil. *Yaopin Huayi* says "Raw licorice is cool and can relieve fever, eliminate carbuncle swelling and sore throat." *Shennong's Classic of Materia Medica* says: "It can still control the evil qi of coldness and heat of viscera, strengthen tendons and bones, generate muscles, timely increase the physical power... and remove toxin." Sheng gan cao (Radix Glycyrrhizae) Reinforcing the healthy qi, expelling the evil, clearing heat and removing toxin, is a multi-functional medicine. Sheng shi gao (Crude Gypsum Fibrosum), Zhang Xichun said it can "cool and disperse, with the force of out-thrusting the external and disperse the tighteness of muscle", is good at clearing the fever of epidemic rash, throat, head and face. Sheng gan cao (Radix Glycyrrhizae) and sheng shi gao (Crude Gypsum Fibrosum) are combined principal medicine. Pei lan (Herba Eupatorii), huo xiang (Herba Agastaches seu Pogostemonis), can resolve turbidity with aroma, outhrust the external and harmonize the middle energizer. Bai zhi (Radix Angelicae Dahuricae) with pungent aroma and warm dispersing function, reacts through Yangming meridian, disinhibit dampness and protect spleen and stomach. Bo he (Herba seu Folium Menthae) opens the orifice with fragrance, can clear headache, pains in nose, throat and larynx. Da huang (Radix et Rhizoma Rhei), can cleanse intestines and stomach, promote blood circulation and resolve blood stasis, purge the turbidity and remove toxin. Bing pian (Borneolum Syntheticum) is used to open the orifice and avoid the filth. She xiang (Moschus) is used to unblock the pass and outhrust the orifice. Zhu sha (Cinnabaris) is used to settle the fright and tranquilize the spirit. The whole prescription uses large amount of sheng gan cao (Radix Glycyrrhizae) and sheng shi gao (Crude Gypsum Fibrosum) as the principal medicine, subordinated by aromatic and purging products, leaving no space to hide the evil of turbid toxin, adjuvented by products of opening the orifice and settling the fright, to ensure the peace of in mind, protecting the place where the evil has not attacked, make effect of clearing turbidity, removing toxin, opening the orifice and settling the fright.

四、危重型，治以开闭固脱，解毒救逆，宜中西医联合治疗
4. To treat the critical disease, we should combine TCM with Western Medicine, using the method of opening the closure, stopping depletion, removing toxin and saving from depletion

浊毒内盛，失治误治，则出现湿、浊、热、毒、瘀、虚并存，浊毒内闭，正气外脱，致脏器损伤，出现多器官功能障碍综合征（MODS），甚或多脏器功能衰竭（MOF）。浊邪害清则神昏、烦躁，热毒炽盛则胸腹灼热，热深厥深则手足逆冷，或阳气外脱则肢冷汗出、呼吸急促。气血相关，气为血之帅，行血统血，全在于气，故当以大补阳气为要。本型当以开闭固脱，解毒救逆为主。对于内闭外脱者，随时要防脱，即扶正防"虚"脱，此外临证还必须辨清"闭"和"脱"之比重，以指导处方中扶正（治虚）药和开闭药之比例。治疗宜中西医联合救治，可酌情予以四逆加人参汤加减、安宫牛黄丸，结合参附注射液或血必净等静脉给药。

Delayed or wrong treatment of internal excessive abundance of turbid toxin, causes the co-existence of dampness, turbidity, heat, toxin, stasis and deficiency, internal obstruction of turbid toxin, external collapse of healthy qi, results in impairing of viscera, onset of multiple organ dysfunction syndrome (MODS), or even multiple organ failure (MOF). When evil of turbidity attacks the clear orifice, dizziness, irritability occur, excessively abundant of heat toxin burns pleuroperitoneum, severe pyretic syncope leads to coldness of hands and feet, or the Yang qi is collapse externally, causes sweating, coldness of limbs and urgent and rapid breath. Qi and blood are related, qi is the commander of blood, fully responsible for promoting and controlling the blood circulation, so the most important measure is to strongly tonify the Yang qi. This type should mainly use the method of opening the closure, stopping depletion, removing toxin and saving from depletion. For patients of internal closure and external collapse, doctors should prevent the collapse in any time, i.e. strengthening the healthy qi and preventing the depletion of "deficiency". In addition, doctors must make clear the the severity of "closure" and "depletion"to guide the medication percentage of healthy qi strengthening medicines and that of closure opening medicines in clinical prescription. The treatment should combine TCM with Western Medicine, use Sini Jia Renshen Decoction, Angong Niuhuang Pill, cooperating with intravenous drip of Shenfu injection and Xuebijing injection according to the disease condition.

五、恢复期治以益气养阴，兼清余毒
5. In the recovery stage,the treatment method is replenishing qi, nourishing Yin, and clearing the residual toxin

此病至恢复期，气阴两伤为基本病机。留一分津液，即有一分生机，故在中期急下以存阴，后期更应以益气养阴为要，兼清浊毒余邪。方用益气养阴败瘟汤，即王氏清暑益气汤去西瓜翠衣、荷梗，加石菖蒲、荷叶等。

In the recovery stage of the disease, dual impairing of qi and Yin is the basic pathogenesis. Leave a part of body fluid, leave the vitality of life. So in the middle stage of the disease, urgent purging is used to leave Yin, in later stage, replenishing qi and nourishing Yin should be emphasized further, and simultaneously clear the remaining evil of turbid toxin. The prescription can choose Decoction of Yiqi

Yangyin Baiwen, i.e. Wang's Qing shu Yiqi Soup, to reduce xi gua cui yi (Exocarpium Citrulli), he geng (Petiolus Nelumbinis), add shi chang pu (Rhizoma Acori Graminei), he ye (Folium Nelumbinis), etc.

第四节 预防调护
Section 4 Prevention and Recuperative Medical Care

一、预防新冠病毒感染的策略
1. Strategies to prevent COVID-19

基于上述病因、病机、治则认识，结合《黄帝内经》"未病先防、既病防变、瘥后防复"的"治未病"思想，李佃贵教授提出了中医预防新冠病毒感染的策略。

Based on the above understanding of the etiology, pathogenesis, treatment principles of the disease, combined with the "Future disease treatment" idea of *The Medical Classic of the Yellow Emperor* "to prevent the disease before the onset, to prevent the transmission and deterioiration of the disease when it occurs, to prevent the recurrence of the disease after recovery", Professor Li Diangui put forward the TCM strategy to prevent COVID-19.

（一）未病先防
1.1 To prevent the disease before the onset

静心气，扶正气，避浊气。
Calm down the mind, strengthen the healthy qi, avoid turbid substance.

1.静心气　本病具有强烈的传染性，心烦意乱、恐慌、焦虑等情绪普遍存在。因此调畅情志是重要的防病之策。

1.1.1 Calm down the mind　As the disease is strongly infectious, the mood of upset, frightening and anxiety are widespread. Therefore, regulating the emotion is an important measure to prevent the disease.

2.扶正气　中医学认为正气存内，邪不可干，邪之所凑，其气必虚，所以通过扶正气，可以有效地预防新冠病毒感染。①节饮食：饮食的结构要好，要荤素搭配，保证营养的全面和均衡。此外，饮食的度要把握好，吃饭以八、九成饱为宜。②适运动：科学合理运动，可振奋人体的阳气，有利于增强机体免疫力，降低病毒感染的风险。适当的运动可增强人体的免疫力和抵抗力。③避风寒：重视环境、气候、季节等寒温变化，适时增减衣物。④慎起居：保持规律的生活节律，起居有常，特别是保持充足的睡眠。

1.1.2 Strengthening healthy qi　Traditional Chinese medicine believes that when healthy qi is sufficiently stored, evil cannot attack. Wherever evil attacks, there must be qi deficiency. Therefore, COVID-19 can be effectively prevented by strengthening healthy qi. a. to manage diet: the structure of the diet should be appropriate, to combine meat with vegetable, to ensure comprehension and balance of nutrition. In addition, the amount of diet should be managed, eat 80% to 90% full is appropriate; b. to keep suitable exercising: scientific and reasonable exercise can activate the physical Yang of the body, enhance the body immunity, reduce the risk of virus infection. Proper exercise can also enhance the human resistance; c. to avoid wind and cold: pay attention to the temperature changes in relation to environment, climate, season, timely increase or decrease clothes; d. to regulate dailylife: keep a regular life rhythm, normalize the allocation of work and rest, especially keep enough sleep.

3.避浊气 《素问·刺法论》言："避其毒气，天牝从来。"针对新冠病毒感染的防治，隔离仍是最重要的预防措施。提倡居家隔离，监测体温、单独居住、每天开窗、正确洗手、佩戴口罩、单独用餐、注意消毒、单独卫浴，以避其毒气。除此之外，还可以制作一些香囊悬挂在身上或屋堂内，以芳香避秽，起到预防作用。比如用河北省新冠病毒感染中医药诊疗方案中推荐的香囊方：藿香、佩兰、金银花、桑叶、菊花、薄荷制为香囊佩戴。或者如《本草纲目》所载：房内用苍术、艾叶、白芷、丁香、硫黄等药焚烧以进行空气消毒辟秽等。

1.1.3 Avoid turbid substance *Simple Conversation-Discussion on Acupuncture Methods* said: "(when the pestilence has occurred, cares should be taken to) avoid its toxic substance. Evil (epidemic) qi usually gets into and out of the body through the nose." Quarantine is still the most important prevention measure against COVID-19. It is advocated to stay at home, monitor body temperature, live alone, open windows every day, wash hands correctly, wear masks, eat separately, pay attention to disinfection, bath separately, to avoid the toxic substance. In addition, as a preventive measure to avoid the toxic substance, you can also make some sachets hanging on the body or in the house. For example, the sachets recommended in Hebei Province: huo xiang (Herba Agastaches seu Pogostemonis), pei lan (Herba Eupatorii), jin yin hua (Lonicerae Japonicae Flos), sang ye (Folium Mori), ju hua (Chrysanthemi Flos), bo he (Menthae Hapocalycis Herba), are used to make sachets for wear. Or as suggested in the *Compendium of Materia Medica*: to burn cang zhu (Rhizoma Atractylodis), ai ye (Folium Artemisiae Argyi), bai zhi (Radix Angelicae Dahuricae), ding xiang (Flos Caryophylli), liu huang (Sulfur) and other drugs in the house to disinfect air.

（二）既病防变

1.2 to prevent the transmission and deterioration of the disease when it occurs

无症状感染者，可服用香苏化浊颗粒以清除体内病毒。重视早发现、早治疗。

Asymptomatic infected persons can take Xiangsu Huazhuo Keli (susulated particles) to remove the virus in the body. Pay attention to detect and treat the disease as early as possible.

（三）瘥后防复

1.3 To prevent recurrence of the disease after recovery

复阳者，重在化浊扶正、补益肺脾，可服用香苏化浊颗粒。肺部影像显示未完全吸收或肺间质纤维化者，可用六君子汤、王氏清暑益气汤补益脾肺。

To treat the patients of rebound positivity, we should focus on turbidity resolving and healthy qi strengthening, reinforcing and replenishing the lung and spleen, using Xiangsu Huazhuo Keli (suturbidity granules). If the lung image shows that the leision has not been fully absorbed or the lung interstitial fibrosis occurs, prescription of Liujunzi Decoction and Wang's Qingshu Yiqi Decoction can be used to tonify and replenish the spleen and lung.

二、预防新冠病毒感染系列方药
2. Series of prescriptions and medicines to prevent COVID-19

（一）预防新冠病毒感染的化浊解毒的代茶饮方
2.1 Tea-style prescriptions to prevent COVID-19

中药代茶饮始于唐宋时期，为我国中药的传统剂型，在疾病的预防、调理、保健中都得到了广泛的应用。其既保留了传统汤剂辨证论治、疗效显著的特点，又克服了传统汤剂煎煮繁琐，携带不便的不足，在众多防疫汤剂中脱颖而出。现给出预防新冠病毒感染的代茶饮方，其组成：黄芪12g，金银花15g，藿香10g，防风10g。方中黄芪益气固表，金银花清热解毒，藿香芳香化浊，防风祛风解表，以上4味药，共奏化浊解毒、益气固表之效。代茶饮中药冲泡饮用前应迅速过水以祛除杂质，予以1500mL左右开水泡药10～30分钟后即可代茶饮用，每日一剂随饮随泡，直至茶饮无味弃去。该方中花叶类中药质地松脆，易破碎，为避免刺激，方便饮用，建议装入小纱袋制成茶包。该代茶饮对于24小时坚守在防疫一线的工作人员和不方便煎煮汤剂的市民来说，有方便易取、可多次饮用的优点，且吸收完全，对疫情防控具有很好的辅助作用。

Traditional Chinese medicine tea drink began in the Tang and Song dynasties, as one of the traditional dosage of traditional Chinese medicine, it has been widely used in disease prevention, regulation and health care. It retains the characteristics of traditional decoction with syndrome differentiation and remarkable efficacy, at the same time, overcomes the shortcoming of traditional decoction as complicated decocting process and inconvenience of carrying, and talently shows its brilliant effect among many epidemic prevention soups. The compostion of the tea drinking prescriptions to prevent COVID-19 is as follows: huang qi (Radix Astragali seu Hedysari) 12g, jin yin hua (Lonicerate Japonivae Flos) 15g, huo xiang (Herba Agastaches seu Pogostemonis) 10g, fang feng (Radix Saposhnikoviae) 10g. In the prescription, huang qi (Radix Astragali seu Hedysari) is used to replenish Qi and strengthening the external surface. Jin yin hua (Lonicerate Japonivae Flos) is used to clear heat and remove toxin. Huo xiang (Herba Agastaches seu Pogostemonis) is used to resolve turbidity with aroma. Fang feng (Radix Saposhnikoviae) is used to dispel wind and release the external. The above 4 drugs collectively make the effect of resolving turbidity, removing toxin, replenishing the qi and consolidating the external. The medicines in the prescription of tea drink should be washed rapidly by water before infusing to remove the impurity substances. Drink it after infusing the medicines in 1500mL of boiled water for 10 to 30 minutes, use it one dose a day. Infuse boiled water into the medicines repeatedly during drinking, abandon it until the tea is tasteless. Medicines of flowers and leaves in the prescription are crisp and easy to break. In order to avoid stimulation and hurt in convenience of drinking, it is recommended to put the medicines into a small gauze bag as tea bags. The tea has the advantages of convenient to drink for many times, and can be fully absorbed especially appropriate for epidemic preventing persons working 24 hours in the front line and the residents of the city who are inconvenient to use the decoction. It can play a good auxiliary role in the epidemic prevention and controlling.

（二）预防新冠病毒感染的化浊解毒香薰方
2.2 Incense method of resolving turbidity and removing toxin to prevent COVID-19

中医防治瘟疫源远流长，运用中药香薰疗法在家庭和社区进行防疫，便是简便廉验的特色疗法，其经济、安全、简便，自古以来既是生活习俗也是养生疗法，因此容易推广。中药香薰疗法利用芳香中药香气的驱虫祛邪、辟秽化浊等作用，其挥发的气味经人体口鼻、皮肤腠理、经络腧穴，通过人体气血经脉的循行而遍及周身，可疏通经络、舒畅气机，使气血调和通畅，以助机体"正气"而达到健康状态。可自制化浊避秽香在屋内焚之（注意防范火灾）。药物组成：艾叶、藿香、白芷、苍术、乳香、甘松、细辛、檀香、降香，制成艾炷，每日焚一炷。

Traditional Chinese medicine has a long history of plague prevention and treatment, using the TCM incense therapy is a simple, convenient, economical and experienced way for epidemic prevention in families and communities. It has been both a living custom and a life-cultivating therapy since ancient times, so it is easy to be popularized. TCM incense therapy uses the fragrance of aromatic Chinese medicine to expel insects, remove evil, prevent filth nd resolve turbidity, the volatile smell passes human mouth and nose, skin and striae, meridians and acupoints, get into everywhere of the body along with the human qi, blood and meridians, can dredge meridians, comfort qi mechanism, regulate the circulation of qi and blood, helping the "healthy qi" to achieve a healthy state. Incense of turbidity resolving and filth avoiding can be made by ourselves to burn in house (Attention shoul be paid to prevent fire). Medicines are as follows: ai ye (Folium Artemisiae Argyi), huo xiang (Herba Agastaches seu Pogostemonis) , bai zhi (Radix Angelicae Dahuricae), cang zhu (Rhizoma Atractylodis), ru xiang ((Resina Boswelliae Carterii seu Masticis), gan song (Rhizoma et Radix Nardostachydis), xi xin (Herba Asari cum Radice), tan xiang (Lignum Santali), jiang xiang (Lignum Dalbergiae Odoriferae), made into moxa cone, burn a cone every day.

（三）预防新冠病毒感染的化浊解毒中药方
2.3 TCM prescription of turbidity resolving and toxin removing for COVID-19 prevention

中医学在防治传染病方面积累了许多宝贵经验，中医治疫，防重于治。李佃贵教授认为本病为浊毒致病，当以化浊解毒、调畅气机、扶正祛邪为要。李佃贵教授给出的预防新冠病毒感染的中药处方如下：广藿香12g，佩兰10g，黄芪15g，炒白术10g，防风9g，金银花15g，芦根15g。用法：水煎煮2次，共取汁400mL，分早晚2次服用，连服5～7天。

Traditional Chinese medicine has accumulated a lot of valuable experience in the prevention and treatment of infectious diseases. Prevention is more important than treatment according to TCM. Professor Li Diangui believes that the disease is caused by turbid toxin, and the treatment should principally resolve turbidity, remove toxin, regulate qi mechanism, strengthen the healthy qi and dispel evil. The prescription for COVID-19 is given by professor Li Diangui as follows: guang huo xiang (Herba Pogostemonis) 12g, pei lan (Herba Eupatorii) 10g, huang qi (Radix Astragali seu Hedysari) 15g, chao bai zhu (fried Rhizoma Atractylodis Macrocephalae) 10g, fang feng (Radix Saposhnikoviae) 9g, jin yin hua (Lonicerate Japonicae Flos) 15g, lu gen (Phragnitis Rhizoma 15). Usage: decoct in water two times, leave 400mL of juice, take twice a day, once in the morning and the other in the evening, take 5-7 days.

（四）感染新冠病毒期间的心理调护

2.4 Psychological recuperative care during COVID-19 infection

此非常时期，我们不仅需要做好隔离与防护，而且还要进行积极的心理健康调护。保持好的心态和免疫力，亦是抗击病毒不可或缺的一部分。在此期间我们应该对新冠病毒感染患者进行心理疏导，主要包括以下几个方面。

In this emergency period, we not only need to do a good job of isolation and protection, but also have a positive psychological health care. Maintaining a good state of mind and immunity is also an indispensable part of the fight against the virus. During this period, we should provide psychological counseling for COVID-19 patients, mainly including the following aspects:

1.要多与家人亲属沟通交流，保持良好的心态，分散注意力，避免心情过度压抑或紧张。保持自信，发挥主观能动性，规律饮食、营养均衡，保证每日睡眠7～9小时，坚持每日适量运动，保持心情愉悦，提升自身机体免疫力。

2.4.1 To communicate more with family members and relatives, maintain a good state of mind, distract the attention, and avoid excessive depression or tension. Maintain self- confidence, activate the subjective initiative, regulate diet, balance nutrition, ensure 7 to 9 hours of sleep a day, insist on moderate daily exercising, keep in a good mood, improve your own body's immunity.

2.及时获悉疫情和健康知识，正确了解疾病的防控知识，规范自身行为，对不理解的信息可向专业人员咨询，不过分解读信息，避免过度焦虑和盲目恐慌。

2.4.2 Be well - informed of the epidemic condition and health knowledge, rightly understand the disease prevention and controlling knowledge, regulate our own behavior. Consult the professionals about the information which we do not understand. Do not over-interpret the information to avoid excessive anxiety and blind panic.

3.保持正常的生活规律，形成健康的生活习惯，尽快适应在疫情常态化下的生活、工作、学习环境的变化，客观、全面而又理性地看待疫情所造成的影响，关注自身、他人以及周围环境积极的一面。

2.4.3 To maintain normal life pattern, and healthy living habit, be adapt to the changes in life, work and learning environment under the normalized epidemic condition as soon as possible. See in an objective, comprehensive and rational view of the impact of the epidemic, focus on the positive side of yourself, others, and your surroundings.

4．社区居（村）委会工作人员要做好对居民的人文关怀，主动帮助其适应特殊阶段生活。在专业部门的指导下，开展心理健康科普宣传，告知居民心理援助热线等求助方式，鼓励居民有需求时及时求助。树立疫情防控人人有责的意识，积极配合落实防控措施。

2.4.4 Staffs of community residence (village) committee should do a good job in humanistic care for the residents, actively help them to be adapt to the special stages of life. Under the guidance of professional departments, carry out scientific popularization of psychological health, inform residents of psychological assistance hotline and other ways for help. Encourage residents to seek psychological help in time when necessary. Establish the awareness that everyone is responsible for epidemic prevention and control, and actively cooperate with the implementation of prevention and control measures.

附录：浊毒论关键词与术语中英文对照表
Appendix: professional key words and expressions in turbid toxin theory

序号	中文	英文
1	浊	turbidity
2	毒	toxin
3	浊毒	turbid toxin
4	浊毒论（浊毒理论）	turbid toxin theory
5	浊毒化	turbid toxin change
6	化浊毒（化浊解毒）	resolve turbidity and remove toxin
7	净化体内环境	purify the inner environment of human body
8	浊毒辨证	turbid toxin syndrome differentiation
9	浊毒体质	turbid toxin constitution
10	理法方药	Principle, method, prescription, medicine
11	君臣佐使	principal, subordinate, adjuvant, guide
12	广义浊毒	broad sense of turbid toxin
13	狭义浊毒	narrow sense of turbid toxin
14	生理之浊	physiological turbidity
15	病理之浊	pathological turbidity
16	湿浊	damp turbidity
17	谷浊	grain turbidity
18	浊化	turbid transmission
19	浊变	turbid change
20	浊毒学说	doctrine of turbid toxin
21	浊毒学派	school of turbid toxin

续表

序号	中文	英文
22	天之浊毒	turbid toxin of heaven
23	地之浊毒	turbid toxin of earth
24	人之浊毒	turbid toxin of human
25	心之浊毒	turbid toxin of mind
26	浊气	turbid substance
27	浊邪	turbid pathogenic factors
28	浊阴	turbid yin
29	浊阳	turbid yang
30	痰浊	turbid phlegm
31	通腑泄浊	to discharge the turbidity by unblocking the Fu-organs
32	芳香化浊解毒	to resolve turbidity and remove toxin with aroma
33	浊毒内蕴	internal accumulation of turbid toxin
34	浊毒壅盛	excessive abundant of turbid toxin
35	浊毒中阻	obstruction of turbid toxin in middle energizer
36	浊毒瘀阻	congestion of turbid toxin
37	热极生毒	Excessive heat generates toxin
38	浊以毒为用	Toxin is the function of turbidity
39	毒以浊为体	Turbidity is the carrier of toxin
40	生克乘侮	generating, restraining, over-restraint, counter-restraint
41	正虚邪实	asthenia healthy qi and sthenia pathogenic factors
42	标本兼治	to treat both the tip and the root
43	急则治标，缓则治本	to treat the tip first in acute disease, to treat the root first in chronic disease